Molecular Pathology Library

Series editor

Philip T. Cagle, MD

Ashraf Khan, MD, FRCPath · Ian O. Ellis, MD,
FRCPath · Andrew M. Hanby, BM, FRCPath
Ediz F. Cosar, MD · Emad A. Rakha, MD,
FRCPath · Dina Kandil, MD
Editors

Precision Molecular Pathology of Breast Cancer

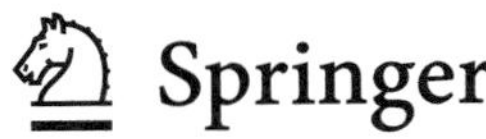

Editors
Ashraf Khan, MD, FRCPath
Department of Pathology
University of Massachusetts Medical
  School
UMassMemorial Medical Center
Worcester, MA
USA

Ian O. Ellis, MD, FRCPath
Department of Histopathology
University of Nottingham
Nottingham
UK

Andrew M. Hanby, BM, FRCPath
Leeds Institute of Cancer and Pathology
St. James University Hospital
Leeds, West Yorkshire
UK

Ediz F. Cosar, MD
Department of Pathology
University of Massachusetts Medical
  School
UMassMemorial Medical Center
Worcester, MA
USA

Emad A. Rakha, MD, FRCPath
Department of Histopathology
University of Nottingham
Nottingham
UK

Dina Kandil, MD
Department of Pathology
University of Massachusetts Medical
  School
UMassMemorial Medical Center
Worcester, MA
USA

ISSN 1935-987X　　　　　　　ISSN 1935-9888　(electronic)
Molecular Pathology Library
ISBN 978-1-4939-4867-3　　　ISBN 978-1-4939-2886-6　(eBook)
DOI 10.1007/978-1-4939-2886-6

Springer New York Heidelberg Dordrecht London

Printed on acid-free paper

Springer Science+Business Media LLC New York is part of Springer Science+Business Media (www.springer.com)

Preface

The past decade has seen an immense growth in our understanding of the molecular basis of cancer, which has made a significant impact on how we manage cancer in this era of personalized medicine. Breast cancer, which is the most common malignancy in women in the western world, has been the vanguard in the application of molecular pathology in its management. Advances in molecular pathology have led to the development of new ancillary studies that are now standard clinical practice for profiling of breast tumors permitting the tailoring of adjuvant treatment. The investigations include diagnostic and predictive biomarkers determined both by immunohistochemistry and more traditional molecular pathology techniques such as FISH. At the advancing research front further potential new targets of therapy within the molecular pathways underpinning current practice are being revealed.

With the fast pace of growth in our knowledge, practicing physicians, including pathologists, are increasingly expected to have a sound understanding of both traditional morphology based interpretation and the molecular pathology of breast cancer. Pathologists are consultants to their clinical colleagues for managing patients with breast cancer, and the role of molecular pathology has become critical in this era of personalized medicine and multidisciplinary cancer care. It is therefore important for pathologists to be familiar with advances in molecular pathology of breast cancer, so they can provide a better, informed, opinion when discussing cases with their clinical colleagues.

This book, which is part of the molecular pathology of cancer series, was put together with the aim of combining histopathologic and cytomorphologic features with changes at the molecular level, and how these latter alterations can play a role in breast cancer management. The editors are experienced practicing diagnostic breast pathologists who apply these molecular pathology techniques routinely in their practice. With the exception of one chapter where we have invited breast radiologist and medical physics experts to write on the molecular basis of breast cancer imaging, all the authors in addition to diagnostic pathologists, include cancer biologists, who focus on the molecular biology of the breast cancer. The editors, who are also the senior author on each chapter, are internationally recognized breast pathologists who bring their own valuable insights into the interface between morphology and molecular pathology.

We are very grateful to all the contributors who have taken time out of their busy schedules to write these chapters. We would also like to take this opportunity to thank the series editor Dr. Philip Cagle for inviting us to write this book and the editorial staff at Springer Publications for all their assistance in making this project possible.

Ashraf Khan
Ian O. Ellis
Andrew M. Hanby
Ediz F. Cosar
Emad A. Rakha
Dina Kandil

Contents

Contributors

Mohammed A. Aleskandarany Department of Histopathology, Division of Cancer and Stem Cells, School of Medicine, The University of Nottingham and Nottingham University Hospitals NHS Trust, Nottingham City Hospital, Nottingham, UK

Jennifer L. Clark Department of Pathology, University of Massachusetts Medical School, UMassMemorial Medical Center, Three Bioetch, One Innovation Drive, Worcester, MA, USA

Ediz F. Cosar Department of Pathology, University of Massachusetts Medical School, UMassMemorial Medical Center, Worcester, MA, USA

Ian O. Ellis Division of Cancer and Stem Cells, Department of Histopathology, School of Medicine, University of Nottingham and Nottingham University Hospitals NHS Trust, Nottingham City Hospital, Nottingham, UK

Yuna Gong Department of Pathology, University of Massachusetts Medical School, UMassMemorial Medical Center, Three Biotech, One Innovation Drive, Worcester, MA, USA

Andrew M. Hanby St. James University Hospital/University of Leeds, Leeds Institute of Cancer and Pathology (LICAP), Leeds, West Yorkshire, UK

Thomas A. Hughes Leeds Institute of Biologial and Clinical Sciences (LIBACS), St. James University Hospital/University of Leeds, Beckett Street, Leeds, West Yorkshire, UK

Lloyd Hutchinson Department of Pathology, University of Massachusetts Medical School, UMassMemorial Medical Center, Worcester, MA, USA

Dina Kandil Department of Pathology, University of Massachusetts Medical School, UMassMemorial Medical Center, Three Biotech, One Innovation Drive, Worcester, MA, USA

Andrew Karellas Department of Radiology, University of Massachusetts Medical School, Worcester, MA, USA

Ashraf Khan Department of Pathology, University of Massachusetts Medical School, UMassMemorial Medical Center, Three Biotech, One Innovation Drive, Worcester, MA, USA

Arthur M. Mercurio Department of Molecular, Cell and Cancer Biology, University of Massachusetts Medical School, Worcester, MA, USA

Rebecca A. Millican-Slater Department of Histopathology, Leeds University Hospitals NHS Trust, Leeds, UK

Marjan Mirzabeigi Department of Pathology, University of Massachusetts Medical School, UMassMemorial Medical Center, Worcester, MA, USA

Abir A. Muftah Department of Histopathology, Division of Cancer and Stem Cells, School of Medicine, The University of Nottingham and Nottingham University Hospitals NHS Trust, Nottingham City Hospital, Nottingham, UK

Abhik Mukherjee Division of Cancer and Stem Cells, Department of Histopathology, School of Medicine, University of Nottingham and Nottingham University Hospitals NHS Trust, Nottingham City Hospital, Nottingham, UK

Claire Nash St. James University Hospital/University of Leeds, Leeds Institute of Cancer and Pathology (LICAP), Leeds, West Yorkshire, UK

Emad A. Rakha Department of Histopathology, Division of Cancer and Stem Cells, School of Medicine, Nottingham University Hospitals NHS Trust, Nottingham City Hospital, The University of Nottingham, Nottingham, UK

Ali Sakhdari Department of Pathology, University of Massachusetts Medical School, UMassMemorial Medical Center, Worcester, MA, USA

Sanjoy Samanta Department of Molecular, Cell and Cancer Biology, University of Massachusetts Medical School, Worcester, MA, USA

Valerie Speirs St. James University Hospital/University of Leeds, Leeds Institute of Cancer and Pathology (LICAP), Leeds, West Yorkshire, UK

James L. Thorne Department of Mathematical and Physical Sciences (MAPS), School of Food Science and Nutrition, Woodhouse Lane, University of Leeds, Leeds, West Yorkshire, UK

Srinivasan Vedantham Department of Radiology, University of Massachusetts Medical School, Worcester, MA, USA

Gopal R. Vijayaraghavan Department of Radiology, University of Massachusetts Medical School, Worcester, MA, USA

Vighnesh Walavalkar Department of Pathology, University of Massachusetts Medical School, UMassMemorial Medical Center, Worcester, MA, USA

Michelle Yang Department of Pathology, University of Massachusetts Medical School, UMassMemorial Medical Center, Worcester, MA, USA

Chapter 1
Molecular Basis of Breast Cancer Imaging

Gopal R. Vijayaraghavan, Srinivasan Vedantham,
Ashraf Khan and Andrew Karellas

Introduction

Over the past decade, annually for women 50 years of age or older, the breast cancer incidence rate in the United States has ranged from 400 to 500 per 100 000 women and the breast cancer mortality rate has ranged from 60 to 80 per 100 000 women [1]. Though there has been a decline in the breast cancer mortality in the past decade it continues to be the second leading cause of death after lung cancer in women over 40 years of age.

Breast cancer continues to be a major health issue among women in the United States. Screening mammogram has significantly contributed to the reduction in mortality. However, screening mammogram has its own limitations. Its sensitivity is 80 % in fatty breasts but is substantially lower in dense breasts [2]. On average nearly 30 % of women reporting for mammograms have dense breasts and 1 in 2 cancers in dense breasts are missed on mammograms due to the masking effect caused by overlapping tissues.

Notwithstanding the limitations of screening mammograms, it is widely considered the most effective tool for the early detection of breast cancer [3], and supplementing mammography with ultrasound and MRI greatly improves the diagnosis of breast cancer. Further improvements in sensitivity and specificity for diagnosis of breast cancer are likely to involve alternative imaging approaches that address

A. Khan (✉)
Department of Pathology, University of Massachusetts Medical School,
UMassMemorial Medical Center, Three Biotech, One Innovation Drive,
Worcester, MA 01605, USA
e-mail: Ashraf.Khan@umassmemorial.org

G.R. Vijayaraghavan · S. Vedantham · A. Karellas
Department of Radiology, University of Massachusetts Medical School,
Worcester, MA 01605, USA

© Springer Science+Business Media New York 2015
A. Khan et al. (eds.), *Precision Molecular Pathology of Breast Cancer*,
Molecular Pathology Library 10, DOI 10.1007/978-1-4939-2886-6_1

the limitations of existing imaging modalities or provide for imaging new contrast mechanisms. An example of the former is digital breast tomosynthesis [4], which can reduce the tissue overlap observed with mammography.

Mammograms and ultrasound images represent anatomic abnormalities that are associated with cancer. Magnetic Resonance Imaging (MRI) with injected contrast media better depicts the physiology of the tumor due to enhancement of tumor-associated angiogenesis and this partly explains its higher sensitivity compared to mammography. Changes at the cellular level that distinguish cancerous cells from benign breast tissue have been explored in newer, innovative imaging techniques. Some of the imaging techniques described are still experimental and not yet considered 'standard of care'. Some of the changes at the cellular level include new blood flow, angiogenesis, expression of protein receptors in breast cancer cells resulting in increased uptake of specific ligands and changes in oxy or deoxy-hemoglobin content of the tumor cells. Radionuclides and optical probes that target specific proteins in the cells are being investigated. Some of these newer modalities can be combined with traditional imaging as part of multimodal imaging to further improve our diagnostic capability [5].

Over the past decade advances in imaging and instrumentation have helped establish molecular breast imaging (MBI) as a useful supplemental tool [6–8]. Cost constraints, tumor size resolution, radiation dose, and sparse availability were some of the cited reasons why these modalities have not gained widespread acceptance [9]. Many of these issues continue to be addressed. Radiation dose from radionuclide-based molecular imaging [10] continues to remain a major impediment compared to established screening mammogram.

Molecular imaging reflects both tumor morphology and physiology and thus has some inherent advantages over conventional mammograms, particularly in a situation of radiographic dense breasts.

MBI techniques currently available include:

1. Breast-specific gamma imaging (BSGI).
2. Positron emission mammography (PEM).
3. Optical imaging with near-infrared spectroscopy.

In addition, imaging tests that can be performed in ex vivo specimens to evaluate cancer margins include:

1. Optical imaging with confocal microscopy.
2. Terahertz imaging.

Breast-Specific Gamma Imaging (BSGI)

While mammography and ultrasound rely on anatomical changes in the breast (calcifications, masses, architectural distortion, or asymmetry), BSGI relies on the physiology (blood flow, mitochondrial activity, and angiogenesis) of the tumor to make the diagnosis.

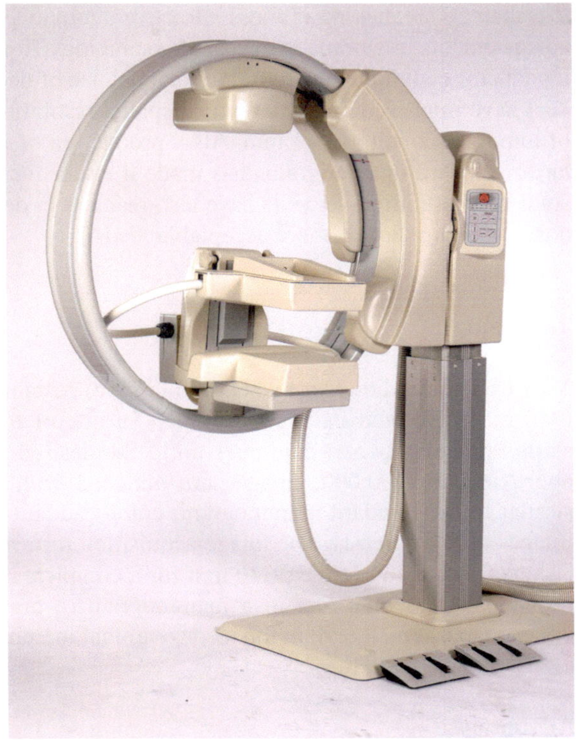

Fig. 1.1 Picture of a molecular breast imaging system. *Courtesy of Jason Koshnitsky, Gamma Medica, Inc., Salem, NH*

A standard two-view mammogram continues to be the gold standard in the evaluation of breast cancers, notwithstanding recent controversies [11]. The sensitivity of mammogram is limited [2]. In dense breasts, small cancers are hidden and can be missed [12, 13]. Breast ultrasound and tomosynthesis have shown the ability to detect some non-palpable breast cancers beyond mammography and address this limitation to a large extent [14, 15]. BSGI also known as molecular imaging of the breast has higher negative predictive value for breast cancers. Figure 1.1 shows a picture of MBI system.

Indications

The indications for performance of a BSGI study include high-risk surveillance, alternative to MRI, palpable breast masses with a negative mammogram and ultrasound, a newly diagnosed breast cancer with occult foci, and in women with breast implants or following direct silicone injection to resolve a difficult question.

Initially studies were performed on a conventional gamma camera and hence there were issues related to optimal positioning of the breast and poor resolution; this technique did not detect small cancers less than 1 cm. The sensitivity was less than 50 %, making it a less attractive alternative [6, 9]. Over the last 20 years advancements in gamma ray detector technology (for example, the use of the semiconductor cadmium zinc telluride) and the use of dedicated dual head breast scanners have improved both energy and spatial resolution. This has enabled detection of tumors as small as 1–3 mm. Also, production of images that are oriented similar to standard mammograms has made it easier for radiologists to interpret these studies. These improvements have also resulted in decreased radiopharmaceuticals doses, making the test more acceptable [7, 16].

Technique

MBI uses the radiotracer technetium (^{99m}Tc) sestamibi in doses of about 20 mCi (740 mBq) injected intravenously (IV) in one of the antecubital veins. Imaging starts immediately and continues up to the desired number of counts per image, approximately 100,000. Images are obtained with breast oriented in a manner similar to the standard mammogram; craniocaudal (CC) and mediolateral (MLO) images of both breasts. The image acquisition time is about 10 min for each view, to a total acquisition time of 40 min for a complete study [9, 17]. The breast compression is less than that in a mammogram (a pressure of 15 lbs/square in. as opposed to 45 lbs/square in. on a conventional mammogram).

Advantages

In addition to its utility as an adjunct diagnostic tool, MBI is an attractive imaging test from the cost point of view because of the wide availability of the radiopharmaceutical and compact size of the imaging equipment. It is a useful problem-solving tool particularly in patients unsuited for MRI, because of metallic implants, renal dysfunction, or claustrophobia. BSGI has high sensitivity, specificity, and positive predictive value (PPV) compared to standard mammograms and ultrasound evaluation [7–9, 16–18]. Figure 1.2 shows an example. Weigert et al. [8] in a multicenter study determining the impact of molecular imaging concluded that statistically BSGI was more accurate (better sensitivity, specificity and PPV) than ultrasound, when findings were discordant from a standard mammogram. Lately, BSGI guided biopsy systems [6, 8] have become available which allows confirmation of pathology results and better correlation with imaging findings.

Limitations

Poor visualization of chest wall and axilla are some of the drawbacks, which can be overcome with additional views. The inability to obtain all of the breast tissue in the field of view (FOV) to a large extent has been alleviated by offering nuclear medicine technologists training in breast positioning by mammographers [9]. In view of potential radiation risks the dose of the injected radiopharmaceutical has

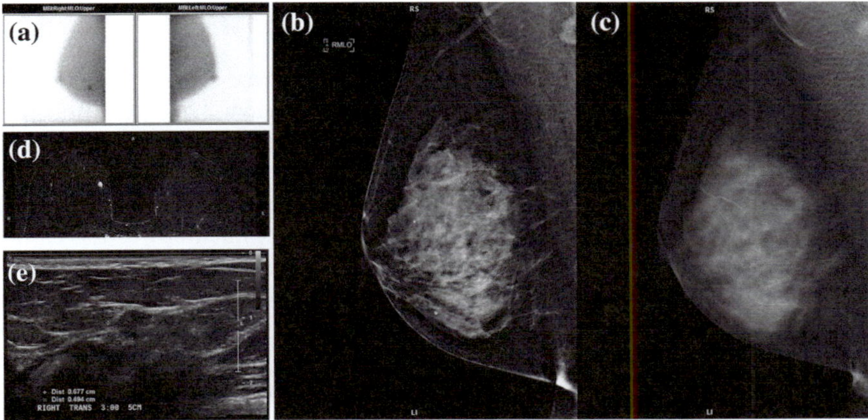

Fig. 1.2 An asymptomatic postmenopausal woman with a prior negative mammogram participated in a research study evaluating the effect of caffeine on Tc99 m sestamibi uptake. Her molecular breast imaging (*MBI*) exam (bilateral MLO) was positive (**a**). There was a focal area of moderate intensity radiotracer uptake in the lower inner right breast at middle depth measuring 1 × 0.7 × 0.8 cm. Subsequent digital mammogram (**b**), and digital breast tomosynthesis (**c**) showed no correlate to the MBI finding. Breast MRI (**d**) depicted a 0.6 × 0.6 × 0.9 cm enhancing round mass with slight irregular margins corresponding to the abnormality identified by MBI (**a**). Second look ultrasound (**e**) followed by ultrasound guided biopsy indicated a 6 mm invasive ductal carcinoma. *Courtesy of Michael K. O'Connor, Ph.D., Mayo Clinic, Rochester, MN*

been steadily decreasing. Initial trials on BSGI used doses of 30 mCi (1110 mBq), currently this has dropped to 20 mCi and some centers use only 10–15 mCi of ^{99m}Tc [7]. Trials at Mayo Clinic in Rochester, MN are experimenting with a dose as low as 4 mCi and by enhancing image quality with digital post-processing. At this dose the radiation dose to the breast is comparable to a standard two-view mammogram. The results from this study will determine if MBI has a role in screening, particularly for the intermediate risk category, where the benefit of MRI is not clearly defined. While one of the earlier limitations of BSGI was the poor sensitivity of molecular imaging in identifying sub-cm tumors, with recent advances, Hruska et al. [16] demonstrated sensitivities up to 80 % for tumors less than 1 cm.

Positron Emission Mammography (PEM)

Positron emission tomography (PET) imaging is a useful diagnostic test in many malignancies, but has not been accepted as standard of care in breast cancers [19]. Dedicated PEM scanners for breast have been developed, providing higher resolution than whole body PET scanners [20]. In PEM and PET imaging, the radiotracer fluoro-deoxyglucose (18-FDG) is used, providing a physiological measure of increased metabolic activity. While a promising tool it also demonstrates 'hot spots' at inflammatory and infective sites resulting in false positives.

Limitations

In order for the test to be sensitive, it is essential that there is good regulation of glucose levels and the blood glucose levels must be below 120 mg/dl. In order to achieve sufficient gamma counts in the image it is necessary for the patient to wait at least 2 h after administration of the radiopharmaceutical before imaging the breast. Also, it is important for the patient to remain quiet and warm to prevent 'hot spots' from unusual muscular activity. One of the limitations of the earlier whole body PET scanners was its inability to pick up sub-cm cancers. This has been addressed to a large extent by the development of new, dedicated breast scanners. Also, low grade tumors and some invasive lobular cancers and ductal carcinoma in situ do not show avid uptake of the radiotracer [19]. Radiation concern continues to be a major limitation [10]. PEM suffers from some of the same limitations associated with positioning as noted in BSGI. Not only does the imaging take 40 min (10 min for each view), but the patient needs to wait about 2 h post tracer injection before the images can be obtained. Like BSGI, the sensitivity in PEM imaging showed a declining trend with smaller sized tumors. In addition, PEM equipment is more expensive than BSGI and requires access to the 18-FDG radiotracer. Hence, PET and PEM are available only in a limited number of clinical practices in the United States.

Advantages

The availability of more recent prototypes of dedicated PEM scanners with its ability to perform imaging guided biopsies has made it an attractive additional imaging tool [19, 21]. PEM sensitivity matched MRI for single lesions and the sensitivity for unsuspected lesion was around 85 % [22, 23]. PEM had higher specificity for unsuspected lesion compared to MRI. PEM imaging is useful in identifying the extent of the tumor and staging, evaluating response to treatment, identifying sites of distant metastases, and distinguishing a scar from recurrence [19, 20, 22, 23].

Research studies over the past 10–15 years have established the role and value of MBI and PEM in breast imaging. While the newer breast molecular imaging modalities have shown promise, they are still only useful as supplemental imaging tools that can increase the radiologists' confidence in detecting breast cancer and cannot supplant established modalities such as screening mammogram, ultrasound, and MR imaging. Additional regulatory approvals are needed for the clinical site to handle radioactivity.

Radiation Risks

Since molecular imaging involves substantial radiation dose to part of the body other than the breast, there is concern about risk of cancer for radiosensitive organs; in the urinary bladder with PEM studies and in the colon with BSGI studies. Hendrick [10] has estimated the lifetime attributable risk (LAR) of a fatal cancer in BSGI studies at standard recommended doses of 20–30 mCi (740–1100 MBq) to be 20–30 times that of a digital mammogram in woman aged 40 years, and 23 times higher with a single PEM study at standard 10 mCi (370 MBq) dose of 18-FDG.

It is also relevant to add that even though considerable advancements have been made in radiotracer-based molecular imaging of the breast, currently it is not a screening tool. Its primary role may be as an adjunct to standard mammography and ultrasound, particularly in women with dense breasts and in the intermediate risk category. In the high-risk women, MRI with its proven track record as the modality with the highest sensitivity for detection is the established modality. Both BSGI and PEM/PET have the advantage of identifying physiological changes that distinguish a cancerous lesion from benign tissue and also identify additional foci in the ipsilateral and contralateral breast. They are also helpful imaging options to monitor response to chemotherapy drugs. Their sensitivity is however known to decrease with smaller sized tumors. A higher incidence of false positive tracer uptake has been noted in fibrocystic lesions, growing fibroadenomas, and fat necrosis. PEM has shown to be useful in distinguishing a scar from recurrence where conventional imaging findings are equivocal.

Optical Imaging with Near Infrared Spectroscopy

Transillumination of the breast using light, referred to as diaphanography, was proposed in 1920s. Variants of this approach were investigated till the early 1990s. However, the approach was not recommended for breast cancer screening [24]. Better understanding of the contrast mechanisms, characterization of absorption and scattering properties of breast tissues at various wavelengths, and techniques for modeling optical photon transport through tissues have facilitated development of quantitative methods for diffuse optical spectroscopic imaging. Diffuse optical imaging using continuous wave, time domain, or frequency domain measurements at near-infrared (NIR) wavelengths can be used to provide noninvasive in vivo quantitation of attenuation and scattering properties of breast tissue. This can be used to determine total hemoglobin content, oxygen saturation (ratio of oxygenated hemoglobin to total hemoglobin), water, and lipid content. Extension of the approach to 3D imaging, similar to computed tomography (CT), has resulted in diffuse optical tomography (DOT) systems. Hand-held diffuse optical spectroscopy imaging systems have been developed and continue to be refined [25, 26]. Stand-alone DOT prototype systems for adjunctive use in diagnostic breast imaging have been developed by academic investigators [27, 28] and by commercial entities (SoftScan®, Advanced Research Technologies, Inc., Montreal, Canada; CTLM®, Imaging Diagnostic Systems, Inc., Fort Lauderdale, USA).

In a study of 90 subjects, DOT showed that the ratio of total hemoglobin in the abnormality to that in the normal contralateral breast was statistically different for malignant tumors [29]. However, the study noted that there may be a resolution threshold of approximately 6 mm. Development of multimodality systems combining NIRS with X-ray imaging has been reported [30–32]. In a study of 189 breasts from 125 subjects including 51 breasts with lesions, a statistically significant increase was observed for total hemoglobin in malignant tumors larger than 6 mm compared to fibroglandular tissue [33]. A hand-held probe combining ultrasound with NIR imaging has been developed, and in a study of 65 subjects with 81 lesions significantly higher concentration of total hemoglobin was observed in malignancies than benign lesions [34].

Development of NIR systems integrated with MRI [35, 36] that incorporates image information from MRI during NIRS reconstruction as well as clinical evaluation of such multimodality systems have shown that malignant tumor exhibit higher concentration of total hemoglobin and lower oxygen saturation. The use of exogenous contrast agents such as indocyanine green as well as tumor-targeted contrast agents that are under development can preferentially enhance lesions and could improve differential diagnosis. Monitoring of neoadjuvant chemotherapy response with a hand-held diffuse optical spectroscopic imaging system in a limited dataset showed that significant changes in oxygenated hemoglobin could be observed approximately 90 days after initiation of therapy [37]. In order to reduce re-excision rates following breast conserving surgery (BCS), NIR-based optical imaging systems to assess tumor margins are being investigated [38, 39]. In summary, the past two decades have witnessed substantial improvement in optical imaging techniques using NIR spectroscopy, and its transition to routine use for some clinical applications is highly probable in the near future.

Optical Imaging with Confocal Microscopy

In the management of early breast cancer, BCS is the standard surgical procedure, where excision of the least volume of breast tissue free of tumor cells at the margins is the goal. However, the current surgical literature [40] estimates positive margins at surgery in the range of 20–70 %. This necessitates revision excision. Currently, the quickest means to evaluate tumor margins is the 'traditional frozen section'. This process is however laborious, time-consuming, does not include the entire tumor surface, and is limited by freezing artifacts of the surgical margins. Cauterization surgery also limits evaluation. Currently, there are many experimental, real-time, imaging options that are being evaluated. There is a need for such techniques to be cost-effective, reproducible, and dependable.

We performed an experimental trial [41–43] of excised lumpectomy specimens at the University of Massachusetts Medical School in collaboration with the Medical Physics department at University of Massachusetts, Lowell, MA. The investigators evaluated lumpectomy specimens from breast cancer patients with polarization techniques after staining the specimen with dilute methylene blue. Wide-field polarization for quick macroscopic survey and small FOV confocal

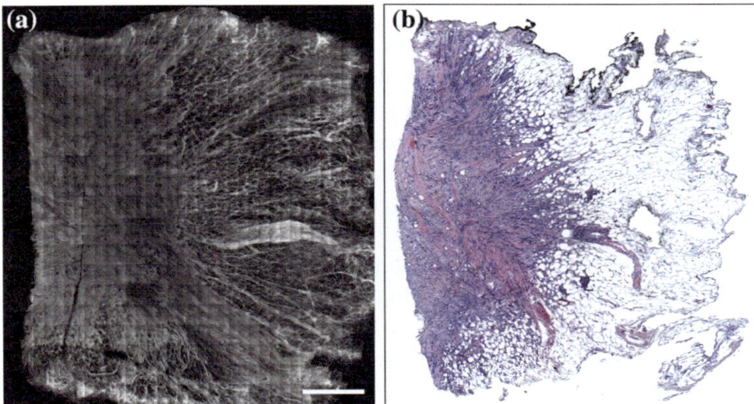

Fig. 1.3 Wide-field fluorescence polarization image (**a**) of a tissue section from a breast lumpectomy specimen with corresponding histopathology at scanning magnification (**b**) showing good demarcation between the benign (*right half*) and malignant (*left half*) breast tissue. *Fluorescence polarization image courtesy Anna Yaroslavsky, Ph.D., University of Massachusetts, Lowell, MA*

microscopy for small FOV with high resolution was performed, images analyzed, and later correlated with findings at Hematoxylin and Eosin (H&E) stained pathology slides evaluated by a trained breast pathologist (Fig. 1.3). The difference in the reflectance and fluorescence polarization values for benign and cancerous tissue was exploited. In these studies, Patel et al. [41–43] observed good correlation between fluorescence polarization values and findings on H&E stained sections of benign and malignant breast tissue on histopathology. The reflectance polarization values did not correlate as well. While the researchers concede to slight misregistration between confocal microscopy images and H&E stained specimens, the ease of use has good future potential to evaluate ex vivo specimens. The instrument could also be used in vivo on patients on the operating table to discern any residual malignant tissue that merits excision. A clinical trial is underway to evaluate the utility of this imaging technique for intraoperative evaluation of margins during BCS.

Terahertz Imaging

Accurate assessment of surgical margins of the excised breast specimen is very important in BCS in order to minimize the likelihood of re-excision. This is particularly relevant in the surgical treatment of invasive breast cancer followed by whole breast radiation therapy [44]. The reference standard for the determination of the tumor margins is by sectioning and imaging the excised specimen by conventional pathology procedures. However, more expedient techniques have been investigated over the years that allow prompt margin assessment at the intraoperative stage, thus affording the opportunity for the surgeon to excise additional tissue if needed. Breast specimen radiography has been used for many years for this purpose. This approach is used routinely in clinical practice but it has certain inherent limitations. Radiography generates planar images of a thick three-dimensional specimen; it provides good contrast for identification of surgical margins on the basis of changes in tissue composition and density, but it is not known to differentiate well between normal tissue and cancer especially when the malignancy does not exhibit prominent morphologic changes in tissue composition and density.

Advanced three-dimensional imaging technologies such as micro-Computed Tomography and micro-MRI have been developed but are limited to research applications due to their complexity and cost. For intraoperative imaging of breast specimens, the trend in recent years has been to identify imaging approaches that can provide improved discrimination between tumor, and surrounding tissue compared to X-ray imaging. Therefore, imaging techniques that are sensitive to the molecular differences between normal and abnormal tissues may improve identification of tumor margins compared to planar X-ray imaging. Interrogation of specimens with certain types of electromagnetic (EM) radiation generates reflected or transmitted signals with intensity and spectral characteristics that may vary substantially between tumors and normal tissue. These radiations include infrared, radiofrequency, or terahertz (10^{12} Hz) radiation and their application may range from detection of the presence of abnormal tissue to assessing their invasive potential [45–47]. In the case of breast surgery, the excised breast specimen is irradiated and the returning signal after absorption, diffuse reflectance, or fluorescence in the tissue is detected and analyzed. Some techniques rely on the detection and analysis in a non-imaging approach while others generate images of the surface of the specimen, which contain intensity and spectroscopic information. One of the newest approaches uses radiation in the terahertz region of the electromagnetic spectrum; this is the part of the spectrum between infrared to microwave with a corresponding wavelength in the region of about 0.05 mm to 1 mm. This type of radiation, also called T-rays, is relatively new to biomedical applications because the development of efficient and compact sources and detectors for biomedical applications has been gradual in the past 20 years. Unlike X-rays that can easily transmit through the entire body, terahertz radiation is readily absorbed by water in the tissue and therefore transmission measurements in thick specimens are not feasible. It penetrates only a few micrometers in the breast specimen depending on the frequency used. The reflected and scattered component of terahertz radiation carries information on composition that can be used to characterize the morphology and composition of tissues. This signal can be used to form an image with compositional topography that represents its molecular status of the specimen at its surface to a depth of a few micrometers below the surface. Tissue contrast can be observed because of differences in attenuation and refractive index of the specimen and these properties have been used to assess the margins of excised breast specimens [48–52]. Therefore, imaging and spectroscopy with terahertz waves is performed in the reflection mode in a scanning beam approach. Images of the specimen can be generated at a spatial resolution, which may vary between about 0.1 and 1.0 mm depending on the imaging system and wavelength. Terahertz images may be combined with images at other wavelengths for improved contrast and delineation of the lesion. Discrimination between normal and malignant tissues can be challenging from the raw images without proper image analysis. Some tissues, glandular and adipose for example, can be easily differentiated in terahertz imaging because of their pronounced differences in their refractive indices. It may be argued that conventional light in the visible spectrum easily discriminates between adipose and other tissues. However, terahertz appears to exhibit certain properties, which may enable detection of features that are characteristic to biochemical changes at the surface of the specimen that are associated with tumors [49].

Terahertz beam reflection, scattering, and spectra from biological specimens generally reveal variations in water composition. Under controlled conditions, Terahertz radiation can also provide characterization based on the concentration of amino acids, and proteins, and other biochemical components [53]. In the case of breast specimens, large differences in the refractive index between fibrous tissue and adipose tissue have been observed due to the large differences in their respective refractive indices and substantial differences have also been observed between fibrous tissue and breast tumors [54]. Such differences and other interactions with tissues can be used to generate images that reveal tumors in a background of healthy tissue in the specimen. In principle, other characteristics such as high levels of protein or amino acids may generate a signal under optimal conditions but at this time a complete accounting of all the components that give rise to contrast between tumors and healthy tissue has not been established.

Other radiations may be used to assess breast surgical specimen margins but at this time, specimen radiography with visual inspection is the most commonly used technique. Interrogation of the specimen with terahertz and other radiations has the potential to provide more specific information on tumor margins assuming that their refractive index and reflection properties are capable of discriminating between normal and malignant tissue. Other techniques for this purpose using optical coherence tomography with infrared radiation are being explored [55].

References

1. DeSantis C, Ma J, Bryan L, Jemal A. Breast cancer statistics, 2013. CA Cancer J Clinic. 2014;64(1):52–62.
2. Mandelson MT, Oestreicher N, Porter PL, White D, Finder CA, Taplin SH, White E. Breast density as a predictor of mammographic detection: comparison of interval and screen detected cancers. J Natl Cancer Inst. 2000;92(13):1081–7.
3. Drukteinis JS, Mooney BP, Floers CI, Gatenby RA. Beyond mammography: new frontiers in breast cancer screening. American J Med. 2013;126(6):472–9.
4. Niklason LT, Christian BT, Niklason LE, Kopans DB, Castleberry DE, OpsahlOng BH, Landberg CE, Slanetz PJ, Giardino AA, Moore R, Albagli D, DeJule MC, Fitzgerald PF, Fobare DF, Giambattista BW, Kwasnick RF, Liu JQ, Lubowski SJ, Possin GE, Richotte JF, Wei CY, Wirth RF. Digital tomosynthesis in breast imaging. Radiology. 1997;205(2):399–406.
5. Herranz M, Ruibal A. Optical imaging in breast cancer diagnosis: the next evolution. J Oncol. 2012;2012:863747.

6. Hruska CB, O'Connor MK. Nuclear imaging of the breast: translating achievements in instrumentation into clinical use. Med Phys. 2013;40(5):050901–23.
7. Rhodes DJ, Hruska CB, Phillips SW, Whaley DH, O'Connor MK. Dedicated dual-head gamma imaging for breast cancer screening in women with mammographically dense breasts. Radiology. 2011;258(1):106–18.
8. Weigert JM, Bertrand ML, Lanzkowsky L, Stern LH, Kieper DA. Results of a multicenter patient registry to determine the clinic impact of breast specific gamma imaging, a molecular breast imaging technique. AJR. 2012;198:W69–75.
9. O'Connor MK, Philips SW, Hruska CB, Rhodes DJ, Collins DA. Molecular breast imaging: advantages and limitations of a scintimammographic technique in patients with small breast tumors. Breast J. 2007;13(1):3–11.
10. Hendrick RE. Radiation doses and cancer risks from breast imaging studies. Radiology. 2010;257(1):246–53.
11. Miller AB, Wall C, Baines CJ, Sun P, To T, Narod SA. Twenty five year follow up for breast cancer incidence and mortality of the Canadian national breast screening study: randomized screening trail. BMJ. 2014;348:g366.
12. Checka CM, Chun JE, Schnabel FR, Lee J, Toth H. The relationship of mammographic density and age: implications for breast cancer screening. AJR. 2012;198:W292–5.
13. Buist DS, Porter PL, Lehman C, Taplin SH, White E. Factors contributing to mammography failure in women aged 40–49 years. J Natl Cancer Inst. 2004;96(19):1432–40.
14. Ciatto S, Houssami N, Bernardi D, Caumo F, Pellegrini M, Brunelli S, Tuttobene P, Bricolo P, Fanto C, Valentini M, Montemezzi S, Macaskill P. Integration of 3D digital mammography with tomosynthesis for population breast-cancer screening (STORM): a prospective comparison study. Lancet Oncol. 2013;14(7):583–9.
15. Giuliano V, Giuliano C. Improved breast cancer detection in asymptomatic women using 3D-automated breast ultrasound in mammographically dense breasts. Clin Imaging. 2013;37(3):480–6.
16. Hruska CB, Phillips SW, Whaley DH, Rhodes DJ, O'Connor MK. Molecular breast imaging: use of a dual-head dedicated gamma camera to detect small breast tumors. AJR. 2008;191:1805–15.
17. Brem RF, Rapelyea JA, Zisman G, Mohtashemi K, Raub J, Teal CB, Majewski S, Welch BL. Occult breast cancer: scintimammography with high-resolution breast-specific gamma camera in women at high risk for breast cancer. Radiology. 2005;237:274–80.
18. Brem RF, Floerke AC, Rapelyea JA, Teal C, Kelly T, Mathur V. Breast specific gamma imaging as an adjunct imaging modality for the diagnosis of breast cancer. Radiology. 2008;247:651–7.
19. Kalles V, Zografos GC, Provatopoulou X, Koulocheri D, Gounaris A. The current status of positron emission mammography in breast cancer diagnosis. Breast Cancer. 2013;20:123–30.
20. Narayanan D, Madsen KS, Kalinyak JE, Berg WA. Interpretation of positron emission mammograpghy and MRI by experienced breast imaging radiologists: performance and observer reproducibility. AJR. 2011;196:971–81.
21. Kalinyak JE, Schilling K, Berg WA, Narayanan D, Mayberry JP, Rai R, Dupree EB, Shusterman DK, Gittleman MA, Luo W, Matthews CG. PET guided breast biopsy. Breast J. 2011;17(2):143–51.
22. Berg WA, Madsen KS, Schilling K, Tartar M, Pisano EA, Larsen LH, Narayanan D, Ozonoff A, Miller JP, Kalinyak JE. Breast cancer: comparative effectiveness of positron emission mammography and MR imaging in presurgical planning for the ipsilateral breast. Radiology. 2011;258:59–72.
23. Berg WA, Madsen KS, Schilling K, Tartar M, Pisano ED, Larsen LH, Narayanan D, Kalinyak JE. Comparative effectiveness of positron emission mammography and MRI in the contralateral breast of women with newly diagnosed breast cancer. AJR. 2012;198:219–32.
24. Centers for Disease. C. Inappropriate use of transillumination for breast cancer screening–Wisconsin, 1990. MMWR. Morb Mortal Wkly Rep. 1991;40(18):293–6.

25. Shah N, Cerussi A, Eker C, Espinoza J, Butler J, Fishkin J, Hornung R, Tromberg BJ. Noninvasive functional optical spectroscopy of human breast tissue. Proc Nat Acad Sci. 2001;98(8):4420–5.
26. Gonzalez J, Decerce J, Erickson SJ, Martinez SL, Nunez A, Roman M, Traub B, Flores CA, Roberts SM, Hernandez E, Aguirre W, Kiszonas R, Godavarty A. Hand-held optical imager (Gen-2): improved instrumentation and target detectability. J Biomed Opt. 2012;17(8):081402–1.
27. McBride TO, Pogue BW, Jiang S, Osterberg UL, Paulsen KD. A parallel-detection frequency-domain near-infrared tomography system for hemoglobin imaging of the breast in vivo. Rev Sci Instrum. 2001;72(3):1817–24.
28. Culver JP, Choe R, Holboke MJ, Zubkov L, Durduran T, Slemp A, Ntziachristos V, Chance B, Yodh AG. Three-dimensional diffuse optical tomography in the parallel plane transmission geometry: evaluation of a hybrid frequency domain/continuous wave clinical system for breast imaging. Med Phys. 2003;30(2):235–47.
29. Poplack SP, Tosteson TD, Wells WA, Pogue BW, Meaney PM, Hartov A, Kogel CA, Soho SK, Gibson JJ, Paulsen KD. Electromagnetic breast imaging: results of a pilot study in women with abnormal mammograms. Radiology. 2007;243(2):350–9.
30. Boverman G, Fang Q, Carp SA, Miller EL, Brooks DH, Selb J, Moore RH. Kopans DB, Boas DA. Spatio-temporal imaging of the hemoglobin in the compressed breast with diffuse optical tomography. Phys Med Biol. 2007;52(12):3619–41.
31. Krishnaswamy V, Michaelsen KE, Pogue BW, Poplack SP, Shaw I, Defrietas K, Brooks K, Paulsen KD. A digital x-ray tomosynthesis coupled near infrared spectral tomography system for dual-modality breast imaging. Opt Express. 2012;20(17):19125–36.
32. Vedantham S, Shi L, Karellas A, Michaelsen KE, Krishnaswamy V, Pogue BW, Paulsen KD. Semi-automated segmentation and classification of digital breast tomosynthesis reconstructed images. In: Conference Proceeding of IEEE Engineering in Medicine and Biology Society, EMBC, 2011. p. 6188–6191.
33. Fang Q, Selb J, Carp SA, Boverman G, Miller EL, Brooks DH, Moore RH, Kopans DB, Boas DA. Combined optical and X-ray tomosynthesis breast imaging. Radiology. 2011;258(1):89–97.
34. Zhu Q, Cronin EB, Currier AA, Vine HS, Huang M, Chen N, Xu C. Benign versus malignant breast masses: optical differentiation with US-guided optical imaging reconstruction. Radiology. 2005;237(1):57–66.
35. Ntziachristos V, Yodh AG, Schnall MD, Chance B. MRI-guided diffuse optical spectroscopy of malignant and benign breast lesions. Neoplasia. 2002;4(4):347–54.
36. Brooksby B, Jiang S, Dehghani H, Pogue BW, Paulsen KD, Kogel C, Doyley M, Weaver JB, Poplack SP. Magnetic resonance-guided near-infrared tomography of the breast. Rev Sci Instrum. 2004;75(12):5262–70.
37. O'Sullivan TD, Leproux A, Chen JH, Bahri S, Matlock A, Roblyer D, McLaren CE, Chen WP, Cerussi AE, Su MY, Tromberg BJ. Optical imaging correlates with magnetic resonance imaging breast density and reveals composition changes during neoadjuvant chemotherapy. Breast Cancer Res. 2013;15(1):R14.
38. Laughney AM, Krishnaswamy V, Rice TB, Cuccia DJ, Barth RJ, Tromberg BJ, Paulsen KD, Pogue BW, Wells WA. System analysis of spatial frequency domain imaging for quantitative mapping of surgically resected breast tissues. J Biomed Opt. 2013 18(3):036012.
39. Dhar S, Lo JY, Palmer GM, Brooke MA, Nichols BS, Yu B, Ramanujam N, Jokerst NM. A diffuse reflectance spectral imaging system for tumor margin assessment using custom annular photodiode arrays. Biomedical optics express. 2012;3(12):3211–22.
40. Jacobs L. Positive margins: the challenge continues for breast surgeons. Ann Surg Oncol. 2008;15(5):1271–2.
41. Patel R, Khan A, Wirth D, Kamionek M, Kandil D, Quinlan R, Yaroslavsky AN. Multimodal optical imaging for detecting breast cancer. J Biomed Optics. 2012;17(6):066008.

42. Patel R, Khan A, Wirth D, Kamionek M, Kandil D, Quinlan R, Yaroslavsky AN. Delineating breast ductal carcinoma using combined dye-enhanced wide-field polarization imaging and optical coherence tomography. Biophoton. 2013;6(9):679–86.
43. Patel R, Khan A, Quinlan R, Yaroslavsky AN. Polarization sensitive multimodal imaging for detecting breast cancer. Cancer Res. 2014;74(17):4685–93.
44. Azu M, Abrahamse P, Katz SJ, Jagsi R, Morrow M. What is an adequate margin for breast-conserving surgery? Surgeon attitudes and correlates. Ann Surg Oncol. 2010;17:558–63.
45. Backman V, Wallace MB, Perelman LT, Arendt JT, Gurjar R, Müller MG, Zhang Q, Zonios G, Kline E, McGilligan JA, Shapshay S, Valdez T, Badizadegan K, Crawford JM, Fitzmaurice M, Kabani S, Levin HS, Seiler M, Dasari RR, Itzkan I, Van Dam J, Feld MS. Nature. 2000;406(6791):35–6.
46. Brown JQ, Vishwanath K, Palmer GM, Ramanujam N. Advances in quantitative UV-visible spectroscopy for clinical and pre-clinical application in cancer. Curr Opin Biotechnol. 2009;20(1):119–31.
47. Brown JQ, Bydlon TM, Kennedy SA, Caldwell ML, Gallagher JE, Junker M, Wilke LG, Barry WT, Geradts J, Ramanujam N. Optical spectral surveillance of breast tissue landscapes for detection of residual disease in breast tumor margins. PLoS ONE. 2013;8(7):e69906.
48. Fitzgerald AJ, Wallace VP, Jimenez-Linan M, Bobrow L, Pye RJ, Purushotham AD, Arnone DD. Terahertz pulsed imaging of human breast tumors. Radiology. 2006;239(2):533–40.
49. Fitzgerald AJ, Pinder S, Purushotham AD, O'Kelly P, Ashworth PC, Wallace VP. Classification of terahertz-pulsed imaging data from excised breast tissue. J Biomed Opt. 2012;17(1):016005.
50. Fitzgerald AJ, Pickwell-MacPherson E, Wallace VP. Use of finite difference time domain simulations and debye theory for modelling the terahertz reflection response of normal and tumour breast tissue. PLoS ONE. 2014;9(7):e99291.
51. Yngvesson SK, St Peter B, Siqueira P, Kelly P, Glick S, Karellas A, Khan A. Feasibility demonstration of frequency domain terahertz imaging in breast cancer margin determination. In: Proceedings of society of photo-optical instrumentation engineers 2012. Optical interactions with tissue and cells XXIII; vol. 8221, 82210N.
52. St Peter B, Yngvesson S, Siqueira P, Kelly P, Khan A, Glick S, Karellas A. Development and testing of a single frequency terahertz imaging system for breast cancer detection. IEEE J Biomed Health Inform. 2013;17(4):785–797.
53. Ajito K, Ueno Y. Thz chemical imaging for biological applications. IEEE Trans Thz Sci Techn. 2011;1(1):293–300.
54. Ashworth PC, Pickwell-MacPherson E, Provenzano E, Pinder SE, Purushotham AD, Pepper M, Wallace VP. Terahertz pulsed spectroscopy of freshly excised human breast cancer. Opt Express. 2009;17(15):12444–54.
55. Savastru D, Chang EW, Miclos S, Pitman MB, Patel A, Iftimia N. Detection of breast surgical margins with optical coherence tomography imaging: a concept evaluation study. J Biomed Opt. 2014;19(5):056001.

Chapter 2
Familial Breast Cancer and Genetic Predisposition in Breast Cancer

Vighnesh Walavalkar, Ashraf Khan and Dina Kandil

Introduction

Breast cancer is the most common non-dermatologic malignancy in women and it is estimated that approximately one in nine women will develop breast cancer over their lifetimes. In the United States, more than 200,000 new cases of breast cancer were reported in 2010 and breast cancer was responsible for approximately 40,000 deaths (15 % of all cancer deaths) in the same calendar year [1]. The etiology behind developing breast cancer is multifactorial, with many risk factors including diet, lifestyle, reproductive factors and hormonal status. However, a very important risk factor is a genetic predisposition and a positive family history. A genetic influence on mammary carcinogenesis has long been implicated and it is estimated that approximately 10 % of breast cancer patients are carriers of gene mutations susceptible for the development of breast cancer [2]. Of these genes, perhaps the most extensively studied are breast cancer 1, early onset (BRCA1), breast cancer 2, early onset (BRCA2) and Tumor protein p53 (TP53) genes. These are associated with a high risk of developing breast cancer in carriers and hence they are referred to as high-penetrance genes. It should be noted, however, that among breast cancer patients with a strong family history; only 40 % have cancers that are thought to be caused by the above-mentioned three genes [3]. This suggests that in the remaining 60 % of cases, apart from sporadic breast cancers, other genetic pathways are likely involved.

V. Walavalkar · A. Khan · D. Kandil (✉)
Department of Pathology, University of Massachusetts Medical School,
UMassMemorial Medical Center, Three Biotech, One Innovation Drive,
Worcester, MA 01605, USA
e-mail: dina.kandil@umassmemorial.org

© Springer Science+Business Media New York 2015
A. Khan et al. (eds.), *Precision Molecular Pathology of Breast Cancer*,
Molecular Pathology Library 10, DOI 10.1007/978-1-4939-2886-6_2

Ataxia Telangiectasia Mutated Gene (ATM), CHEK2, BRIP1, PALB2, RAD50, PTEN, CDH1, STK11, etc. are examples of genes that are thought to play important roles in breast cancer pathways. In fact, it has now been shown that these moderate penetrance genes along with many low penetrance single nucleotide polymorphisms (SNPs) [4] interact with one another as well as influence pathways involving BRCA1 and BRCA2. Studies have suggested that these genes are involved in complex genetic pathways, some of which are closely related and ultimately are associated with the development of breast cancer. This chapter gives an overview of some of these genes along with the clinicopathologic features of the cancers associated with them. This will be summarized in Table 2.1. We will also briefly touch upon clinical syndromes associated with breast cancer, genetic testing, preventive strategies and certain aspects of management of familial breast cancer in the United States. A summary of these clinical syndromes are presented in Table 2.2.

Genetics of Breast Cancer

High-Penetrance Genes

Breast Cancer 1, Early Onset (BRCA1)

BRCA1 is a large gene located on the long (q) arm of chromosome 17 at position 21 (17q21). BRCA1 is a tumor suppressor gene, which is expressed in response to genomic instability and is influenced by estrogen. Its main function is related to DNA repair including homologous recombination, nucleotide excision repair, and spindle regulation. It also acts as a gatekeeper of cell-cycle progression mainly through checkpoint control [5]. Recent studies have described complex and innovative mechanisms for the localization of BRCA1 to DNA-breaks, including an emerging ubiquitylation-dependent cascade and an association with BRCA2 and genes in the Fanconi anemia pathway [6]. Thus, BRCA1 acts as a regulator of genome stability and its main function is to respond to various types of DNA damage via a complex interaction with BRCA2 and other genes.

Numerous mutations in BRCA1 have been described. The majority of which are point mutations and small insertions/deletions leading to truncated forms of the BRCA1 protein [7]. Large genomic deletions including whole exon deletions have also been detected using more sophisticated methods such as multiplex ligation-dependent probe amplification (MLPA) [8]. Some mutations appear to be more common in certain ethnic groups (founder mutations). The most commonly described is the c.5266dupC mutation (also known as 5382insC or 185delAG), which is seen in up to 2 % of the Ashkenazi Jewish population. However, recent studies have suggested that this mutation may be prevalent in some other ethnic groups where genetic screening of BRCA1 is not routinely performed [9].

Approximately 1 in 1000 individuals in the female population carries a pathogenic mutation in BRCA1. BRCA1 cancers account for approximately 10 %

Table 2.1 A summary of genes associated with the development of breast cancer

Gene	Chromosomal location	Function	Mode of inheritance	Lifetime risk of developing breast cancer	Other major cancer risk	Clinical syndrome association
TP53	17p13.1	Regulates expression of many genes by anti-proliferative mechanisms inducing cell cycle arrest and apoptosis	Autosomal dominant	85–90 %	Soft tissue (sarcomas), bone (osteosarcoma), CNS tumors (choroid plexus tumors), adrenal gland[a]	Li-Fraumeni syndrome, Li-Fraumeni-like syndrome
ATM	11q22-q23	Upstream regulator of proteins involved in double-stranded DNA repair, including BRCA1, TP53, and CHEK2	Autosomal dominant and recessive	~20 % or less	Lymphoproliferative disorders	Ataxia-telangiectasia
CHEK2	22q12.1	Encodes for a threonine/serine kinase that prevents cell proliferation by phosphorylation of proteins involved in checkpoint control	Autosomal dominant and recessive	~20 % or less	Colorectal, prostate	–
BRIP1	17q22.2	Encodes for a DNA helicase that performs BRCA1-dependent DNA repair and checkpoint control	Autosomal dominant and recessive	~20 % or less	Ovary, cervix	Fanconi anemia
PALB2	16p12.2	Acts as a functional bridging molecule linking the DNA repair functions of BRCA1 and BRCA2	Autosomal dominant and recessive	~20 % or less	Pancreas	Fanconi anemia

(continued)

Table 2.1 (continued)

Gene	Chromosomal location	Function	Mode of inheritance	Lifetime risk of developing breast cancer	Other major cancer risk	Clinical syndrome association
CDH1	16q22.1	Encodes for a cell adhesion molecule called E-cadherin	Autosomal dominant	50–60 %	Stomach	Hereditary diffuse gastric cancer syndrome
PTEN	10q23.3	Down-regulates the phosphatidylinositol-3-kinase (PI3K) signal transduction cascade and acts as a tumor suppressor and growth regulator	Autosomal dominant	25–50 %	Thyroid (except medullary carcinoma), endometrium, colon, rectum	Cowden syndrome
STK11	19p13.3	Encodes for serine threonine kinase	Autosomal dominant	~30 %	Colorectal, gastric, pancreatic, ovary	Peutz-Jeghers syndrome
RAD50	5q31	Part of MRN complex along with MRE11 and NBS1, which facilitates double-strand DNA break repair	Unknown	Unknown	Unknown	Ataxia-telangiectasia-like disorder, Nijmegen breakage syndrome (NBS) and NBS-like disorder

[a]Additional risk in TP53 mutations include: gastrointestinal tract cancers (esophageal, gastric and colorectal), genitourinary cancers (renal, Wilms tumor, endometrial, ovarian, prostate), melanoma, thyroid, and lymphoproliferative disorders

Table 2.2 Clinical syndromes associated with breast cancer

	Gene(s) involved	Clinical manifestations	Cancer prevention strategy	Cancer management
Hereditary breast and ovarian cancer syndrome[a]	BRCA1, BRCA2	Early onset of breast and ovarian cancer. Also high risk for early onset prostate, pancreas, skin (melanoma), gastrointestinal tract cancers	• Genetic counseling and standard genetic testing with full gene sequencing and large genomic alterations analysis • Patient awareness and routine monthly self breast exam from 18 years of age onwards • Biannual clinical breast exam from 25 years of age onward • Annual bilateral mammogram and MRI starting at age 25 • Discuss ovarian cancer screening (transvaginal ultrasound and serum CA125 testing every 6 months) • Discuss risks and benefits of chemoprevention • Risk-reducing mastectomies and salpingoophorectomies • Prostate cancer screening in men after age 40	• Individualized chemotherapeutic regimen with poly(ADP-ribose) polymerase inhibitors ± platinum or other combination therapy • Bilateral mastectomies and salpingoophorectomy
Li-Fraumeni and Li-Fraumeni-like syndrome[a]	TP53	Autosomal dominant cancer predisposition syndrome associated with early onset of breast cancer, choroid plexus carcinomas, adrenocortical carcinoma, soft tissue sarcoma and osteosarcomas. Also high risk for many other visceral malignancies and lymphoproliferative disorders	• Genetic counseling and testing • Patient awareness and routine monthly self breast exam from 18 years of age onwards • Biannual clinical breast exam from 25 years of age (or as early as 18 years) onward • Annual bilateral mammogram and MRI from 25 years of age (or as early as 18 years) onward • Colonoscopy every 2–5 years starting 25 years of age onward • Annual skin and neurologic exam	• Surgical management preferred ± individualized chemotherapeutic regimen • Radiation therapy often used as last option as there is a questionable risk for therapy induced secondary malignancy

(continued)

Table 2.2 (continued)

	Gene(s) involved	Clinical manifestations	Cancer prevention strategy	Cancer management
Cowden syndrome[a]	PTEN	Autosomal dominant cancer predisposition syndrome with early onset of breast, thyroid, endometrium, and colorectal cancers. Also characterized by multiple hamartomas, facial trichilemmomas, acral keratoses and oral papillomatous papules	• Genetic counseling and testing • Patient awareness and monthly breast exams • Discuss annual mammography ± MRI • Discuss increased surveillance for endometrial, thyroid, and colorectal cancers, although there is no consensus screen strategy • Discuss prophylactic mastectomies and hysterectomy	• Individualized treatment strategy
Peutz-Jeghers syndrome	STK11	Rare autosomal dominant condition characterized by hamartomatous polyps in the GI tract, mucocutaneous pigmentation and increased risk for breast, colorectal, gastric, pancreatic, and ovarian cancer	• Patient awareness, genetic counseling and testing • No established guidelines on cancer prevention, patients may be followed on an individualized basis	• Individualized treatment strategy
Ataxia-telangiectasia (AT), AT-like disorder, Nijmegen breakage syndrome (NBS) and NBS-like disorder	ATM, RAD50, NBS1, MRE11 and MRN complex	AT is an autosomal recessive disorder characterized by progressive neurologic impairment, cerebellar ataxia, ocular telangiectasia, variable immunodeficiency, defective organogenesis and an increased risk of developing visceral malignancies and lymphoproliferative disorders	• Patient awareness, genetic counseling, and testing • No established guidelines on cancer prevention, patients may be followed on an individualized basis	• Individualized treatment strategy

(continued)

Table 2.2 (continued)

	Gene(s) involved	Clinical manifestations	Cancer prevention strategy	Cancer management
Fanconi anemia	BRIP1, PALB2, BRCA2 and other FANC group of genes	X-linked recessive disorder characterized by bone marrow failure, developmental abnormalities, and increased risk for ovarian, prostate, pancreas, skin gastrointestinal tract, and cervix cancers. Clinical features include skin pigmentation, short stature, upper limb, and eye malformations	• Patient awareness, genetic counseling and testing • No established guidelines on cancer prevention, patients may be followed on an individualized basis	• Individualized treatment strategy • Cells with mutated FANC genes show profound sensitivity to DNA interstrand cross-linking agents (cisplatin and mitomycin C) • Radiation and PARP inhibitors may play a role
Hereditary diffuse gastric cancer syndrome	CDH1	Autosomal dominant cancer predisposition syndrome with increased risk for developing breast and gastric cancers	• Patient awareness, genetic counseling, and testing • No established guidelines on cancer prevention, patients may be followed on an individualized basis	• Individualized` treatment strategy

[a]NCCN Guidelines Version 1.2014: breast and/or ovarian cancer genetic assessment

of all familial cancers; [10–12] and a mutation in BRCA1 confers a 70–85 % lifetime risk of developing breast cancer [11–13]. BRCA1 mutations also are associated with a 50 % increased risk of developing ovarian cancer, especially high-grade serous carcinoma [14]. The risk for developing both breast and ovarian cancer in BRCA1 patients is age dependant, and the age at which these cancers present is much younger than that of the general population [11, 14]. Tumors developing in patients with BRCA1 mutations are usually triple-negative (negative for ER, PR, and HER2), high-grade invasive ductal carcinomas. However, approximately 5–25 % of BRCA1 breast carcinomas can be ER positive and a small percentage can show low-grade nuclear histology. Gene expression profiling studies show that BRCA1 associated breast carcinomas tend to cluster with sporadic triple-negative cancers [15–18]. BRCA1 breast cancers share many morphologic features with medullary-like carcinoma and basal-like carcinoma, with pushing margins, a prominent lymphocytic infiltrate, high-grade nuclear atypia and brisk mitosis (see Chap. 11) [15, 16]. Further, immunohistochemical expression of basal cytokeratins such Cytokeratin (CK) 5/6, CK14, CK17 and epidermal growth factor receptor (EGFR) which define BLBC are also identified in many BRCA1 related tumors [19]. BRCA1 carcinomas also tend to show high expression of cell proliferation marker Ki-67 as well as p53 and p16 positivity as compared to sporadic cancers [20].

Breast Cancer 2, Early Onset (BRCA2)

BRCA2 is a large gene located on the long (q) arm of chromosome 13 at position 12.3 (13q12.3). BRCA2 belongs to a family of genes involved in the Fanconi anemia pathway; which also includes partner and localizer of BRCA2 (PALB2) and BRCA1 interacting protein C-terminal helicase 1 (BRIP1) which are discussed later in the chapter.

As in BRCA1, BRCA2 is also involved in DNA repair. Its role however is not as well understood as that of BRCA1. It is now thought that BRCA2 facilitates homologous recombination and double-strand break repair through its interaction with RAD51. The BRCA2 protein forms a stable complex with the RAD51 protein and directs it to sites of DNA damage [21]. 21 BRCA2 also plays a role in the Fanconi anemia pathway of breast cancer through its interaction with other FANC (Fanconi anemia, complementation groups) genes such as BRIP1 and PALB2. A defect in any one of the proteins along the Fanconi anemia pathway prevents cancer cells from repairing interstrand crosslinks, predisposing them to chromosomal instability. It is suggested that BRCA2 protein helps to prevent these interstrand crosslinks by its ability to facilitate homologous recombination [22, 23].

Similar to BRCA1, hundreds of mutations have been described in BRCA2, the majority being point mutations leading to frameshifts and production of an abnormally truncated BRCA2 protein. Founder mutations in BRCA2 have been described in certain ethnic groups such as the c.5946delT (6174delT) mutation in the Ashkenazi Jewish population [3, 11].

Approximately 1 in 800 individuals in the female population carry a pathogenic mutation in BRCA2. Similar to BRCA1, BRCA2 cancers account for approximately

10 % of familial cancers; [10–12] and a mutation in BRCA2 confers a 50–85 % lifetime risk of developing breast cancer [11–13]. There is an approximate 30 % risk for BRCA2 patients to develop ovarian cancer [14]. Males who are carriers of germline mutations in BRCA2 have an increased risk of developing breast cancer, approximately 10 % greater than men in the general population [24]. BRCA2 also confers an increased risk for the development of other cancers. Compared to non-carriers, men with BRCA2 mutations have a three-fold risk of developing prostate cancer and; according to recent studies; these tumors are often of a higher grade (Gleason score >7) and have an increased risk of recurrence [25]. Germline BRCA2 gene mutations are also responsible for approximately 5–20 % of familial pancreatic cancers [26, 27]. Additionally, there is some evidence for an increased risk of gastrointestinal tract cancers, melanomas, bone tumors and even rarely pharyngeal carcinomas in BRCA2 families [28, 29]. BRCA2 associated breast cancers are generally heterogeneous and unlike BRCA1, there is no specific phenotype that has proven to be predictive of BRCA2 status. Clinical features of BRCA1 and BRCA 2 genes and their associated cancers are compared in Table 2.3.

Table 2.3 Comparison of BRCA1 and BRCA2

Gene	BRCA1	BRCA2
Chromosomal location	17q21	13q12.3
Function	DNA repair including homologous recombination, nucleotide excision repair, and spindle regulation	Homologous recombination and double-strand break repair through its interaction with RAD51
Mode of inheritance	Autosomal dominant	Autosomal dominant
Lifetime risk of developing breast cancer	70–85 %	50–85 %
Other major cancer risk	Ovary	Ovary, male breast, prostate, pancreas, skin (melanoma), gastrointestinal tract
Clinical syndrome association	Hereditary breast and ovarian cancer syndrome	Hereditary breast and ovarian cancer syndrome, Fanconi anemia
Typical phenotype	High-grade ductal carcinomas, often with 'basal phenotype' (medullary appearance, pushing edges, lymphocytic infiltrate, high nuclear grade, and brisk mitotic activity). Tumors are often triple negative	No specific phenotype, ductal carcinoma NOS
Cancer management	Individualized chemotherapeutic regimen with poly (ADP-ribose) polymerase (PARP) inhibitors ± platinum-based therapy. Bilateral mastectomies and salpingoophorectomy	Individualized chemotherapeutic regimen with poly (ADP-ribose) polymerase (PARP) inhibitors ± platinum-based therapy. Bilateral mastectomies and salpingoophorectomy

Tumor Protein P53 (TP53)

TP53 is a tumor suppressor gene located on the short (p) arm of chromosome 17 at position 13.1 (17p13.1). It is the most commonly altered gene in human cancer; being mutated in more than 50 % of all cancers.

TP53 encodes a transcription factor which responds to numerous cellular mechanisms to regulate expression of target genes, and does so primarily by anti-proliferative mechanisms inducing cell cycle arrest and apoptosis.

Thousands of mutations in TP53 have been described in a variety of human cancers. The majority of which are missense substitutions; and other alterations include frameshift insertions and deletions, nonsense mutations, and silent mutations [30]. An exhaustive and comprehensive list of over 25,000 germline, somatic and experimentally induced mutations in TP53 along with information on the functional impact of mutant p53 proteins is available online at the International Agency for Research on Cancer (IARC) TP53 Database [31].

Rare germline mutations in TP53 cause Li-Fraumeni and Li-Fraumeni-like syndrome, which are autosomal dominant genetic disorders characterized by an increased likelihood of developing a number of different malignancies. Somatic mutations in tumors are very common and occur in more than 50 % of all human cancers. In patients with a TP53 mutation, the lifetime risk for developing any cancer is almost 100 %. This risk is age dependant, with approximately 35–50 % developing by age 30, and 80–90 % by age 60 [32]. The majority of cancers seen in affected families are breast cancer (most common), soft tissue sarcomas, osteosarcomas, central nervous system tumors (especially choroid plexus tumors) and adrenocortical carcinomas. Other cancers seen in patients with TP53 mutations are gastrointestinal malignancies (esophageal, gastric, and colorectal), genitourinary malignancies (bladder, renal, Wilms tumor, endometrial, ovarian, germ cell tumors, prostate), melanoma, thyroid cancers, and lymphoproliferative disorders. Due to its general low prevalence, TP53 mutations account for less than 1 % of familial breast cancers [10]. There is no specific phenotype seen in TP53 mutated breast cancers.

Moderate Penetrance Genes

Ataxia Telangiectasia Mutated Gene (ATM)

The ATM gene is located on the long (q) arm of chromosome 1, between positions 22 and 23 (11q22-q23). A large number of mutations involving the ATM gene have been identified, which are responsible for approximately 2 % of familial breast cancers [33].

The ATM protein acts as an important upstream regulator of proteins involved in double-stranded DNA repair, including BRCA1, TP53, and CHEK2. ATM mediates checkpoint regulation and homologous repair by phosphorylation of these proteins. Most mutations in this gene lead to truncated forms of the ATM protein which increases the susceptibility for developing genomic instability, especially during exposure to ionizing radiation [34]. Mutations in ATM lead to ataxia-telangiectasia, an autosomal recessive disorder characterized by progressive neurologic impairment, cerebellar ataxia, ocular telangiectasia, variable immuno-deficiency, defective organogenesis and an increased risk of developing visceral malignancies, and lymphoproliferative disorders. A link between ATM mutations and breast cancer has been suspected for many years. Recent studies of patients with ataxia-telangiectasia have suggested that female relatives have a two to five fold increase in risk of developing breast cancer [35–37]. There are no known his-tologic phenotypes of breast cancer that predict an ATM mutation, and the clinical usefulness of testing for ATM mutations in breast cancer patients is uncertain at this time.

CHEK2 (Checkpoint Kinase 2 Gene)

The CHEK2 gene is located on the long (q) arm of chromosome 22 at position 12.1 (22q12.1). CHEK2 is a tumor suppressor gene, and mutations in this gene have been identified in a number of human malignancies including breast, pros-tate, and colon cancers [38].

CHEK2 encodes a threonine/serine kinase involved in the same pathways as TP53 and BRCA1. In response to DNA damage, this protein prevents cell prolifer-ation by phosphorylation of proteins involved in checkpoint control, thus blocking cellular entry into mitosis [39]. Mutations in CHEK2 were originally investigated as a cause of Li-Fraumeni like syndrome [40], however, many subsequent studies have shown that CHEK2 mutations are directly associated with the development of breast cancer. Although numerous mutations in CHEK2 have been described, perhaps the most important is a founder mutation, 1100delC, discovered in peo-ple of North European descent. The 1100delC mutation is present in ~1 % of European families and in up to 5 % of breast cancer families of North European descent. Individuals heterozygous for this mutation have a two to three fold increased risk of developing breast cancer [41, 42]. In women with estrogen recep-tor–positive breast cancer, 1100delC heterozygosity is also associated with a three to four fold risk of developing a second breast cancer [43]. Many more CHEK2 mutations have been described, but their clinical significance are still unknown.

BRCA1 Interacting Protein C-Terminal Helicase 1 (BRIP1)

The BRIP1 gene is located on the long (q) arm of chromosome 17 at position 22.2 (17q22.2). BRIP1 belongs to the Fanconi anemia pathway of genes, which also includes PALB2 (discussed ahead) and BRCA2.

BRIP1 encodes for a DNA helicase that interacts with BRCA1 and has BRCA1-dependent DNA repair and checkpoint functions. Biallelic mutations in

BRIP1 result in the chromosome instability disorder Fanconi anemia, while heterozygous inactivating mutations have been reported to confer an increased susceptibility to breast cancer in monoallelic carriers [44, 45]. These account for less than 0.5 % of all breast cancers. Patients with BRIP1 mutations have approximately a 20 % lifetime risk of developing breast cancer. Frameshift mutations in BRIP1 have been described which may be associated with an increased risk of developing ovarian cancers in some European populations [46]. Most recently, BRIP1 has been implicated in the genetic susceptibility for developing cervical cancer [47].

Partner and Localizer of BRCA2 Gene (PALB2)

The PALB2 gene is located on the short (p) arm of chromosome 16 at position 12.2 (16p12.2). As discussed above, PALB2 belongs to the FANC group of genes in the Fanconi anemia pathway of breast cancer.

PALB2 encodes for a protein that is involved in double-stranded DNA break repair. Studies have suggested that PALB2 acts as a functional bridging molecule linking the DNA repair functions of BRCA1 and BRCA2; as well as stimulating the recombinant functions of RAD51, and hence is critical in the maintenance of genomic stability [48–50]. PALB2 mutations account for a minority of breast cancer (less than 0.5 %). Similar to BRIP1 mutations, PALB2 mutations confer an approximate 20 % overall lifetime risk of developing breast cancer. Recently, PALB2 germline truncating mutations have also been implicated in the development of pancreatic cancer [51].

Other Genetic Mutations Conferring an Increased Risk of Developing Breast Cancer

Germline mutations of **CDH1 [cadherin 1, type 1, E-cadherin (epithelial) located at 16q22.1]** are associated with Hereditary Diffuse Gastric Cancer, which is an autosomal dominant cancer predisposition syndrome. CDH1 encodes for a cell adhesion molecule called E-cadherin. Patients with germline CDH1 mutations have a very high risk of developing gastric cancer but are also at an increased risk of developing breast cancer including both ductal and lobular carcinomas [52, 53]. Lobular carcinomas that arise in CDH1 mutation carriers as well as sporadic cases show similar phenotypes; i.e., both are characterized by a loss of E-cadherin expression at the cell membrane which can be demonstrated by immunohisto-chemistry. CDH1 mutations account for a small fraction of familial breast cancers (<2 %); and female carriers have an approximate 50 % lifetime risk of developing breast cancer [54]. Studies have estimated the cumulative risk of developing gastric cancer by age 80 years to be ~65 % for men and ~80 % for women [55].

STK11 (serine/threonine kinase 11, located at 19p13.3) mutations lead to Peutz-Jeghers syndrome, a rare autosomal dominant condition associated with the development of hamartomatous polyps throughout the gastrointestinal tract and mucocutaneous pigmentation. These patients are at increased risk of developing gastrointestinal as well as breast cancers. Women who are STK11 mutation carriers have an approximate 30 % lifetime risk of developing breast cancer. These tumors are often bilateral and sometimes develop at an early age [56].

PTEN (phosphatase and tensin homolog), located at 10q23.3) mutations are associated with the development of the autosomal dominant Cowden syndrome, characterized by multiple hamartomas in different organs, increased risk of cancers, facial trichilemmomas, acral keratoses and oral papillomatous papules. PTEN functions by down-regulating the phosphatidylinositol-3-kinase (PI3K) signal transduction cascade and acts as a tumor suppressor and growth regulator [57]. Many types of mutations in the PTEN gene have been identified in patients with Cowden syndrome. Breast cancer is the most common cancer seen in Cowden syndrome and females who carry mutations in the PTEN gene have a 25–50 % lifetime risk of developing breast cancer [58]. Cowden syndrome is responsible for less than 1 % of familial breast cancers. Other cancers seen in patients with PTEN mutations include thyroid cancers (non-medullary), colon, rectal, and endometrial carcinomas.

RAD50 (RAD50 homolog gene, located at 5q31) is a gene that has been implicated in the development of breast cancer. RAD50 interacts with two other genes, **MRE11 (meiotic recombination 11, located at 11q21)** and **NBS1 [Nijmegen breakage syndrome 1 (also called Nibrin), located at 8q21]**, to form the **MRN complex** which acts as the primary sensor of double-stranded DNA breaks. The MRN complex facilitates double-strand DNA break repair by activating ATM kinase (discussed above). Mutations of MRE11, NBS1, and RAD50 give rise to cancer predisposition syndromes: ataxia-telangiectasia-like disorder, Nijmegen breakage syndrome (NBS) and NBS-like disorder, respectively [59, 60]. A founder mutation in RAD50 (687delT) has been discovered in breast cancer families of Finnish descent, but as this mutation is rare and has not been discovered in non-familial populations, its actual role in breast cancer development is still under scrutiny [61].

The risk of breast cancer in **Lynch Syndrome** (Hereditary Non-Polyposis Colorectal Cancer Syndrome) is uncertain due to conflicting data, and currently the National Comprehensive Cancer Network (NCCN) has no guidelines on risk assessment or screening for breast cancer in patients with Lynch Syndrome [62].

In recent years, well-validated studies have implicated a number of **SNPs** in various genes (e.g.,: **FGFR2, TOX3/TNRC9, MRPS30, MAP3K1, NOTCH2, RAD51L1** etc.) to be associated with a slightly increased or decreased risk of developing breast cancer [4, 63–70]. SNPs in these genes are considered to be of low penetrance in the development of familial breast cancer and their clinical significance is currently uncertain. These genes are however important in understanding the biology of breast cancer development and may play a key role in discovering potential therapeutic targets in the future.

Clinical testing for moderate penetrance genes is difficult and controversial due to the rarity of these mutations and the lack of clinical data on how to manage patients with positive results. There is obvious clinical concern that patients who test positive for one of these genetic mutations may seek unnecessary treatment; and that those who test negative may be left with a false sense of security which may preclude routine preventive strategies. Many studies suggest that these genes, along with other low-penetrant alleles implicated in the development of breast cancer, act in interrelated pathways and therefore testing for these mutations in patients with a strong family histories may be justified [4, 5, 71]. Genetic surveillance of patients in the correct clinical context, (appropriate ethnic background and those with significant family histories), may help to stratify patients into a high-risk group that may benefit from increased radiographic surveillance, chemoprevention, or risk-reducing surgery. Genetic testing for rare mutations that have not been proven to be pathogenic or of clinical utility should be discouraged as their true significance it still unknown. Clinical features of the genes implicated in breast cancer and their associated cancer predisposition syndromes are summarized in Tables 2.2 and 2.3.

Genetic Testing and Management of Familial Breast Cancer in the United States

Guidelines for Genetic Testing in the United States

Strong family history, early onset of breast cancer, ethnic background, and possibly histologic phenotype, are important criteria determining the need for genetic testing. In the United States, there are two main regulatory groups that have established guidelines for genetic testing in breast cancer patient; the NCCN and the United States Task Force Preventive Services (USTFPS), both of which have similar recommendations [72, 73]. The NCCN recommends referral to a cancer genetics professional if: an individual with breast cancer has a family member with a known mutation in a breast cancer susceptibility gene, an early onset of breast cancer, a triple-negative breast cancer, a male breast cancer, two breast primaries in the same individual; or in an unaffected individual who has a history of a first or second degree relative with cancers that are known to be associated with familial cancer syndromes. If the patient meets criteria for screening, then the NCCN recommends full sequencing of BRCA1 and BRCA2 for point mutations along with further testing for large genomic alterations. If the patient has a known family mutation, then it is appropriate to screen for that mutation in lieu of full sequencing. If a patient is suspected to have Li-Fraumeni or Li-Fraumeni-like syndrome and meets criteria for Classic Li-Fraumeni syndrome [74] or fulfills modified Chompret Criteria for Germline TP53 Mutation Screening, [75] then full sequencing of TP53 along with deletion/duplication analysis is recommended.

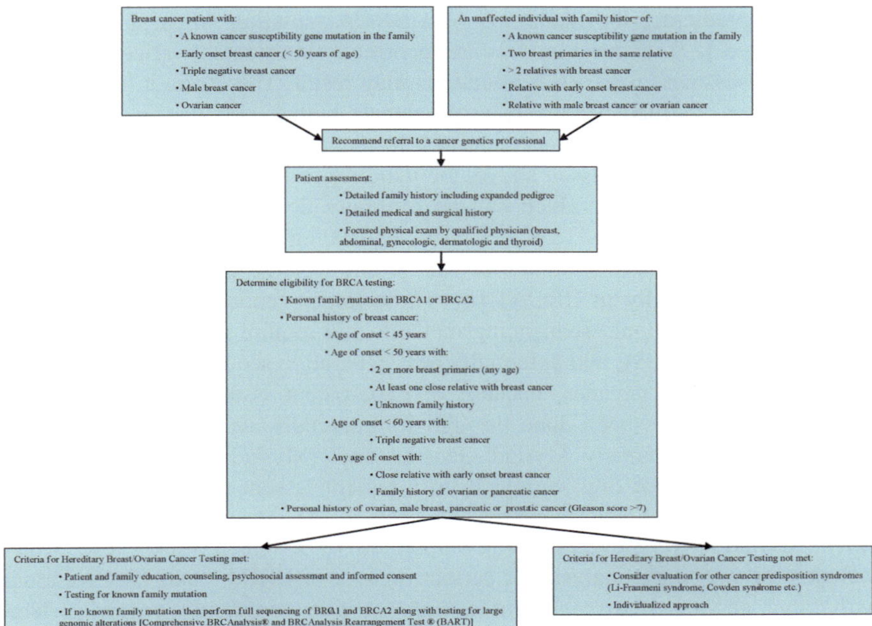

Fig. 2.1 Summary of recommendations regarding genetic testing for BRCA1 and 2

Again, if the patient has a known family mutation [31], then it is appropriate to screen for that mutation first. Patients who meet criteria for Cowden syndrome [76] should have full sequencing of the PTEN gene including deletion/duplication and promoter analysis. Studies have shown that genetic counseling by a cancer genetics professional reduces patient stress, improves the estimation, and likelihood of actual cancer risk as well as reduces unintentional or unnecessary testing [73]. The NCCN does not have specific recommendation for other rare familial cancer predisposition syndromes and recommends an individualized multidisciplinary approach in the management of these patients. Guidelines for genetic testing for BRCA mutations are summarized in Fig. 2.1.

Modality of BRCA Testing

There are several predictive models based on statistical methods, pedigree, and outcome data that are used by genetic counselors to determine the likelihood or risk of mutations in BRCA1 or BRCA2. These models include BRCAPRO, Myriad, the Finnish, the National Cancer Institute, the University of Pennsylvania, and Yale University models. Recent studies have shown these models have equal efficacy in predicting the likelihood of a BRCA mutation when applied in the proper context [77]. If these models are incorrectly interpreted, varied results and false risk assessment for BRCA mutations may result. Therefore, it is imperative to ensure that qualified healthcare professionals with experience in genetics are included in the multidisciplinary approach to make decisions on whether BRCA testing is needed. As discussed above, the majority of BRCA1 and BRCA2 mutations are point mutations which can be routinely detected by traditional DNA sequencing methodologies (e.g.,: Sanger sequencing). Apart from these point mutations, <1 % of BRCA mutations can be due to large genomic deletions and duplications, especially in BRCA1 [8]. These larger genomic alterations cannot be detected by traditional sequencing methods and require more complex testing modalities (e.g.,: MLPA, and potentially next generation sequencing).

For the last two decades, because of gene-patent issues, BRCA testing in the United States has been done through commercially available tests from one genetic laboratory, namely Myriad Genetics Inc. (Myriad Genetics, Salt Lake City, UT). A blood or oral sample from a patient is sent to their central reference laboratory and results are reported back to the consulting healthcare provider. Myriad now provides the Comprehensive BRCAnalysis® test, which includes full sequence analysis for certain regions of BRCA1 and BRCA2 along with large genomic rearrangement testing for five commonly occurring large genomic rearrangements of the BRCA1 gene. Testing for a few commonly occurring point mutations is also available (e.g.,: 187delAG and 5385insC in BRCA1; 6174delT in BRCA2). In an effort to identify other large genomic alterations not detected by Comprehensive BRCAnalysis®, Myriad has offered a test called the BRCAnalysis Rearrangement Test (BART)® in 2006. BART allows assessment of all coding exons, flanking intron regions and their promoters in BRCA1 and BRCA 2, either by quantitative endpoint polymerase chain reaction (PCR) analysis or microarray comparative genomic hybridization analysis (microarray-CGH) [78, 79]. Therefore, patients who were tested before 2006 by Comprehensive BRCAnalysis® only and had subsequent negative results may benefit from repeat testing along with BART to ensure large genomic alterations are not missed [72].

The Gene-patent controversy surrounding Myriad, who in association with others, located and sequenced BRCA1 and BRCA2 almost 20 years ago, has ended in June 2013 when a landmark decision in gene patenting was reached in response to a case filed by the Association of Molecular Pathology. The Supreme Court upheld that, "A naturally occurring DNA segment is a product of nature and is not patent eligible merely because it has been isolated, but cDNA is patent eligible because it is not naturally occurring." thus possibly ending the monopoly of Myriad Genetics in the field of BRCA testing [80, 81]. Since then, several companies (Gene by Gene, Ltd.; Counsyl, Inc.; Quest Diagnostics; gnostics; GeneDx; Invitae Corporation; Laboratory Corporation of America Holdings; etc.) have announced plans of developing a commercially available BRCA test in the United States and other countries.

Prevention Strategies and Clinical Management of Familial Breast Cancer

Patient awareness and education are of paramount importance in the overall management of familial breast cancer. A multidisciplinary approach in patient care including input from oncologists, surgeons, radiation oncologists, radiologists, pathologists, genetic counselors, and clinical psychologists is recommended. Women in breast cancer families should perform monthly self-breast exams starting from 18 years of age, and have biannual clinical breast exams by a physician starting from 25 years of age onward. Current NCCN guidelines suggest that annual mammograms along with magnetic resonance imaging (MRI) starting from the age of 25 are appropriate screening options in women with known mutations in breast cancer susceptibility genes [72]. Digital mammography (with or without tomosynthesis) and MRI can be performed at the same time, or as some studies have suggested are more accurate and cost-effective in detecting suspicious lesions when performed alternatively at 6 month intervals [82–84]. Since MRI is more sensitive in detecting architectural distortion in breast tissue as compared to conventional mammography, theoretic harms of intensive screening include: increased false-positive imaging studies (resulting in unnecessary biopsies); unnecessary additional imaging (e.g.,: targeted ultrasound after MRI). unnecessary surgical treatment; patient anxiety and increased financial burden on patients and hospitals. A recent large study showed significantly higher false-positive and lower false-negative rates for MRI compared with mammography [85]. Studies have shown that women who undergo intensive radiographic screening have no increased pain, discomfort, or anxiety when compared to women undergoing routine screening [85]. Studies looking at the clinical utility of extensive radiographic surveillance in familial breast cancer families are conflicting and therefore its role in preventing breast cancer is currently uncertain [73].

Breast cancer risk-reducing medications should also be discussed with patients who are BRCA mutation carriers. Chemoprevention of breast cancer with estrogen receptor antagonists and selective estrogen receptor modulators is not common in the United States owing to their well-known thromboembolic side effects. Tamoxifen and Raloxifene are two drugs that have been widely studied for their potential use in breast cancer prevention and are currently FDA approved for this use (for a period of up to 5 years). Since BRCA-associated cancers are usually hormone receptor-negative, there are no studies looking at the role of these drugs in BRCA mutation carriers specifically. However, there are large studies investigating their role in women with varied risks [73]. The National Surgical Adjuvant Breast and Bowel Project Breast Cancer Prevention Trial (NSABP P-1) [86–88] demonstrated that tamoxifen reduced the risk of estrogen receptor positive breast cancers in the population studied. The benefits of tamoxifen chemoprevention were thought to outweigh the risks associated with its use. The main risks of tamoxifen use as mentioned above, were found to be thromboembolic events such as stroke and deep-vein thrombosis, as well as cataracts. There was also a moderate increased risk of developing endometrial cancer reported with tamoxifen use but was not statistically significant. The NSABP Study of Tamoxifen and Raloxifene (STAR) P-2 [89] trial compared tamoxifen to raloxifene in the prevention of invasive breast cancer and found that tamoxifen had a greater efficacy than raloxifene in reducing invasive breast cancer, but was associated with a higher risk of complications.

The NCCN also recommends discussing the option of risk-reducing surgery, i.e.,: prophylactic mastectomy and bilateral salpingo-oopherectomy, in patients who are at a high risk for developing breast cancer including those who are BRCA mutation carriers. Prophylactic mastectomies have been reported to reduce the overall risk of developing breast cancer by approximately 90 %, [90] and a significantly decreased rate of breast cancer specific death. In patients with breast cancers, risk-reducing salpingoophorectomies are associated with also an approximate 90 % reduction in breast cancer specific death and a very high reduction in the risk for gynecologic cancers [91]. In patients without breast cancer, risk-reducing salpingoophorectomies provide a significantly reduced risk of developing a primary breast cancer and this benefit is thought to be more so for BRCA2 mutation carriers as compared to BRCA1 mutation carriers.

The treatment of BRCA associated cancers is complex and difficult due to the relative rarity of these cancers. Knowing that the mechanism of carcinogenesis in cells that have BRCA mutations is related to defective homologous recombination DNA repair, the role of DNA cross-linking agents such as carboplatin, cisplatin, and mitomycin-C have been widely studied. These agents cause DNA damage, which would normally be repaired via an intact BRCA mediated process. Therefore, these agents may potentially cause irreversible fatal DNA damage and chromosomal instability in BRCA mutated cancers cells leading to suppression of tumor growth [92]. Poly(ADP-ribose) polymerase 1 (PARP) inhibitors are also currently being investigated for their potential role in the treatment of BRCA associated breast cancers. PARP is a nuclear protein which localizes to the site of DNA damage and initiates double-stranded DNA break repair by recruiting repair proteins. Therefore, PARP inhibitors such as iniparib may help to prevent DNA repair in BRCA mutated cancer cells leading to cell death. Studies are beginning to reveal that PARP inhibitors may also be potentially useful in other BRCA associated cancers such as ovarian and pancreatic cancers. Clinical trials using PARP inhibitors as a single agent or in combination therapy with other drugs are currently underway for many types of cancers (see Chap. 11).

Key Points

- Approximately 10 % of breast cancer patients are carriers of gene mutations susceptible for the development of breast cancer.
- BRCA1, BRCA2, and TP53 genes are associated with a high risk of developing breast cancer in carriers and hence are referred to as high-penetrance genes.

- ATM, CHEK2, BRIP1, PALB2, RAD50, PTEN, CDH1, STK11, etc. are examples of moderate penetrance genes, while SNPs are considered low penetrance.

References

1. Jemal A. et al. Cancer Statistics, 2010. CA Cancer J Clin. 2010;60(5):277–300.
2. Claus EB, Schildkraut JM, Thompson WD, Risch NJ. The genetic attributable risk of breast and ovarian cancer. Cancer. 1996;77(11):2318–24.
3. Ford D, et al. Genetic heterogeneity and penetrance analysis of the BRCA1 and BRCA2 genes in breast cancer families. The Breast Cancer Linkage Consortium. Am J Hum Genet. 1998;62(3):676–89.
4. Turnbull C, et al. Genome-wide association study identifies five new breast cancer susceptibility loci. Nat Genet. 2010;42(6):504–7.
5. Roy R, Chun J, Powell SN. BRCA1 and BRCA2: different roles in a common pathway of genome protection. Nat Rev Cancer. 2011;12(1):68–78.
6. Huen MS, Sy SM, Chen J. BRCA1 and its toolbox for the maintenance of genome integrity. Nat Rev Mol Cell Biol. 2010;11(2):138–48.
7. Mazoyer S. Genomic rearrangements in the BRCA1 and BRCA2 genes. Hum Mutat. 2005;25(5):415–22.
8. Hogervorst FB, Nederlof PM, Gille JJ, McElgunn CJ, Grippeling M, Pruntel R, et al. Large genomic deletions and duplications in the BRCA1 gene identified by a novel quantitative method. Cancer Res. 2003;63(7):1449–53.
9. Hamel N, Feng BJ, Foretova L, Stoppa-Lyonnet D, Narod SA, et al. On the origin and diffusion of *BRCA1* c.5266dupC (5382insC) in European populations. Eur J Hum Genet. 2011;19(3):300–6.
10. Lalloo F, Varley J, Ellis D, et al. Family history is predictive of pathogenic mutations in BRCA1, BRCA2 and TP53 with high penetrance in a population based study of very early onset breast cancer. Lancet. 2003;361:1101–2.
11. Evans DG, Shenton A, Woodward E, Lalloo F, Howell A, Maher ER. Penetrance estimates for BRCA1 and BRCA2 based on genetic testing in a clinical cancer genetics service setting. BMC Cancer. 2008;8(1):155.
12. Ford D, Easton DF, Stratton M, et al. Genetic heterogeneity and penetrance analysis of the BRCA1 and BRCA2 genes in breast cancer families. The Breast Cancer Linkage Consortium. Am J Hum Genet. 1998;62(3):676–89.
13. Chen S, Iversen ES, Friebel T, et al. Characterization of BRCA1 and BRCA2 mutations in a large United States sample. J Clin Oncol. 2006;24(6):863–71.
14. Antoniou A, Pharoah PDP, Narod S, et al. Average risks of breast and ovarian cancer associated with mutations in *BRCA1* or *BRCA2* detected in case series unselected for family history: a combined analysis of 22 studies. Am J Hum Genet. 2003;72(5):1117–30.
15. Lakhani SR, Gusterson BA, Jacquemier J, Sloane JP, Anderson TJ, et al. The pathology of familial breast cancer: histological features of cancers in families not attributable to mutations in BRCA1 or BRCA2. Clin Cancer Res. 2000;6(3):782–9.
16. Lakhani SR, Jacquemier J, Sloane JP, Gusterson BA, Anderson TJ, et al. Multifactorial analysis of differences between sporadic breast cancers and cancers involving BRCA1 and BRCA2 mutations. J Natl Cancer Inst. 1998;90(15):1138–45.
17. Perou CM, Sorlie T, Eisen MB, van de Rijn M, Jeffrey SS, Rees CA, et al. Molecular portraits of human breast tumours. Nature. 2000;406(6797):747–52.
18. Sorlie T, Perou CM, Tibshirani R, Aas T, Geisler S, Johnsen H, et al. Gene expression patterns of breast carcinomas distinguish tumor subclasses with clinical implications. Proc Natl Acad Sci USA. 2001;98(19):10869–74.

19. Nielsen TO, Hsu FD, Jensen K, Cheang M, Karaca G, Hu Z, et al. Immunohistochemical and clinical characterization of the basal-like subtype of invasive breast carcinoma. Clin Cancer Res. 2004;10(16):5367–74.
20. Rakha EA, Elsheikh SE, Aleskandarany MA, Habashi HO, Green AR, Powe DG, et al. Triple-negative breast cancer: distinguishing between basal and nonbasal subtypes. Clin Cancer Res. 2009;15(7):2302–10.
21. Jensen RB, et al. Purified human BRCA2 stimulates RAD51- mediated recombination. Nature. 2010;467(7316):678–83.
22. Tischkowitz M, Xia B. PALB2/FANCN: recombining cancer and Fanconi anemia. Cancer Res. 2010;70(19):7353–9.
23. Howlett NG, et al. Biallelic inactivation of BRCA2 in Fanconi anemia. Science. 2002;297(5581):606–9.
24. Tai YC, Domchek S, Parmigiani G, Chen S. Breast cancer risk among male BRCA1 and BRCA2 mutation carriers. J Natl Cancer Inst. 2007;99(23):1811–4.
25. Gallagher DJ, Gaudet MM, Pal P, Kirchhoff T, Balistreri L, et al. Germline BRCA mutations denote a clinicopathologic subset of prostate cancer. Clin Cancer Res. 2010;16(7):2115–21.
26. Hahn SA, Greenhalf B, Ellis I, et al. BRCA2 germline mutations in familial pancreatic carcinoma. J Natl Cancer Inst. 2003;95:214–21.
27. Canto MI, Harinck F, Hruban HR, Offerhaus GJ, Poley JW, et al. International Cancer of the Pancreas Screening (CAPS) Consortium summit on the management of patients with increased risk for familial pancreatic cancer. Gut. 2013;62(3):339–47.
28. van Asperen CJ, Brohet RM, Meijers-Heijboer EJ, et al. Cancer risks in BRCA2 families: estimates for sites other than breast and ovary. J Med Genet. 2005;42(9):711–9.
29. Moran A, O'Hara C, Khan S, Shack L, Woodward E, et al. Risk of cancer other than breast or ovarian in individuals with BRCA1 and BRCA2 mutations. Fam Cancer. 2012;11(2):235–42.
30. Petitjean A, Achatz MI, Borresen-Dale AL, Hainaut P, Olivier M. TP53 mutations in human cancers: functional selection and impact on cancer prognosis and outcomes. Oncogene. 2007;26:2157–65.
31. Olivier M, Eeles R, Hollstein M, Khan MA, Harris CC, Hainaut P. The IARC TP53 database: new online mutation analysis and recommendations to users. Hum Mutat. 2002;19:607–14.
32. Gonzalez KD, et al. Beyond Li Fraumeni syndrome: clinical characteristics of families with p53 germline mutations. J Clin Oncol. 2009;27(8):1250–6.
33. Paglia LL, Lauge A, Weber J, Champ J, Cavaciuti E, Russo A, et al. ATM germline mutations in women with familial breast cancer and a relative with haematological malignancy. Breast Cancer Res Treat. 2010;119(2):443–5233.
34. Shiloh Y. ATM and related protein kinases: safeguarding genome integrity. Nat Rev Cancer. 2003;3:155–68.
35. Swift M, Reitnauer PJ, Morrell D, Chase CL. Breast and other cancers in families with ataxia-telangiectasia. N Engl J Med. 1987;316(21):1289–94.
36. Thompson D, Duedal S, Kirner J, McGuffog L, Last J, et al. Cancer risks and mortality in heterozygous ATM mutation carriers. J Natl Cancer Inst. 2005;97(11):813–22.
37. Renwick A, et al. ATM mutations that cause ataxia-telangiectasia are breast cancer susceptibility alleles. Nat Genet. 2006;38(8):873–5.
38. Cybulski C, et al. CHEK2 is a multiorgan cancer susceptibility gene. Am J Hum Genet. 2004;75(6):1131–5.
39. Stolz A, et al. The CHK2-BRCA1 tumour suppressor pathway ensures chromosomal stability in human somatic cells. Nat Cell Biol. 2010;12(5):492–9.
40. Bell DW, et al. Heterozygous germ line hCHK2 Mutations in Li-Fraumeni syndrome. Science. 1999;286(5449):2528–31.
41. Weischer M, Bojesen SE, Ellervik C, et al. CHEK2*1100delC genotyping for clinical assessment of breast cancer risk: Meta-analyses of 26,000 patient cases and 27,000 controls. J Clin Oncol. 2008;26:542–8.

42. Zhang B, Beeghly-Fadiel A, Long J, et al. Genetic variants associated with breast-cancer risk: comprehensive research synopsis, meta-analysis, and epidemiological evidence. Lancet Oncol. 2011;12:477–88.

43. Weischer M, Nordestgaard BG, Pharoah P, et al. CHEK2*1100delC heterozygosity in women with breast cancer associated with early death, breast cancer-specific death, and increased risk of a second breast cancer. J Clin Oncol. 2012;30(35):4308–16.

44. Cantor S, Drapkin R, Zhang F, Lin Y, Han J, Pamidi S, Livingston DM. The BRCA1-associated protein BACH1 is a DNA helicase targeted by clinically relevant inactivating mutations. Proc Natl Acad Sci USA. 2004;101(8):2357–62.

45. Seal S, Thompson D, Renwick A, et al. Truncating mutations in the Fanconi anemia J gene BRIP1 are low-penetrance breast cancer susceptibility alleles. Nat Genet. 2006;38(11):1239–41.

46. Rafnar T, Gudbjartsson DF, Sulem P, et al. Mutations in BRIP1 confer high risk of ovarian cancer. Nat Genet. 2011;43(11):1104–7.

47. Ma XD, Cai GQ, Zou W, Huang YH, Zhang JR, Wang DT, Chen BL. First evidence for the contribution of the genetic variations of BRCA1-interacting protein 1 (BRIP1) to the genetic susceptibility of cervical cancer. Gene. 2013;524(2):208–13.

48. Zhang F, et al. PALB2 functionally connects the breast cancer susceptibility proteins BRCA1 and BRCA2. Mol Cancer Res. 2009;7(7):1110–8.

49. Sy SM, Huen MS, Chen J. PALB2 is an integral component of the BRCA complex required for homologous recombination repair. Proc Natl Acad Sci USA. 2009;106(17):7155–60.

50. Dray E, et al. Enhancement of RAD51 recombinase activity by the tumor suppressor PALB2. Nat Struct Mol Biol. 2010;17(10):1255–9.

51. Jones S, et al. Exomic sequencing identifies PALB2 as a pancreatic cancer susceptibility gene. Science. 2009;324(5924):217.

52. Pharoah PD, Guilford P, Caldas C. Incidence of gastric cancer and breast cancer in CDH1 (E-cadherin) mutation carriers from hereditary diffuse gastric cancer families. Gastroenterology. 2001;121(6):1348–53.

53. Suriano G, Yew S, Ferreira P, Senz J, Kaurah P, Ford JM, et al. Characterization of a recurrent germ line mutation of the E-cadherin gene: implications for genetic testing and clinical management. Clin Cancer Res. 2005;11(15):5401–9.

54. Kaurah P, MacMillan A, Boyd N, Senz J, De Luca A, Chun N, et al. Founder and recurrent CDH1 mutations in families with hereditary diffuse gastric cancer. JAMA. 2007;297(21):2360–72.

55. Pharoah PD, Guilford P, Caldas C. International Gastric Cancer Linkage Consortium. Incidence of gastric cancer and breast cancer in CDH1 (E-cadherin) mutation carriers from hereditary diffuse gastric cancer families. Gastroenterology. 2001;121(6):1348–53.

56. Boardman LA, Thibodeau SN, Schaid DJ, et al. Increased risk for cancer in patients with the Peutz-Jeghers syndrome. Ann Intern Med. 1998;128(11):896–9.

57. Gage M, Wattendorf D, Henry LR. Translational advances regarding hereditary breast cancer syndromes. J Surg Oncol. 2012;105(5):444–51.

58. Nusbaum R, Vogel KJ, Ready K. Susceptibility to breast cancer: hereditary syndromes and low penetrance genes. Breast Dis. 2006;27:21–50.

59. Stracker TH, Petrini JH. The MRE11 complex: starting from the ends. Nat Rev Mol Cell Biol. 2011;12(2):90–103.

60. Williams RS, Williams JS, Tainer JA. Mre11-Rad50-Nbs1 is a keystone complex connecting DNA repair machinery, double-strand break signaling, and the chromatin template. Biochem Cell Biol. 2007;85(4):509–20.

61. Heikkinen K, et al. RAD50 and NBS1 are breast cancer susceptibility genes associated with genomic instability. Carcinogenesis. 2006;27(8):1593–9.

62. NCCN Guidelines Version 1.2014 Lynch Syndrome. http://www.nccn.org/professionals/physician_gls/pdf/genetics_colon.pdf. Accessed 20 Mar 2014.

63. Easton DF, Pooley KA, Dunning AM, et al. Genome-wide association study identifies novel breast cancer susceptibility loci. Nature. 2007;447(7148):1087–93.
64. Stacey SN, Manolescu A, Sulem P, et al. Common variants on chromosomes 2q35 and 16q12 confer susceptibility to estrogen receptor positive breast cancer. Nat Genet. 2007;39(7):865–9.
65. Cox A, Dunning AM, Garcia-Closas M, et al. A common coding variant in CASP8 is associated with breast cancer risk. Nat Genet. 2007;39(3):352–8.
66. Ahmed S, Thomas G, Ghoussaini M, et al. Newly discovered breast cancer susceptibility loci on 3p24 and 17q23.2. Nat Genet. 2009;41(5):585–90.
67. Milne RL, Benítez J, Nevanlinna H, et al. Risk of estrogen receptor positive and negative breast cancer and single-nucleotide polymorphism 2q35-rs13387042. J Natl Cancer Inst. 2009;101(14):1012–8.
68. Thomas G, Jacobs KB, Kraft P, et al. A multistage genome-wide association study in breast cancer identifies two new risk alleles at 1p11.2 and 14q24.1 (RAD51L1). Nat Genet. 2009;41(5):579–84.
69. Stacey SN, Manolescu A, Sulem P, et al. Common variants on chromosome 5p12 confer susceptibility to estrogen receptor-positive breast cancer. Nat Genet. 2008;40(6):703–6.
70. Zheng W, Long J, Gao YT, et al. Genome-wide association study identifies a new breast cancer susceptibility locus at 6q25.1. Nat Genet. 2009;41(3):324–8.
71. Byrnes GB, Southey MC, Hopper JL. Are the so-called low penetrance breast cancer genes, ATM, BRIP1, PALB2 and CHEK2, high risk for women with strong family histories? Breast Cancer Res. 2008;10(3):208.
72. NCCN Guidelines Version 1.2014 Breast and/or Ovarian Cancer Genetic Assessment. http://www.nccn.org/professionals/physician_gls/pdf/genetics_screening.pdf. Accessed 20 Mar 2014.
73. Nelson HD, Fu R, Goddard K, Mitchell JP, Okinaka-Hu L, Pappas M, Zakher B. Risk assessment, genetic counseling, and genetic testing for BRCA-related cancer: systematic review to update the U.S. preventive services task force recommendation (Internet). Rockville (MD): Agency for Healthcare Research and Quality (US); 2013.
74. Li FP, Fraumeni JF Jr, Mulvihill JJ, et al. A cancer family syndrome in twenty-four kindreds. Cancer Res. 1988;48(18):5358–62.
75. Tinat J, Bougeard G, Baert-Desurmont S, et al. 2009 version of the Chompret criteria for Li Fraumeni syndrome. J Clin Oncol. 2009;27(26):e108–9.
76. Pilarski R, Burt R, Kohlman W, Pho L, Shannon KM, Swisher E. Cowden syndrome and the PTEN hamartoma tumor syndrome: systematic review and revised diagnostic criteria. J Natl Cancer Inst. 2013;105(21):1607–16.
77. Parmigiani G, Chen S, Iversen ES Jr, et al. Validity of models for predicting BRCA1 and BRCA2 mutations. Ann Intern Med. 2007;147:441–50.
78. Nelson HD, Fu R, Goddard K, Mitchell JP, Okinaka-Hu L, Pappas M, Zakher B. Risk assessment, genetic counseling, and genetic testing for BRCA-related cancer: systematic review to update the U.S. Preventive services task force recommendation (Internet). Rockville (MD): Agency for Healthcare Research and Quality (US); 2013.
79. MyriadGeneticsLaboratories. http://www.myriad.com/lib/technical-specifications/BRACAnalysis-Technical-Specifications.pdf. Accessed 20 Mar 2014.
80. United States Supreme Court. http://www.supremecourt.gov/opinions/12pdf/12-398_1b7d.pdf. Accessed 20 Mar 2014.
81. State of Utah Federal Court. https://ecf.utd.uscourts.gov/cgi-bin/show_public_doc?214md2510-7. Accessed 20 Mar 2014.
82. Lowry KP, Lee JM, Kong CY, et al. Annual screening strategies in BRCA1 and BRCA2 gene mutation carriers: a comparative effectiveness analysis. Cancer. 2012;118(8):2021–30.
83. Cott Chubiz JE, Lee JM, Gilmore ME, Kong CY, et al. Cost-effectiveness of alternating magnetic resonance imaging and digital mammography screening in BRCA1 and BRCA2 gene mutation carriers. Cancer. 2013;119(6):1266–76.

84. Le-Petross HT, Whitman GJ, Atchley DP, et al. Effectiveness of alternating mammography and magnetic resonance imaging for screening women with deleterious BRCA mutations at high risk of breast cancer. Cancer. 2011;117(17):3900–7.
85. Spiegel TN, Esplen MJ, Hill KA, et al. Psychological impact of recall on women with BRCA mutations undergoing MRI surveillance. Breast. 2011;20(5):424–30.
86. Hermsen BB, Olivier RI, Verheijen RH, et al. No efficacy of annual gynaecological screening in BRCA1/2 mutation carriers: an observational follow-up study. Br J Cancer. 2007;96:1335–42.
87. Bourne TH, Campell S, Reynolds KM, et al. Screening for early familial ovarian cancer with transvaginal ultrasonography and colour blood flow imaging. BMJ. 1993;306(3884):1025–9.
88. Fisher B, Costantino J, Wickerham DL, et al. Tamoxifen for the prevention of breast cancer: current status of the national surgical adjuvant breast and bowel project P-1 study. J Natl Cancer Inst. 2005;97(22):1652–62.
89. Vogel VG, Costantino JP, Wickerham DL, et al. Update of the national surgical adjuvant breast and bowel project study of tamoxifen and raloxifene (STAR) P-2 trial: preventing breast cancer. Cancer Prev Res (Phila). 2010;3(6):696–706.
90. Hartmann LC, Sellers TA, Schaid DJ, et al. Efficacy of bilateral prophylactic mastectomy in BRCA1 and BRCA2 gene mutation carriers. J Natl Cancer Inst. 2001;93(21):1633–7.
91. Domchek SM, Friebel TM, Singer CF, et al. Association of risk-reducing surgery in BRCA1 or BRCA2 mutation carriers with cancer risk and mortality. JAMA. 2010;304(9):967–75.
92. Turner N, Tutt A, Ashworth A. Targeting the DNA repair defect of BRCA tumours. Curr Opin Pharmacol. 2005;5:388–93.

Chapter 3
Modelling the Molecular Pathology of Breast Cancer Initiation

Claire Nash, Andrew M. Hanby and Valerie Speirs

Introduction

With the advancement of technologies such as next-generation sequencing and gene expression microarrays, scientists are now uncovering a plethora of genetic mutations and alterations within breast cancers. This advancement has highlighted the vast heterogeneity of breast cancers genetically, for example one recent study showed that breast cancer could be classified into at least 10 different molecular subtypes [1], with one of these subtypes being broken down further to reveal six subtypes of triple negative breast cancers [2]. Subtypes are often defined by expression of human epidermal growth factor receptor-2 (HER2) or oestrogen receptor (ER), and in many studies these correlate with patient outcome [3].

Recognising this diversity is a prerequisite in understanding breast cancer progression and invasion since the process may vary as a consequence of this diversity. Notwithstanding these advances, how benign breast tissue progresses to malignancy is a field that is relatively less explored. This area has recently been recognised internationally by a panel of expert breast cancer scientists and healthcare professionals to be of great importance to our understanding of breast cancer progression and the development of preventative treatments [4]. Nearly all adult female breast samples contain a mix of benign changes under the umbrella term of fibrocystic change. Most of these entities within this grouping are likely to be harmless, however, subsets may well be precursors to breast cancer, but how they are formed and which ones will progress to tumours are fields that are not well understood.

C. Nash · A.M. Hanby (✉) · V. Speirs
St. James University Hospital/University of Leeds, Leeds Institute
of Cancer and Pathology (LICAP), Beckett Street, LS9 7TF Leeds, West Yorkshire, UK
e-mail: a.m.hanby@leeds.ac.uk

© Springer Science+Business Media New York 2015
A. Khan et al. (eds.), *Precision Molecular Pathology of Breast Cancer*,
Molecular Pathology Library 10, DOI 10.1007/978-1-4939-2886-6_3

Histological and epidemiological evidence over the past century has resulted in the proposal of a linear model of breast cancer progression. In this model an initiating event occurs in the luminal epithelium of normal breast and results in the formation of 'benign' non-obligate precursor lesions. In one scenario, lesions such as flat epithelial atypia (FEA) develop and gain a growth advantage with expansion of this population with an increased chance of a further 'hit' and the progression to more advanced lesions such as atypical ductal hyperplasia (ADH) and ultimately ductal carcinoma in situ (DCIS). When these cells gain the ability to breach the basement membrane, this gives rise to infiltrating [5]. This deduction supported by the observation that lesions such as FEA, ADH, and DCIS occur in the same breast [6], have overlapping morphological and immunohistochemical features [7, 8] and share similar genomic alterations [9–11] indicating an evolutionary continuum.

Precursor lesions for high grade DCIS have been elusive. It is now thought that low grade IDC and high grade IDC have distinct pathways of progression, which has led to the categorisation of low grade neoplasia family and high grade neoplasia families. The high grade neoplasia family possesses uniquely different genomic [12] and immunohistochemical [8, 11] profiles to the low grade neoplasia family. In reality it is intuitive that the heterogeneity in invasive cancers detailed at the start of the introduction, above, will be underpinned similarly by variety in the pathways by which they develop.

In each of these evolutionary pathways molecular drivers underpinning the progression of the different pathways or indeed determining 'forks' between subtypes are likely to exist. In order to understand how these might work or, indeed confirm or deny whether something is a driver for this process experimental data is needed.

In order to explore this field, models that allow experimentation in a controlled laboratory environment, and that accurately recapitulate the heterogeneity of normal human breast tissues, benign lesions and tumours in vivo are required and key methodologies in unravelling the molecular pathology of breast cancer in all its diverse forms. Over the past few decades, several in vitro laboratory models of normal breast and breast tumours have been developed but whether they are suitable for studying early breast tumour initiating events in breast is unclear. The aim of this chapter is to present many of the different in vitro models available for research into breast cancer initiation and the understanding of the general molecular pathology of this disease.

Two-Dimensional (2D) Cell Line Models

Types and Techniques

Over the past century, several breast cancer cell lines have been established. These have proven to be valuable experimental tools with many examples of research carried out with breast cancer cell lines leading to the production of new therapies for patient benefit. Studies have shown that the molecular subtypes of breast cancer outlined by Perou et al. [13] can be also delineated in panels of breast cancer cell lines. Although not examined so far, the lines available may further prove to represent the more extended heterogeneity documented by Curtis et al. [1].

Immortalised cell lines are readily available and provide a potentially infinite source of breast tumour cells. In theory this makes them a reproducible, reliable and inexpensive tool for experimentation in the laboratory. In addition, cell line cultures are amenable to genetic manipulation by standard RNA interference and gene overexpression laboratory techniques making them ideal for studying complex intracellular signalling mechanisms in great detail.

However, there are pitfalls in the interpretation of data derived from experimentation on such cells. The majority of long-established breast cancer cell lines have been derived from tumour metastases and pleural effusions and thus the line available are likely to over-represent more aggressive tumours. In addition, many of these cell lines have been virally immortalised and may therefore not be a true representative of cells in vivo. A study by Forozan et al. in 2000 used comparative genomic hybridisation on 38 common breast cancer cell lines to determine how cell lines differed from their original uncultured tumour counterparts at a genomic level [14]. This study highlighted that cultured cell lines contained many amplification sites not found in the primary tissue. This suggests that cell immortalisation and in vitro culture change the genetic profile from in vivo tissue.

Perhaps a more suitable alternative to cell lines is the use of primary cell cultures derived directly from patient tumour samples. These have the advantage in that they have had less time to transform and drift from their original in vivo phenotype than long-term immortalised cell lines. However, primary culture poses challenges such as finite life span in vitro, donor-to-donor variability making experiments hard to reproduce and the availability of patient tissue.

One other major limitation of 2D in vitro cell culture regardless of the source of cells is that the intercellular interactions between cells and interactions with cells and their environment in vivo are lost. It is increasingly recognised that the culture of cells in 2D on plastic cannot recapitulate in vivo conditions with a loss of polarity and extracellular signalling affecting cell morphology and behaviour [15]. In addition, cells are highly sensitive to their environment. Even carefully selected culture media has the capacity to induce inappropriate pathway activation and change the phenotype of cells in 2D culture [16]. Therefore, there has been a move to developing more sophisticated model systems that incorporate the surrounding three-dimensional cell microenvironment discussed later in this chapter.

Suitability of 2D Cultures to Model Breast Cancer Initiation

Since cell line models are easy to visualise, genetically manipulate and analyse at a molecular level; these may be ideally suited to the study of early genomic alterations associated with FEA and ADH [9–11] in close detail. The study of early breast cancer initiating events leading to these lesions will rely on the ability to accurately mimic the morphology, immunoprofile and genetic profile of normal disease-free breast epithelium.

Despite the large number of breast cancer cell lines available, there is a scarcity of normal luminal epithelial cell lines. The MCF10A cell line has customarily been chosen as a representative of normal luminal epithelium due to their ultrastructural similarities to luminal epithelium in vivo and expression of breast epithelial cytokeratins and sialomucins [17, 18]. However, the propensity of MCF10A cells to adopt a basal phenotype has been described by several research groups [17, 19] and is reported to be highly sensitive to changes in culture conditions [20]. This suggests they may not stably reflect the morphology and phenotype of normal luminal epithelium in vivo. In addition, MCF10A cells have been demonstrated to contain several genomic alterations compared with normal diploid cells such as gains in 5q, 8p, 13q and 19q and losses in 3p, 9p, 16p and 22q [21]. This suggests that these cells are not genetically "normal" making it challenging for researchers to investigate which genetic alterations drive development of FEA or ADH lesions from normal tissues. One other less commonly used alternative is the HB2 cell line which was originally isolated from breast milk [22] and also has luminal epithelial characteristics. Work in our laboratory [unpublished] has demonstrated a more stable morphology and phenotype of HB2 cells, perhaps providing a viable luminal epithelial alternative to MCF10A cells. However, like MCF10A cells, a recent study has also highlighted the presence of several changes in chromosomal number and structure in these cells [23].

These observations suggest that although MCF10A cells and HB2 cells can largely recapitulate the morphology and phenotype of "normal" luminal breast epithelium in vivo, they are not genetically "normal" and therefore inject a note of caution in the interpretation of results of experimental work using them. This could perhaps be overcome through the use of primary cell cultures; however, work in our laboratory has proven isolation of pure normal luminal epithelium challenging and largely unsuccessful [unpublished].

As with normal cell lines, cell lines originating from DCIS lesions are scarce. These are limited to MCF10DCIS.com cells [24] and SUM225 cells [25]. However, out of these cell lines, only SUM225 cells have been isolated from human breast DCIS tissue. MCF10DCIS.com cells were originally developed through the xenograft implantation of the premalignant MCF10AT cell line into immunocompromised mice [24]. These represent high grade comedo DCIS. SUM225 cells originally isolated from chest wall recurrence of DCIS and are HER2 positive [25]. Since invasive breast tumours are a heterogeneous group, this diversity extends to the precursor DCIS and it is improbable that the two DCIS cell lines available to researchers could capture this heterogeneity. The high grade nature of these cells lines limits their use to the study of the high grade neoplasia. To the best of the authors' knowledge, there are no cell lines available that represent low grade DCIS or early breast lesions.

These data highlight the need for the development of new normal, FEA, ADH and DCIS cell lines for the study of breast cancer initiation and early benign lesions in the laboratory, perhaps through primary cell culture. These may prove valuable in elucidating the complex intracellular mechanisms and genomic alterations associated with early breast lesions. However, cell lines grown in 2D in this way do not take into account the 3D architecture or microenvironmental influences that occur in vivo. For this reason, cell lines such as these would need to be incorporated into 3D in vitro systems to better recapitulate in vivo breast tissue.

Three-Dimensional (3D) Models

Types and Techniques

For several decades, a simple approach to culturing cells in 3D has been taken whereby single cell types have been cultured in 3D but have proven remarkably similar to aspects of differentiated tissues [26, 27]. The simplest form of 3D in vitro model developed takes advantage of the fact that many cell types have the propensity to aggregate together. This can be achieved through various methods including rotary cell culture [28] and hanging drop cell culture [29] and typically result in cell spheroids. These can be mono- or multicellular depending on the research question. However, typically, these are used for modelling growth and invasion of solid tumours [30, 31] perhaps proving more suitable for high-throughput screens [32] and anti-cancer drug screening and testing [33]. Nevertheless, the use of spheroids has also revolutionised research into mammary stem cell biology which are easily analysable and quantifiable [34–36]. This could provide an opportunity to investigate the cancer initiating potential of mammary stem cells and the cell of origin theory, an aspect of the breast cancer initiation field still under close debate. However, spheroid cultures are limited in that they still lack influence from the surrounding extracellular matrix (ECM) and may not accurately reflect tissue in vivo.

Alternatively, cells can be cultured in 3D in the presence of in vivo-like ECM. Two methods are commonly used to generate 3D acini-like structures. The "embedding" technique involves completely embedding epithelial cells in an ECM matrix. Epithelial cells are pre-aggregated through centrifugation or rotary culture and then suspended in liquid ECM solution and then gels left to set or, single cells can be suspended in the ECM solution before setting permitting organisation of the cells in 3D matrix. Once embedded, gels are layered with culture media and can either be left fixed to the bottom of the cell culture plastic, or, be freed and allowed to float in culture media [37] or suspended using Transwell® inserts [38]. Another commonly used method is the "overlay" technique whereby cells are seeded onto a bed of ECM gel and may be layered with culture media with diluted ECM [39].

There are several ECM materials available for this purpose but the most commonly used are natural ECM materials sourced from mice. The reconstituted basement membrane preparation Matrigel™ or Type I Collagen are preferred for 3D culture. Culture of breast epithelial cells in 3D Matrigel™ has seen the formation of acini-like structures [40] with evidence of milk protein expression [41]. However, materials such as Matrigel™ should be used with caution. Levels of growth factors within Matrigel™ can vary, and components such as collagen IV can differ in subunit composition to in vivo components [42] potentially increasing susceptibility to remodelling and proteolysis not commonly found in vivo. Matrigel™ may also provide tumour cells with additional survival and proliferative signals facilitating tumorigenesis [43]. Although these caveats can be overcome by use of growth factor reduced Matrigel™, there are alternative ECM materials to Matrigel™ that may be more appropriate for the culture of breast cells in vitro. As demonstrated by our group and reported by Parmar and Cunha [44], the main constituent of normal breast stroma consists predominantly of collagen I. The remodelling and mechanical tension of collagen I have been proven to influence breast tumour cell invasion [45] and the morphology of breast cells [46, 47]. An increase in collagen density has also been linked to increased risk of breast cancer [48, 49]. It therefore seems prudent that the influence of collagen I matrix be accounted for in 3D in vitro models of breast and may provide a more physiologically relevant environment for culture of breast cells. Production of successful acini- and duct-like structures akin to those cultured in Matrigel™ has already been achieved [50, 51] through culture of mammary epithelial cells in collagen I perhaps making collagen I a viable and more appropriate choice of ECM matrix for 3D models of breast.

However, although an improvement on 2D culture, 3D culture is not without its disadvantages. One of the biggest challenges with the use of 3D in vitro cultures is the subsequent analysis of observations. Biochemical analysis is problematic due to difficulties in separating cells from the surrounding ECM [52]. Imaging of these cultures requires specialised and often not readily available equipment due to the necessity of an excellent signal-to-noise ratio, optical sectioning ability, good spatial resolution and ample penetration of thick specimens [53]. In addition, collagen ECM causes considerable background fluorescence making visualisation of collagen-based cultures even more challenging [54]. This can be overcome by use of multiphoton microscopy [55] or optical coherence/projection tomography [56, 57] but can be both expensive and time-consuming. However, recent technological advances have been made and have proven that 3D co-culture models can not only be cultured for long periods of time (up to 23 days) but can also be imaged in real time to observe cell-to-cell interactions [58].

The obvious limitation of all 3D in vitro models is the lack of a complex in vivo system complete with blood supply, immune infiltrates and regulation by hormonal cues. This limits these models to the study of cell interactions and signalling pathways. In order to study tumour progression and metastasis, animal models are required.

Suitability of 3D Cultures to Model Breast Cancer Initiation

The resemblance of 3D in vitro cultures to mammary acini morphology and biology provides new opportunities to study cancer initiation mechanisms which may not have been possible with 2D cultures. The establishment of 3D culture systems

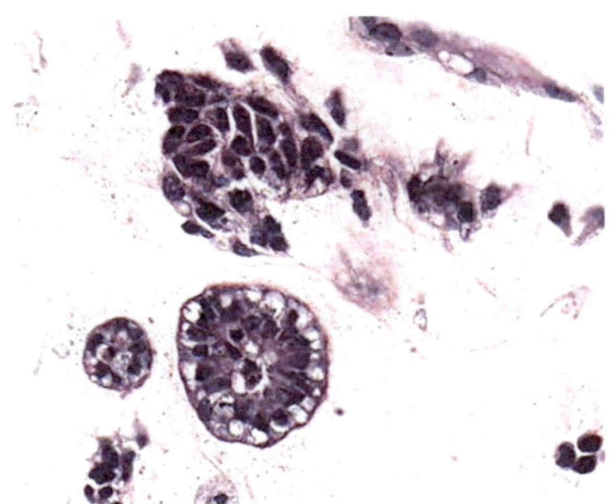

Fig. 3.1 H&E section from a mixed culture of fibroblast, breast epithelial cells and myoepithelial cells grown in a 3D collagen 1 matrix. Note particularly the organisation of clear myoepithelial cells around lumenal cells with the recapitulation of the histology of an acinus, towards the mid/bottom of this photomicrograph. The group of epithelial cells superior to it are not encompassed by myoepithelial cells and lack this organisation

that accurately resemble disease-free breast tissue architecture (Fig. 3.1) may hold the key to investigating the subtle changes that occur during the development of benign lesions discussed such as FEA, ADH and DCIS.

As discussed, the most commonly used representative of normal luminal breast epithelium is MCF10A cells. Culture of these cells in Matrigel^{TM} has yielded some impressive acini-like structures which are polarised, contain hollow lumens and produce basement membrane proteins [40, 59]. This has also been recapitulated in collagen I matrix [60]. Branching 3D duct-like structures have also been achieved through culture of HB2 cells in collagen I [51]. However, while culture of these cells in 3D matrix has resulted in structures akin to in vivo breast acini and ducts which cannot be achieved through culture in 2D, in vivo breast architecture is much more complex including a variety of other cell types that influence epithelial architecture. This has led to a rise in 3D co-culture with stromal cells with co-culture with fibroblasts most commonly reported [38, 47, 60] and examples of combinations of fibroblasts and adipocytes also demonstrated [61, 62]. It has emerged that fibroblasts regulate epithelial cell invasion [63] secreting various growth factors such as MMPs [64], which have been proven through use of 3D co-cultures. Markedly, some of these effects are only evident upon culture in collagen I [65]. Myoepithelial cells also play a key role in normal in vivo breast. Given their tumour suppressive nature [66, 67] and their capacity to maintain luminal cell polarity [68], it seems apt to include these cells in normal in vitro models of breast; however, to date studies incorporating these cells are lacking.

It stands to reason that luminal epithelial organisation is maintained by a delicate balance between the opposing functions of fibroblasts and myoepithelial cells. It seems apt that both these cell types are included in a 3D in vitro model of normal breast with luminal epithelial cells to accurately reflect the in vivo environment. One such tri-culture model has been achieved previously by Holliday et al. [38] but this used aberrant luminal epithelial cells thus representing DCIS. In our laboratory, we have developed a tri-culture model of normal breast that incorporates HB2 cells, myoepithelial cells and fibroblasts isolated from breast reduction mammoplasty samples in the physiologically relevant matrix collagen I. We have demonstrated that each individual cell type retained an in vivo phenotype and that combined shared morphology and phenotype with normal breast reduction mammoplasty acini. In addition, we have proved through overexpression of HER2 that formation of structures that accurately reflect DCIS in vivo can be achieved. What is more, we have proved that these structures are quantifiable by standard inexpensive laboratory techniques [unpublished].

However, despite better recapitulating the in vivo breast environment, models such as these are still reliant on cell line culture which may already represent aberrant breast epithelium. As discussed previously, the use of new primary cell cultures that represent the morphology, immunoprofile and genetic profile of normal and earlier benign breast lesions would be necessary to accurately model breast cancer initiation in the laboratory. The culture of primary breast epithelial cells in 3D Matrigel™ has been achieved previously [69] but has been limited to a single cell population. In order to accurately recapitulate the in vivo breast environment, multiple primary cell types would need to be isolated, characterised to ensure they accurately represented their in vivo counterparts, labelled to enable tracking and then cultured together in 3D ECM. The finite life span of primary cell cultures in vitro would make this challenging for researchers with further genetic and proteomic manipulation even more difficult.

Conclusion

In summary, when cultured under the right conditions, current available representative cell lines of normal and DCIS breast epithelium could provide valuable insight into the morphological, phenotypical and architectural changes that occur in the development from normal breast to benign lesions and cancer initiation. The use of cell lines grown in 2D offers the opportunity to study the complex intracellular mechanisms that may drive these processes in great detail while culture in 3D can perhaps better mimic the pathology and immunoprofile of these lesions in a more physiologically relevant setting. However, in order to recapitulate the genomic alterations that appear to drive the transition from normal breast to DCIS, better primary cell cultures would need to be developed.

Key Points

- To understand the molecular pathology of breast cancer initiation and progression, appropriate models that allow experimentation in a controlled laboratory environment and reflect the heterogeneity of breast cancer are necessary.

- Many cell lines used in breast cancer been virally immortalised and may therefore not be a true representative of cells in vivo.
- To the best of the authors' knowledge, there are no cell lines available that represent low grade DCIS or early breast lesions.
- A limitation of all 3D in vitro models is the lack of a complex in vivo system complete with blood supply, immune infiltrates and regulation by hormonal cues.
- In order to more faithfully recapitulate breast-like structures in a 3D matrix co-cultures with other cell types, notably fibroblasts and myofibroblasts, is necessary.

References

1. Curtis C, et al. The genomic and transcriptomic architecture of 2000 breast tumours reveals novel subgroups. Nature. 2012;486(7403):346–52.
2. Lehmann BD, et al. Identification of human triple-negative breast cancer subtypes and preclinical models for selection of targeted therapies. J Clin Investig. 2011;121(7):2750–67.
3. Sørlie T, et al. Gene expression patterns of breast carcinomas distinguish tumor subclasses with clinical implications. Proc Natl Acad Sci U.S.A. 2001;98(19):10869–74.
4. Eccles SA, et al. Critical research gaps and translational priorities for the successful prevention and treatment of breast cancer. Breast Cancer Res. 2013;15:5.
5. Wellings SR, Jensen HM, Marcum RG. An atlas of subgross pathology of the human breast with special reference to possible precancerous lesions. J Natl Cancer Inst. 1975;55(2):231–73.
6. Carley AM, et al. Frequency and clinical significance of simultaneous association of lobular neoplasia and columnar cell alterations in breast tissue specimens. Am J Clin Pathol. 2008;130(2):254–8.
7. Abdel-Fatah TM, et al. High frequency of coexistence of columnar cell lesions, lobular neoplasia, and low grade ductal carcinoma in situ with invasive tubular carcinoma and invasive lobular carcinoma. Am J Surg Pathol. 2007;31(3):417–26.
8. Abdel-Fatah TM, et al. Morphologic and molecular evolutionary pathways of low nuclear grade invasive breast cancers and their putative precursor lesions: further evidence to support the concept of low nuclear grade breast neoplasia family. Am J Surg Pathol. 2008;32(4):513–23.
9. Dabbs DJ, et al. Molecular alterations in columnar cell lesions of the breast. Mod Pathol. 2006;19(3):344–9.
10. Moinfar F, et al. Concurrent and independent genetic alterations in the stromal and epithelial cells of mammary carcinoma: implications for tumorigenesis. Cancer Res. 2000;60(9):2562–6.
11. Simpson PT, et al. Columnar cell lesions of the breast: the missing link in breast cancer progression? A morphological and molecular analysis. Am J Surg Pathol. 2005;29(6):734–46.
12. Aubele MM, et al. Accumulation of chromosomal imbalances from intraductal proliferative lesions to adjacent in situ and invasive ductal breast cancer. Diagn Mol Pathol. 2000;9(1):14–9.
13. Perou CM, et al. Molecular portraits of human breast tumours. Nature. 2000;406(6797):747–52.
14. Forozan F, et al. Comparative genomic hybridization analysis of 38 breast cancer cell lines: a basis for interpreting complementary DNA microarray data. Cancer Res. 2000;60(16):4519–25.
15. Weigelt B, Bissell M. Unraveling the microenvironmental influences on the normal mammary gland and breast cancer. Semin Cancer Biol. 2008;18(5):311–21.

16. Matthay MA, et al. Transient effect of epidermal growth factor on the motility of an immortalized mammary epithelial cell line. J Cell Sci. 1993;106(Pt 3):869–78.
17. Soule HD, et al. Isolation and characterization of a spontaneously immortalized human breast epithelial cell line, MCF-10. Cancer Res. 1990;50(18):6075–86.
18. Tait L, Soule HD, Russo J. Ultrastructural and immunocytochemical characterization of an immortalized human breast epithelial cell line, MCF-10. Cancer Res. 1990;50(18):6087–94.
19. DiRenzo J, et al. Growth factor requirements and basal phenotype of an immortalized mammary epithelial cell line. Cancer Res. 2002;62(1):89–98.
20. Yusuf R, Frenkel K. Morphologic transformation of human breast epithelial cells MCF-10A: dependence on an oxidative microenvironment and estrogen/epidermal growth factor receptors. Cancer Cell Int. 2010;10(1):30.
21. Marella NV, et al. Cytogenetic and cDNA microarray expression analysis of MCF10 human breast cancer progression cell lines. Cancer Res. 2009;69(14):5946–53.
22. Bartek J, et al. Efficient immortalization of luminal epithelial cells from human mammary gland by introduction of simian virus 40 large tumor antigen with a recombinant retrovirus. Proc Natl Acad Sci U.S.A. 1991;88(9):3520–4.
23. Caradonna F, Luparello C. Cytogenetic characterization of HB2 epithelial cells from the human breast. In Vitro Cell Dev Biol Anim. 2014;50(1):48–55.
24. Miller FR, et al. MCF10DCIS.com xenograft model of human comedo ductal carcinoma in situ. J Natl Cancer Inst. 2000;92(14):1185–6.
25. Forozan F, et al. Molecular cytogenetic analysis of 11 new breast cancer cell lines. Br J Cancer. 1999;81(8):1328–34.
26. Bissell MJ, Radisky D. Putting tumours in context. Nat Rev Cancer. 2001;1(1):46–54.
27. Cukierman E, Pankov R, Yamada KM. Cell interactions with three-dimensional matrices. Curr Opin Cell Biol. 2002;14(5):633–9.
28. Zwezdaryk KJ, et al. Rotating cell culture systems for human cell culture: human trophoblast cells as a model. J Vis Exp. 2012;18:59.
29. Foty R. A simple hanging drop cell culture protocol for generation of 3D spheroids. J Vis Exp. 2011;51:2720. doi: 10.3791/2720.
30. Naber HP. Spheroid assay to measure TGF-beta-induced invasion. J Vis Exp. 2011;16(57):3337.
31. Nagelkerke A, et al. Hypoxia stimulates migration of breast cancer cells via the PERK/ATF4/LAMP3-arm of the unfolded protein response. Breast Cancer Res. 2013;15(1):R2.
32. Ivascu A, Kubbies M. Rapid generation of single-tumor spheroids for high-throughput cell function and toxicity analysis. J Biomol Screen. 2006;11(8):922–32.
33. Zhang X, et al. Development of an in vitro multicellular tumor spheroid model using microencapsulation and its application in anticancer drug screening and testing. Biotechnol Prog. 2005;21(4):1289–96.
34. Smart CE, et al. In vitro analysis of breast cancer cell line tumourspheres and primary human breast epithelia mammospheres demonstrates inter- and intrasphere heterogeneity. PLoS ONE. 2013;8(6):e64388.
35. Farnie G, et al. Novel cell culture technique for primary ductal carcinoma in situ: role of Notch and epidermal growth factor receptor signaling pathways. J Natl Cancer Inst. 2007;99(8):616–27.
36. Shaw FL, et al. A detailed mammosphere assay protocol for the quantification of breast stem cell activity. J Mammary Gland Biol Neoplasia. 2012;17(2):111–7.
37. Leeper AD, et al. Long-term culture of human breast cancer specimens and their analysis using optical projection tomography. J Vis Exp. 2011;29(53).
38. Holliday DL, et al. Novel multicellular organotypic models of normal and malignant breast: tools for dissecting the role of the microenvironment in breast cancer progression. Breast Cancer Res. 2009;11(1):R3.
39. Debnath J, Brugge JS. Modelling glandular epithelial cancers in three-dimensional cultures. Nat Rev Cancer. 2005;5(9):675–88.

40. Debnath J, Muthuswamy SK, Brugge JS. Morphogenesis and oncogenesis of MCF-10A mammary epithelial acini grown in three-dimensional basement membrane cultures. Methods. 2003;30(3):256–68.
41. Streuli CH, Bailey N, Bissell MJ. Control of mammary epithelial differentiation: basement membrane induces tissue-specific gene expression in the absence of cell-cell interaction and morphological polarity. The Journal of Cell Biology. 1991;115(5):1383–95.
42. Wisdom BJ, et al. Type IV collagen of Engelbreth-Holm-Swarm tumor matrix: identification of constituent chains. Connect Tissue Res. 1992;27(4):225–34.
43. Vaillant F, Lindeman G, Visvader J. Jekyll or Hyde: does Matrigel provide a more or less physiological environment in mammary repopulating assays? Breast Cancer Res. 2011;13(3):108.
44. Parmar H, Cunha GR. Epithelial-stromal interactions in the mouse and human mammary gland in vivo. Endocr Relat Cancer. 2004;11(3):437–58.
45. Provenzano P, et al. Collagen reorganization at the tumor-stromal interface facilitates local invasion. BMC Med. 2006;4(1):38.
46. Provenzano PP, et al. Matrix density-induced mechanoregulation of breast cell phenotype, signaling and gene expression through a FAK-ERK linkage. Oncogene. 2009;28(49):4326–43.
47. Dhimolea E, et al. The role of collagen reorganization on mammary epithelial morphogenesis in a 3D culture model. Biomaterials. 2010;31(13):3622–30.
48. Maskarinec G, et al. Mammographic density as a predictor of breast cancer survival: the Multiethnic Cohort. Breast Cancer Res. 2013;15(1):R7.
49. Alowami S, et al. Mammographic density is related to stroma and stromal proteoglycan expression. Breast Cancer Res. 2003;5(5):R129–35.
50. Krause S, et al. A novel 3D in vitro culture model to study stromal-epithelial interactions in the mammary gland. Tissue Eng Part C Methods. 2008;14(3):261–71.
51. Berdichevsky F, et al. Branching morphogenesis of human mammary epithelial cells in collagen gels. J Cell Sci. 1994;107(12):3557–68.
52. O'Brien LE, et al. Morphological and biochemical analysis of Rac1 in three-dimensional epithelial cell cultures. Methods Enzymol. 2006;406:676–91.
53. Dickinson ME. Multimodal imaging of mouse development: tools for the postgenomic era. Dev Dyn. 2006;235(9):2386–400.
54. Kubow KE, Horwitz AR. Reducing background fluorescence reveals adhesions in 3D matrices. Nat Cell Biol. 2011;13(1):3–5.
55. Zipfel WR, Williams RM, Webb WW. Nonlinear magic: multiphoton microscopy in the biosciences. Nat Biotechnol. 2003;21(11):1369–77.
56. Huang D, et al. Optical coherence tomography. Science. 1991;254(5035):1178–81.
57. Sharpe J, et al. Optical projection tomography as a tool for 3D microscopy and gene expression studies. Science. 2002;296(5567):541–5.
58. Sameni M, et al. MAME models for 4D live-cell imaging of tumor: microenvironment interactions that impact malignant progression. J Vis Exp. 2012;17(60):3661.
59. Petersen OW, et al. Interaction with basement membrane serves to rapidly distinguish growth and differentiation pattern of normal and malignant human breast epithelial cells. Proc Natl Acad Sci U.S.A. 1992;89(19):9064–8.
60. Krause S, et al. A novel 3D in vitro culture model to study stromal-epithelial interactions in the mammary gland. Tissue Eng Part C: Methods. 2008;14(3):261–71.
61. Shekhar MPV, Werdell J, Tait L. Interaction with endothelial cells is a prerequisite for branching ductal-alveolar morphogenesis and hyperplasia of preneoplastic human breast epithelial cells: regulation by estrogen. Cancer Res. 2000;60(2):439–49.
62. Wang X, et al. Preadipocytes stimulate ductal morphogenesis and functional differentiation of human mammary epithelial cells on 3D silk scaffolds. Tissue Eng Part A. 2009;15(10):3087–98.
63. Olsen C, et al. Human mammary fibroblasts stimulate invasion of breast cancer cells in a three-dimensional culture and increase stroma development in mouse xenografts. BMC Cancer. 2010;10(1):444.

64. Egeblad M, Werb Z. New functions for the matrix metalloproteinases in cancer progression. Nat Rev Cancer. 2002;2(3):161–74.
65. Gilles C, et al. Implication of collagen type 1-induced membrane-type 1 matrix metalloproteinase expression and matrix metalloproteinase-2 activation in the metastatic progression of breast carcinoma. Lab Invest. 1997;76(5):651–60.
66. Barsky SH. Myoepithelial mRNA expression profiling reveals a common tumor-suppressor phenotype. Exp Mol Pathol. 2003;74(2):113–22.
67. Jones JL, et al. Primary breast myopithelial cells exert an invasion-suppressor effect on breast cancer cells via paracrine down-regulation of MMP expresssion in fibroblasts and tumour cells. J Pathol. 2003;201(4):562–72.
68. Gudjonsson T, et al. Normal and tumor-derived myoepithelial cells differ in their ability to interact with luminal breast epithelial cells for polarity and basement membrane deposition. J Cell Sci. 2002;115(1):39–50.
69. Jeanes AI, Maya-Mendoza A, Streuli CH. Cellular microenvironment influences the ability of mammary epithelia to undergo cell cycle. PLoS ONE. 2011;6(3):e18144.

Chapter 4
Molecular Pathology of Precancerous Lesions of the Breast

Abhik Mukherjee, Ian O. Ellis and Emad A. Rakha

Introduction

Evidence has now emerged that low- and high-grade breast cancers (BCs) evolve through distinct evolutionary pathways and not through various steps of dedifferentiation [1–4] and differences between these tumours are maintained throughout the process of tumour initiation, development and progression. This is reflected in the molecular biology of precancerous lesions of the breast, which includes the low-grade lesions, as part of the 'low grade neoplasia family', as well as the high-grade lesions. At the lower end of the spectrum, the coexistence of low-grade precursor lesions with invasive low-grade BCs that defy justification by chance alone [5, 6] as well as their overlapping morphological, and immunohistochemical and genetic features [5–9] provide evidence that these lesions represent a continuum in terms of BC development and progression. Their low proliferative activity and characteristic features are fundamentally different from those observed in precursors of a histological higher grade BC [6]. When high-grade precursors progress to invasive cancer, the latter is usually of high-grade, sharing the same genetic aberrations. This chapter explores the fundamental differences in molecular profiles of the two spectrums of precancerous lesions of the breast, low and high grade.

A. Mukherjee · I.O. Ellis · E.A. Rakha (✉)
Division of Cancer and Stem Cells, Department of Histopathology,
School of Medicine, University of Nottingham and Nottingham
University Hospitals NHS Trust, Nottingham City Hospital, Nottingham, UK
e-mail: emad.rakha@nottingham.ac.uk

© Springer Science+Business Media New York 2015
A. Khan et al. (eds.), *Precision Molecular Pathology of Breast Cancer*,
Molecular Pathology Library 10, DOI 10.1007/978-1-4939-2886-6_4

Low-Grade Precursor Lesions

Salient Histopathological Features

These clonal intraductal lesions originate from the terminal duct-lobular unit (TDLU) and show low-cytonuclear atypia with or without intraluminal proliferation (summarised from [10, 11]). Columnar cell lesion (CCL), flat epithelial atypia (FEA), atypical ductal hyperplasia (ADH), atypical lobular hyperplasia (ALH), lobular carcinoma in situ (LCIS) and low-grade ductal carcinoma in situ (DCIS) are included in this category. Columnar Cell Lesions (CCLs) are characterised by distended acini lined by columnar epithelial cells with apical snouts. There may be associated epithelial hyperplasia (cellular stratification >2 cell layers but no complex architectural patterns). When CCL shows cytonuclear atypia, it is designated as flat epithelial atypia (FEA). FEA typically lacks well-developed architectural atypia (micropapillae, tufts, fronds, rigid bridges and punched out spaces: features of ADH /low-grade DCIS). In FEA, the nuclei are uniform, rounded and evenly spaced. CCLs are more frequent with tubular carcinoma (TC) and invasive cribriform carcinoma (ICC) (92 and 60 %, respectively) [5, 6, 12, 13]. Low-grade DCIS shows intraductal proliferation of evenly spaced, usually small monomorphic cells with hyperchromatic nuclei but inconspicuous nucleoli. Cells are arranged in cribriform and micropapillary patterns, with the cribriform pattern being predominant. The solid pattern is rare within this category of DCIS. Mitosis and necrosis are also infrequent. ADH is cytologically and architecturally similar to low-grade DCIS but its extent is limited (a 2–3 mm focal lesion confined to one or two duct spaces). ADH is a recognised risk indicator and a non-obligate precursor of low-grade DCIS and invasive BCs, though the risk of invasive carcinoma developing is smaller compared to DCIS [14].

Lobular neoplasia (LN), on the other hand, refers to non-invasive proliferative low-grade lesions consisting of a monomorphic population of generally small and discohesive cells that fill and expand the TDLU. LN encompasses both ALH and LCIS, which are morphologically similar but ALH represents an early/less well-developed lesion with partial involvement of acini. The morphological distinction of ALH and LCIS is however, somewhat arbitrary, depending on extent. There are rare variants of LCIS that show more aggressive features. These include pleomorphic and mass-forming necrotizing LCIS. LN can behave both as a high-risk lesion and a non-obligate precursor to BC [10, 11].

Molecular Features

Loss of heterozygosity (LOH) and comparative genomic hybridization (CGH) studies have established that low-grade and high-grade BCs are dissimilar at the DNA level. Low-grade precursors display a lower level of genomic instability with fewer chromosomal aberrations and exhibit recurrent losses of 16q and gains of 1q and 16p [2, 3], which often arise from an unbalanced chromosomal translocation involving chromosomes 1 and 16. Frequent loss of 16q has been demonstrated in all varieties of the low-grade neoplasia family viz. CCL [9], FEA [7], ADH [15] and low-grade DCIS [16]. The loss of 16q, which is a frequent (>70 %) event, involves the whole chromosomal arm in contrast to high-grade precursors where it is infrequent (<20 %) and occurs through a different process (LOH with mitotic recombination) [1–3, 17]. Although the loss of 16q is observed in both low-grade ductal and lobular precursors, the target genes differ in these two lesions. The gene involved in loss of 16q in LN is CDH1 (E-cadherin), which maps to 16q22.1. E-cadherin is now well characterised as a tumour suppressor gene in LN as evident by CDH1 mutation and loss of E-cadherin protein. Such mutations are rare in DCIS. Within the lobular neoplasia family, although the morphological boundary of ALH and LCIS is nebulous, evidence suggests that LCIS harbours greater copy number alterations [18] and possesses a higher risk of invasive BC development than ALH.

To characterise the LOH in DCIS, microsatellite-length polymorphisms at seven loci (AluVpa, ESR, D11S988, D13S267, D16S398, D17S1159 and D17S855) have been investigated from microdissected paraffin sections of DCIS cases [19]. Allelic loss or imbalance, reflecting LOH has been found to be commoner in invasive ductal carcinoma (IDC) rather than in DCIS. LOH in DCIS was most frequent at the D16S398 (26 %) locus. LOH at this locus was commoner in low- and intermediate-grade DCIS than in high-grade DCIS. Overall, microsatellite instability (MSI) at only one locus was more frequent in DCIS (28 %) than in IDC (6 %) ($p < 0.001$). The occurrence of MSI at multiple loci was similar in frequency in both DCIS (6 %) and in IDC (3 %). Together, these observations indicate that chromosomal losses of 16q may occur in low- and intermediate-grade DCIS and MSI involving multiple loci is uncommon in both IDC and DCIS.

Phenotypic Characteristics

More recent studies using cDNA expression array technology have confirmed that the core intrinsic molecular subgroups, including luminal, HER2 and basal, found in invasive breast cancer [20, 21] are replicated in DCIS, although at different frequencies [22] showing that the molecular heterogeneity of invasive carcinomas exists among in-situ lesions as well. Low-grade precursors are morphologically and immuno-phenotypically uniform (i.e. strongly positive for oestrogen receptor (ER) and luminal cytokeratins (CK) within lesional cells, but negative for basal CKs). Immunohistochemical studies usually demonstrate strong diffuse ER-positivity, PR-positivity and HER2-negativity within these lesions along-with low Ki67 labelling, and lack of expression of p53, p-cadherin and basal CKs (i.e. CK5/6 and CK14). Luminal CKs (CK19 and CK8/18), androgen receptor, Bcl-2 and cyclin D1 are often positive. In a recent study, [23] 112 cases of a series of

314 DCIS cases were classified as low grade. On phenotyping with routine ER, PR and HER2 staining, 71, 24, 9 and 8 cases distributed, respectively, to Luminal A, Luminal B, HER2 and triple negative subtypes. The overall % of low-grade DCIS within each of these phenotypic types was as follows: 52, 26, 18 and 20 %. This shows that the Luminal A subtype predominates in low-grade DCIS.

High Grade Precursor Lesions

Salient Histopathological Features

High-grade DCIS features (summarised from [10]) highly atypical cells within the duct space arranged in solid, cribrifrom or micropapillary patterns. The nuclei exhibit pleomorphism, are poorly polarised, often with irregular contour. Nucleoli are prominent and the chromatin is coarse and clumped. Mitotic figures, though common, are not a necessity for diagnosis. A frequently observed feature is comedo necrosis, where abundant necrotic debris in the lumina is surrounded by pleomorphic tumour cells. Necrotic intraluminal debris is often associated with amorphous microcalcifications. However, like mitoses, comedo necrosis is not obligatory for diagnosis. If typical morphological features are present even in a single space, this is deemed sufficient for diagnosis. High-grade DCIS may be diagnosed even if a single flat layer of highly atypical cells line a duct space, the 'flat/clinging' DCIS [7]. Cancerisation of lobule (involvement of the lobule by ductal epithelial cells) is more frequent with high-grade DCIS than with low-grade DCIS.

Molecular Features

High-grade DCIS is distinct from low-grade DCIS not only on morphology but also by phenotype and molecular genetics. They are usually aneuploid and rarely harbour the low-grade signature pattern (16q loss/1q gain) [24–27]. Whereas well-differentiated DCIS exhibits loss of 16q and 17p, high-grade tumours harbour significant losses of other allelic chromosomal arms including 1p, 1q, 6q, 9p, 11p, 11q, 13q and 17q as shown by array CGH studies [28]. In addition, high-grade DCIS displays gains at 17q, 11q and 13q [29]. Intermediate-grade DCIS shows features of both high- and low-grade DCIS, showing 16q loss but higher incidence of gains of 1q and losses of 11q in comparison to low-grade DCIS, but lacking the frequent amplifications at 17q12 and 11q13 that may occur in high-grade DCIS [16]. The average number of genetic imbalances in intermediate-grade DCIS though are higher than in low-grade DCIS. Flat type high-grade DCIS (clinging type DCIS) exhibits LOH at 11q, 16q and 17q in approximately 50, 60 and 40 %, respectively [7]. Other studies for LOH reveal that certain loci viz. D11S988 and D17S1159 are more frequently involved in high-grade DCIS.

Especially, LOH at D11S988 was commoner in those cases with no evidence of comedo necrosis [19].

Certain specific genes have been identified to be amplified or inactivated in DCIS. cDNA micro-array technology has shown that the angio-associated migratory cell protein, a multifunctional protein with a putative role in motility and angiogenesis, is up-regulated in DCIS of high grade and in the presence of necrosis [30]. Another research group [31] identified upregulation of lactoferrin in DCIS, and downregulation of the oxytocin receptor and hevin (a cell adhesion related glycoprotein), though no correlation was identified with DCIS grade. *HER*2 is well recognised as being amplified in DCIS, with increased overexpression correlating with increasing nuclear grade [32] and will be further discussed in the next section on phenotype. Amplification of cyclin D1, a cell cycle regulator, has also been observed in DCIS [33] with overexpression being common in intermediate- and high-grade disease. Inactivating mutations of p53 are also observed in high-grade DCIS [32]. Another tumour suppressor gene apparently inactivated in DCIS is the IGF-II-receptor gene (on 6q) [33].

Phenotypic Features

The immunohistochemical profile of high-grade DCIS has been studied in various series. In a recent study of 314 cases DCIS [23], 202 cases were histologically of high grade. Phenotyping on the basis of ER, PR and HER2 staining, 63, 64, 44, 32 cases distributed respectively to Luminal A, Luminal B, HER2 and triple negative subtypes. The overall percentage of high-grade DCIS within each of these phenotypic classes was as follows: 48, 74, 88 and 80 %. In contrast to the low-grade DCIS of the series (discussed earlier), HER2 positives and triple negatives were more prevalent within high grades. Some studies [34] have investigated the phenotype of special histological variants of DCIS like cystic hyper-secretory DCIS. A special variant of DCIS with colloid-like luminal secretions, this subtype was found to be either intermediate or high grade and usually ER positive but HER2 negative and occasionally androgen receptor positive. Other studies have probed the distribution of intrinsic types of breast cancer in the context of whether DCIS shows associated invasion or not [23, 35–37]. In a study of 99 cases of pure DCIS and 96 cases of co-existing DCIS/IDC [36], there was a high rate of co-expression of CKs, ER-α, PR, HER2 and EGFR between DCIS and its co-existing IDC. The rate of discordance among biomarker expression was low and was present more commonly with high-grade DCIS/IDC. HER2, EGFR, CK5/6 and CK14 expression was associated with high-grade DCIS while ER and PR expression was observed low-grade cases. There was no difference in luminal CKs 8/18 expression between high- and low-grade categories. A recent immunohistochemistry based study [23] with 5 markers (ER, PR, HER2, CK5 and EGFR), revealed that for high-grade DCIS without accompanying invasive cancer, the distribution of phenotypic surrogates was as follows: luminal A (57.1 %), luminal B (11.9 %),

HER2 (16.7 %), basal-like phenotype (0 %) and un-classified (14.3 %). For cases associated with invasive carcinoma, luminal cancers were also predominant viz. luminal A (58.2 %) and luminal B (12.7 %). HER2 positives were at a frequency of (7.6 %), but there were more basal-like (7.6 %) DCIS and in these cases the invasive component mirrored this phenotype. These results are in contrast to another study [37] which demonstrated differences in the occurrences of luminal A, luminal B, and HER2 phenotypes, but no difference in the basal-like phenotype with associated invasive malignancies. In another study [38] of 146 samples of DCIS and adjacent invasive malignancy, CK5/6 showed different distribution in DCIS and IDC, presenting a significant association with the triple negative phenotype in IDC, but a negative association within DCIS. A triple-positive profile (ER/PR/HER2 positive) and CK5/6 expression were negatively associated with invasion. In the low-grade DCIS subgroup, only CK5/6 expression exhibited a negative association with the probability of invasion. Given the variability especially in relation to the basal-like markers, further studies are warranted to establish the relationships between pure DCIS and co-existing DCIS/IDC.

Another area of substantial research interest has been HER2 expression and its significance in DCIS. In a series [39] of 103 pure DCIS and 38 cases of DCIS with <5 mm invasive carcinoma, pure high-grade, ER-negative DCIS with comedo necrosis showed a high frequency of HER2 overexpression. For DCIS with accompanying invasion, HER2 expression in the invasive component was higher than in DCIS. In a Chinese single institution study [40], 183 pure DCIS, and 43 patients of DCIS with invasion were studied where the HER2-positive subtype accounted for 27.9 % of the cases. Though on univariate analyses higher histological grade (Grades 2 and 3), and HER2 positive status were associated with invasion, on multivariate analysis only the HER2-positive status retained significance. In invasive cases, on further stratification of the accompanying DCIS as extensive or small (in relation to the total tumour area using a 25 % cut-off), HER2-positivity was associated with the cohort showing extensive DCIS. HER2 overexpression is also a typical feature of DCIS associated with Paget's disease of the nipple.

In addition to the core findings above, the molecular biology of high-grade DCIS has been explored within BRCA mutation carriers [41]. DCIS in BRCA1 mutation carriers were high grade with high proliferation index and basal type by phenotype with low ER/PR/HER2 expression, but frequent CK5/6, CK14 and EGFR expression. On the other hand, within BRCA2 mutation carriers, DCIS exhibited the luminal phenotype in spite of being high grade. In BRCA1 and BRCA2 mutation carriers there was a high concordance between DCIS lesions and their concomitant invasive counterpart with regard to expression of individual markers as well as molecular subtype. The same research group has demonstrated that within both categories of BRCA mutation carriers, the hypoxia-related proteins HIF-1alpha, CAIX and Glut-1 are expressed in both DCIS and accompanying invasive cancer [42], and indicate the possible role of hypoxia in breast carcinogenesis and progression in these patients.

While phenotyping into intrinsic subtypes of BC, there is yet an unmet need to identify through molecular techniques, lesions that transit to IDC from DCIS. Gene expression analyses followed by hierarchical clustering comparing pure DCIS, pure invasive cancers and cases of mixed diagnosis establishes that cases group by intrinsic subtype, not by diagnosis [43]. Even DCIS of high histological grade are heterogeneous in their transcriptomes, clustering into either a ER negative/HER2 positive group or a predominantly ER + group, termed DCIS I (invasive like) and II, respectively, by the authors. Within the DCIS I subtype, differentially expressed genes, independent of grade, ER and HER2 status, include among others, genes related to immune function, epithelial mesenchymal transition and IL12 pathways. These were validated on another previous dataset which had also generated a gene signature to distinguish between DCIS and IDC as well as poor and well-differentiated DCIS [44]. In spite of the small numbers, the results aim to address the gap in knowledge in this field. Genes differentially expressed between non-invasive type II DCIS and IDC also included genes involved in epithelial mesenchymal transition including several matrix metalloproteinases [43]. Such studies indicate that being high grade alone does not always create the potential for invasion for DCIS and other molecular characteristics of the lesion and its interface may be vital.

Overall from various series, it may be summarised that high-grade DCIS with large nuclear size and comedo necrosis strongly associate with DNA aneuploidy, high proliferative activity, low expression of steroid receptors, and overexpression of HER2 and p53. This contrasts with both low-grade DCIS and LCIS, which are predominantly diploid with low proliferation indices, and rare expression of HER2 or p53.

Other Molecular Characteristics

The role of DNA methylation in DCIS has been explored [45] for a panel of well-characterised genes using methylation-sensitive high resolution melting (MS-HRM) in formalin-fixed, paraffin-embedded (FFPE) sections. The RASSF1A gene was most frequently methylated (90 % of samples) and this feature was significantly associated with comedo necrosis. The methylation profile revealed a highly methylated cluster that was significantly associated with high nuclear grade, amplified HER2 but negative ER/PR status. High nuclear grade was specifically associated with the methylation of APC and CDH13 genes while methylation of CDH13 and RARβ genes were associated with HER2-amplification.

Given the amplification of cyclin D1 in high-grade DCIS, other proteins interacting with cyclin D1 have been investigated by immunohistochemistry [46]. One such protein, matricellulin (CCN1), shows greater cytoplasmic expression in high and intermediate-grade DCIS than in low-grade DCIS (H-scores of 170, 160 vs. 60). Membranous β-catenin expression also correlated with the grade of intraepithelial carcinoma [46]. These proteins probably play a role in cell cycle progression through cyclin D1.

Clinical Implications of the Molecular Characteristics of DCIS

The molecular features described above elucidate the heterogeneity of DCIS. As prognosis varies within the low and high grades [47], it is imperative to understand the clinical implications of the molecular features of DCIS. Studies have indicated that luminal B and HER2 subtypes of DCIS had a propensity for local recurrence compared to the luminal A and triple negative phenotypes [48]. Of these, HER2 positive status was significantly correlated with local recurrence on multivariate analysis, especially invasive recurrence. This contrasts with another series [49] where DCIS cases with HER2 positivity treated by breast-conserving surgery alone had a higher risk of DCIS recurrence but not invasive recurrence. Instead, a two-fold increased risk of invasive recurrence was observed in DCIS that expressed p16+/Cox-2+/Ki-67+. However, the variation between the two series can be attributed to the fact that the interpretation of immunohistochemistry for borderline HER2 positivity (score 2+) was different in the two series. The [49] series reported this as positive in all cases and hence the results are to be interpreted with caution. This also stresses the need for conformity to further deconstruct the molecular portraits of recurrence. More data will emerge from mature results of the NSABP B-43, a prospective randomised phase III trial [50] comparing the effects of whole breast irradiation with or without trastuzumab in HER2-positive pure DCIS cases treated by lumpectomy. The analysis of HER2 in this large series is centralised and stringent with preliminary results indicating a 34.9 % HER2 positivity of DCIS in the series, much lower than a previously reported rate of 50 %. On completion, the trial will help formulate better treatment for HER2-positive DCIS and also consolidate the prognostic strength of HER2 in pre-invasive breast malignancy. Other prognostication attempts [51] on a large population-based cohort using the St Gallen criteria has failed to demonstrate a prognostic value for the intrinsic subtypes of DCIS for up to 10 years post-diagnosis. After 10 years, triple negative DCIS posed a higher risk of recurrence in this study. Given all these conflicting results, there is no doubt that further prognostic fine-tuning is much desired. Such an attempt has been made through the Van Nuys Prognostic Index (VNPI) after integration of either genomic grade (GGI) or proliferation index (Ki-67) [52]. DCIS samples were divided into three VNPI risk groups, low, intermediate and high risk based on nuclear grade ± necrosis alongwith tumour size, excision margin width and age. For VNPI-GGI, nuclear grade was replaced by a genomic grade index (GGI) and for VNPI-Ki67, combined with Ki67 expression. The majority of the recurrent cases were classified in VNPI intermediate and high-risk groups. While VNPI-Ki-67 did not improve the prognostic value of VNPI, VNPI-GGI more accurately identified high-risk DCIS patients with early relapses within 5 years. Such prognostication tools need further validation in DCIS clinical trials.

Conclusion

Low-and high-grade breast neoplasia pathways are being understood better currently, given the plethora of emerging molecular data. While the basic molecular tenets of low- and high-grade neoplasia precursors in BC have been characterised, more will unfold in the near future. The gaps in knowledge mainly relate to prognostication and the development of tailored therapeutic options. Also, the biology of progression from pre-invasive to invasive cancer needs to be investigated further to delineate targets. The progress of understanding in invasive BC has been aided both by genetic analysis as well as simple biomarker analysis. The same will probably hold true for preinvasive lesions. While biomarker research in invasive cancers have been speeded and economised by tissue micro-array technology, this may prove technically challenging in DCIS. The way forward in a technically progressive era may be through digital platforms such as virtual TMAs [53] in both research and clinical settings.

Key Points

- Precancerous/pre-invasive breast lesions are either low- or high-grade and represent distinct clonal evolutionary pathways.
- The low-grade lesions include FEA, ADH and low-grade DCIS within the ductal subtype and ALH to LCIS within the lobular subtype.
- The low-grade lesions have fewer chromosomal aberrations and exhibit recurrent losses of 16q and gains of 1q and 16p. They are predominantly diploid, luminal by phenotype and rarely express HER2 and p53.
- The prototype high-grade lesion is high-grade DCIS.
- High-grade DCIS is characterised by DNA aneuploidy and harbours losses of multiple chromosome alleles and gains in 17q, 11q and 13q. HER2-positive and triple-negative subtypes predominately cluster within this category.
- HER2 positivity and triple negativity have been variably related to invasion and recurrence in DCIS.
- Further molecular characterisation is necessary to identify subsets that are likely to progress to invasive neoplasia and therefore would benefit from additional treatment.

References

1. Roylance R, et al. Allelic imbalance analysis of chromosome 16q shows that grade I and grade III invasive ductal breast cancers follow different genetic pathways. J Pathol. 2002;196(1):32–6.
2. Roylance R, et al. Comparative genomic hybridization of breast tumors stratified by histological grade reveals new insights into the biological progression of breast cancer. Cancer Res. 1999;59(7):1433–6.

3. Cleton-Jansen AM, et al. Different mechanisms of chromosome 16 loss of heterozygosity in well- versus poorly differentiated ductal breast cancer. Genes Chromosomes Cancer. 2004;41(2):109–16.

4. Natrajan R, et al. Loss of 16q in high grade breast cancer is associated with estrogen receptor status: Evidence for progression in tumors with a luminal phenotype? Genes Chromosomes Cancer. 2009;48(4):351–65.

5. Abdel-Fatah TM, et al. High frequency of coexistence of columnar cell lesions, lobular neoplasia, and low grade ductal carcinoma in situ with invasive tubular carcinoma and invasive lobular carcinoma. Am J Surg Pathol. 2007;31(3):417–26.

6. Abdel-Fatah TM, et al. Morphologic and molecular evolutionary pathways of low nuclear grade invasive breast cancers and their putative precursor lesions: further evidence to support the concept of low nuclear grade breast neoplasia family. Am J Surg Pathol. 2008;32(4):513–23.

7. Moinfar F, et al. Genetic abnormalities in mammary ductal intraepithelial neoplasia-flat type ("clinging ductal carcinoma in situ"): a simulator of normal mammary epithelium. Cancer. 2000;88(9):2072–81.

8. Oyama T, et al. Atypical cystic lobule of the breast: an early stage of low-grade ductal carcinoma in-situ. Breast Cancer. 2000;7(4):326–31.

9. Simpson PT, et al. Columnar cell lesions of the breast: the missing link in breast cancer progression? A morphological and molecular analysis. Am J Surg Pathol. 2005;29(6):734–46.

10. Pathology Reporting of Breast Disease. A Joint document incorporating the third edition of the NHS breast screening programme's guidelines for pathology reporting in breast cancer screening and the second edition of The Royal College of Pathologists' minimum dataset for breast cancer histopathology. NHSBSP Publication No 58, January 2005. p. 50–59. Available from: http://www.rcpath.org/Resources/RCPath/Migrated%20Resources/Documents/P/PathologyReportingOfBreastDisease-CORRECTED-lowres.pdf.

11. Rakha EA. The low nuclear grade breast neoplasia family. Diagnostic Histopathology. 2012;18(3):124–32.

12. Rajan S, et al. What is the significance of flat epithelial atypia and what are the management implications? J Clin Pathol. 2011;64(11):1001–4.

13. Rakha EA, et al. Tubular carcinoma of the breast: further evidence to support its excellent prognosis. J Clin Oncol. 2010;28(1):99–104.

14. Rakha EA, et al. Characterization and outcome of breast needle core biopsy diagnoses of lesions of uncertain malignant potential (B3) in abnormalities detected by mammographic screening. Int J Cancer. 2011;129(6):1417–24.

15. O'Connell P, et al. Analysis of loss of heterozygosity in 399 premalignant breast lesions at 15 genetic loci. J Natl Cancer Inst. 1998;90(9):697–703.

16. Buerger H, et al. Comparative genomic hybridization of ductal carcinoma in situ of the breast-evidence of multiple genetic pathways. J Pathol. 1999;187(4):396–402.

17. Buerger H, et al. Ductal invasive G2 and G3 carcinomas of the breast are the end stages of at least two different lines of genetic evolution. J Pathol. 2001;194(2):165–70.

18. Mastracci TL, et al. Genomic alterations in lobular neoplasia: a microarray comparative genomic hybridization signature for early neoplastic proliferationin the breast. Genes Chromosomes Cancer. 2006;45(11):1007–17.

19. Ando Y, et al. Loss of heterozygosity and microsatellite instability in ductal carcinoma in situ of the breast. Cancer Lett. 2000;156(2):207–14.

20. Perou CM, et al. Molecular portraits of human breast tumours. Nature. 2000;406(6797):747–52.

21. Sorlie T, et al. Gene expression patterns of breast carcinomas distinguish tumor subclasses with clinical implications. Proc Natl Acad Sci U.S.A. 2001;98(19):10869–74.

22. Vincent-Salomon A, et al. Integrated genomic and transcriptomic analysis of ductal carcinoma in situ of the breast. Clin Cancer Res. 2008;14(7):1956–65.

23. Williams KE, et al. Molecular Phenotypes of DCIS predict overall and invasive recurrence. Ann Oncol. 2015;26:1019–1025.

24. Aubele M, et al. Extensive ductal carcinoma In situ with small foci of invasive ductal carcinoma: evidence of genetic resemblance by CGH. Int J Cancer. 2000;85(1):82–6.
25. Aubele MM, et al. Accumulation of chromosomal imbalances from intraductal proliferative lesions to adjacent in situ and invasive ductal breast cancer. Diagn Mol Pathol. 2000;9(1):14–9.
26. Bombonati A, Sgroi DC. The molecular pathology of breast cancer progression. J Pathol. 2011;223(2):307–17.
27. Ma XJ, et al. Gene expression profiles of human breast cancer progression. Proc Natl Acad Sci U S A. 2003;100(10):5974–9.
28. Fujii H, et al. Genetic progression, histological grade, and allelic loss in ductal carcinoma in situ of the breast. Cancer Res. 1996;56(22):5260–5.
29. Chuaqui RF, et al. Analysis of loss of heterozygosity on chromosome 11q13 in atypical ductal hyperplasia and in situ carcinoma of the breast. Am J Pathol. 1997;150(1):297–303.
30. Adeyinka A, et al. Analysis of gene expression in ductal carcinoma in situ of the breast. Clin Cancer Res. 2002;8(12):3788–95.
31. Luzzi V, Holtschlag V, Watson MA. Expression profiling of ductal carcinoma in situ by laser capture microdissection and high-density oligonucleotide arrays. Am J Pathol. 2001;158(6):2005–10.
32. Tsuda H, Fukutomi T, Hirohashi S. Pattern of gene alterations in intraductal breast neoplasms associated with histological type and grade. Clin Cancer Res. 1995;1(3):261–7.
33. van de Vijver MJ. Ductal carcinoma in situ of the breast: histological classification and genetic alterations. Recent Results Cancer Res. 1998;152:123–34.
34. D'Alfonso TM, et al. Cystic hypersecretory (in situ) carcinoma of the breast: a clinicopathologic and immunohistochemical characterization of 10 cases with clinical follow-up. Am J Surg Pathol. 2014;38(1):45–53.
35. Perez AA, et al. Immunohistochemical profile of high-grade ductal carcinoma in situ of the breast. Clinics (Sao Paulo). 2013;68(5):674–8.
36. Steinman S, et al. Expression of cytokeratin markers, ER-alpha, PR, HER-2/neu, and EGFR in pure ductal carcinoma in situ (DCIS) and DCIS with co-existing invasive ductal carcinoma (IDC) of the breast. Ann Clin Lab Sci. 2007;37(2):127–34.
37. Tamimi RM, et al. Comparison of molecular phenotypes of ductal carcinoma in situ and invasive breast cancer. Breast Cancer Res. 2008;10(4):R67.
38. Aguiar FN, et al. Basal cytokeratin as a potential marker of low risk of invasion in ductal carcinoma in situ. Clinics (Sao Paulo). 2013;68(5):638–43.
39. Horimoto Y, et al. Significance of HER2 protein examination in ductal carcinoma in situ. J Surg Res. 2011;167(2):e205–10.
40. Liao N, et al. HER2-positive status is an independent predictor for coexisting invasion of ductal carcinoma in situ of the breast presenting extensive DCIS component. Pathol Res Pract. 2011;207(1):1–7.
41. van der Groep P, et al. Molecular profile of ductal carcinoma in situ of the breast in BRCA1 and BRCA2 germline mutation carriers. J Clin Pathol. 2009;62(10):926–30.
42. van der Groep P, et al. HIF-1alpha overexpression in ductal carcinoma in situ of the breast in BRCA1 and BRCA2 mutation carriers. PLoS ONE. 2013;8(2):e56055.
43. Muggerud AA, et al. Molecular diversity in ductal carcinoma in situ (DCIS) and early invasive breast cancer. Mol Oncol. 2010;4(4):357–68.
44. Hannemann J, et al. Classification of ductal carcinoma in situ by gene expression profiling. Breast Cancer Res. 2006;8(5):R61.
45. Pang JM, et al. Methylation profiling of ductal carcinoma in situ and its relationship to histopathological features. Breast Cancer Res. 2014;16(5):423.
46. Saglam O, et al. Matricellular protein CCN1 (CYR61) expression is associated with high-grade ductal carcinoma in situ. Hum Pathol. 2014;45(6):1269–75.
47. Sue GR, Chagpar AB. Predictors of recurrence in patients diagnosed with ductal carcinoma in situ. Am Surg. 2015;81(1):48–51.

48. Han K, et al. Expression of HER2neu in ductal carcinoma in situ is associated with local recurrence. Clin Oncol (R Coll Radiol). 2012;24(3):183–9.
49. Kerlikowske K, et al. Biomarker expression and risk of subsequent tumors after initial ductal carcinoma in situ diagnosis. J Natl Cancer Inst. 2010;102(9):627–37.
50. Siziopikou KP, et al. Preliminary results of centralized HER2 testing in ductal carcinoma in situ (DCIS): NSABP B-43. Breast Cancer Res Treat. 2013;142(2):415–21.
51. Zhou W, et al. Molecular subtypes in ductal carcinoma in situ of the breast and their relation to prognosis: a population-based cohort study. BMC Cancer. 2013;13:512.
52. Altintas S, et al. Fine tuning of the Van Nuys prognostic index (VNPI) 2003 by integrating the genomic grade index (GGI): new tools for ductal carcinoma in situ (DCIS). Breast J. 2011;17(4):343–51.
53. Quintayo MA, et al. Virtual tissue microarrays: a novel and viable approach to optimizing tissue microarrays for biomarker research applied to ductal carcinoma in situ. Histopathology. 2014;65(1):2–8.

Chapter 5
Breast Cancer Stem Cells: Role in Tumor Initiation, Progression, and Targeted Therapy

Sanjoy Samanta, Ashraf Khan and Arthur M. Mercurio

Introduction

Despite significant advances in the diagnosis, prognosis and treatment of breast cancer, tumor recurrence, and resistance to therapy are lingering problems that continue to drive morbidity and mortality. Resolving these problems demands a better understanding of breast cancer biology that is often complicated by the fact that breast tumors are not homogenous structures. Tumor cells within a given tumor differ in morphology, karyotype, proliferative capacity, expression of cytogenetic markers, metastatic ability, and sensitivity to therapeutic agents, features that are referred to collectively as tumor heterogeneity [1–3]. Tumor heterogeneity is not a unique feature of breast cancer; almost all other cancers (both solid tumors and leukemias) are heterogeneous. The most convincing evidence supporting tumor heterogeneity is that all cells within a tumor are not capable of initiating a new tumor when transplanted into immunocompromised mice as well as into syngeneic recipients [4, 5].

To understand the cause of tumor heterogeneity, it is important to understand the genesis of cancer. Two major hypotheses have been put forward to explain the process of tumorigenesis: the clonal evolution model and the cancer stem cell

A. Khan (✉)
Department of Pathology, University of Massachusetts Medical School,
UMassMemorial Medical Center, Three Biotech, One Innovation Drive,
Worcester, MA 01605, USA
e-mail: Ashraf.Khan@umassmemorial.org

S. Samanta · A.M. Mercurio
Department of Molecular, Cell and Cancer Biology, University of Massachusetts Medical
School, Worcester, MA, USA

© Springer Science+Business Media New York 2015
A. Khan et al. (eds.), *Precision Molecular Pathology of Breast Cancer*,
Molecular Pathology Library 10, DOI 10.1007/978-1-4939-2886-6_5

(CSC) model. The clonal evolution model states that tumor cells with a growth advantage (acquired by random mutations over time) are selected and expand, with cells in the dominant population having similar proliferative capacity [6]. On the other hand, the CSC model states that tumors harbor a small population of cells that have stem-like properties, proliferate extensively, self-renew and drive the process of tumorigenesis [7–10]. These two models are not mutually exclusive because CSCs themselves undergo clonal evolution [11]. In this review, we focus on the CSC model of breast tumor propagation and its implications.

Cancer Stem Cells (CSCs)

According to the CSC model, tumor cells are organized hierarchically, similar to normal tissue, and that the CSC is at the top of the hierarchy [10, 12, 13]. The consensus definition of a CSC is "a cell within a tumor that possesses the capacity to self-renew and to cause the heterogeneous lineages of cancer cells that comprise the tumor" [14]. CSCs are defined experimentally by their ability to initiate a new tumor when transplanted into immunocompromised mice (xenograft) and they must be able to generate all different cell types of the original tumor. For this reason, CSCs are often termed *tumor initiating cells* (TICs) or *tumorigenic* cancer cells. Self-renewal is the process by which a stem cell divides asymmetrically or symmetrically to generate one or two daughter stem cells that have the developmental potential of the mother cell [15]. Stem cells self-renew to expand their number during development, maintain a pool in adult tissues and restore this pool after injury. The self-renewal ability of CSCs is determined functionally by serial transplantation, i.e., their ability to form new tumors in secondary and subsequent mice. CSCs can divide symmetrically to produce two identical cells that have the potential to self-renew and possess the ability to differentiate into all other heterogeneous cells of the tumor, which in most cases constitute the bulk of the tumor [8]. CSCs can also divide asymmetrically to generate one identical self-renewing cell and a progenitor cell that does not possess the ability to self-renew or has limited self-renewal ability but can differentiate to other cell types [16].

The CSC concept was pioneered in leukemia fueled by the accessibility of clinical specimens and the need for a better understanding of bone marrow transplantation [17, 18]. Studies on acute myeloid leukemia (AML) in the 1990s provided the first evidence for the existence of CSCs [12, 19]. This work demonstrated that a rare subset of leukemic cells, comprising 0.01–1 % of the total population and displaying a $CD34^+CD38^-$ cell surface phenotype, was able to induce leukemia when transplanted into immunodeficient mice.

Evidence for the existence of CSCs in solid tumors came initially from studies on breast cancer. In 2003, Al-Hajj and colleagues demonstrated that $CD44^+/CD24^{-/low}/Lin^-$ human breast cancer cells were much more tumorigenic compared to other tumor cells when transplanted in immunodeficient mice (CD44 is a cell surface receptor for hyaluronan and CD24 is a cell surface glycoprotein) [20].

Moreover, tumors formed by these CD44$^+$/CD24$^{-/low}$/Lin$^-$ cells exhibited the heterogeneity of the original human tumor. The CD44$^+$/CD24$^{-/low}$/Lin- cells were also capable of serial transplantation, providing evidence that they have characteristics of CSCs. It is important to note that not every cell with the CD44$^+$/CD24$^{-/}$low/Lin-phenotype is a CSC because it has not been demonstrated that a *single cell* with this phenotype can form a tumor in immunodeficient mice. Moreover, tumor initiation potential of CD44$^+$/CD24$^{-/low}$/Lin$^-$ cells can be enriched significantly by separating the CD44$^+$/CD24$^{-/low}$/Lin$^-$ cells further based on ESA (epithelial surface antigen/EpCAM) expression: ESA$^+$CD44$^+$/CD24$^{-/low}$/Lin$^-$ cells are much more tumorigenic compared to ESA$^-$ CD44$^+$/CD24$^{-/low}$/Lin$^-$ cells [20].

Approaches Used to Enrich for Breast CSCs

Several approaches used to enrich for breast CSCs are described below. Note that these approaches enrich for CSCs and do not result in the isolation of pure populations of these cells. Ongoing efforts are aimed at achieving this latter goal. The assay of choice for determining CSC function is to assess the ability of a population of cell to initiate new tumors in immunocompromised mice that recapitulate the original tumor and can be passaged serially. Although this assay is used widely, it is limited by several factors including the fact that the host immune system, which is known to have a significant role in tumorigenesis, is compromised [21].

Mammosphere Assay

This assay is based on the fact that when cells are grown under non-adherent condition in serum-free medium supplemented with growth factors (typically epidermal growth factor (EGF) or basic-fibroblast growth factor (bFGF) or both) and a specialized supplement (B27), most of the cells die within days of culture and only stem cells or progenitor cells survive and form spherical structures called mammospheres [22]. Mammospheres are highly enriched with undifferentiated cells (mostly progenitors) and can be passaged serially [22]. Moreover, these mammosphere-derived cells are capable of regenerating a mammary ductal tree in vitro [22], providing evidence for the existence of stem cells. Human breast cancer cells also form mammospheres and these mammosphere-derived cells are much more tumorigenic when transplanted into immunodeficient mice compared to adherent cells [23]. Mammosphere culture of the human breast cancer cell line MCF7 was shown to increase the CD44$^+$CD24$^-$ population eight fold compared to adherent culture [24]. Nevertheless, the use of mammosphere cultures to enrich for breast CSCs has limitations including the fact that the number of mammospheres formed is not a reliable indicator of CSC frequency [25]. Moreover, mammosphere data are often over-interpreted, based on the incorrect assumption that every mammosphere must originate from a CSC. A mammosphere can also be formed by a committed progenitor cell that has potential to differentiate but possesses limited proliferation ability and lacks self-renewal ability for extended period of times [26].

Side Population Discrimination

The 'side population discrimination' assay is a flow-cytometry based assay performed to discriminate stem cells and non-stem cells. The assay is based on the differential ability of cells to efflux the Hoechst dye (Hoechst 33342) through a family of ATP-binding cassette (ABC) transporter proteins that are expressed on the cell surface [27]. Hoechst 33342 is a cell permeable [28] fluorescent dye that binds preferentially to AT-rich sequences in nucleic acids [29]. Hoechst 33342, when excited with an ultraviolet (UV) light, emits fluorescence that can be detected in two different channels of flow cytometer: *Hoechst Blue* (detected using 450/50 nm band pass filter) and *Hoechst red* (detected using 675/20 nm long pass filter). When cells are analyzed, a population emerges as a 'tail' toward lower Hoechst blue signal and is termed as side population (SP) [30]. The existence of the SP was first demonstrated in 1996 using mouse bone marrow cells and this population cells was shown to be highly enriched for hematopoietic stem cells [31]. Existence of the SP in human and mouse mammary epithelium was first demonstrated by Alvi and colleagues in 2003 [32]. They observed that human mammary epithelium contains approximately 0.18 % ($\pm$ 0.23 %) and mouse mammary epithelium contains approximately 0.45 % ($\pm$ 0.22 %) SP cells. SP cells have been detected in many cancers and shown to have increased self-renewal ability and tumor initiating capacity when transplanted in immunodeficient mice [33–38]. Although SP cells have been detected in several breast cancer cell lines, they have only been isolated from one primary human breast cancer sample [39].

Aldeflour Assay

This is a biochemical assay that measures the enzymatic activity of aldehyde dehydrogenases (ALDHs), a family of evolutionary conserved enzymes that consists of 19 isoforms, which are localized in the cytoplasm, nucleus, and mitochondria [40]. Their primary physiological function is to oxidize intracellular aldehydes, produced by a variety of metabolic processes, to carboxylic acids [40]. This assay is based on the fact that stem cells have high ALDH activity [41]. The assay typically uses flow cytometry to analyze and quantify aldeflour positive cells in presence of an ALDH inhibitor, diethylaminobenzaldehyde (DEAB) [42–44]. This assay was first utilized for the isolation of leukemia CSCs when it was demonstrated that ALDH$^+$ cells, isolated from AML, regenerated the disease much more efficiently compared to ALDH$^-$ cells in immunocompromised mice [45]. Subsequently,

Ginestier et al. isolated ALDH$^+$ cells from breast cancer and showed that these cells were much more tumorigenic compared to ALDH$^-$ cells and possessed self-renewal ability [46]. Moreover, tumors generated by ALDH$^+$ cells exhibit the phenotypic diversity of original tumor [46, 47]. ALDH$^+$ cells isolated from normal mammary epithelium were also shown to have stem cell properties [46].

Surface Markers

Human breast CSCs have been isolated *prospectively* using previously mentioned markers (CD44$^+$/CD24$^{-/low}$ and ESA$^+$) and cells isolated using these markers exhibit properties of stem cells as evidenced by their ability to initiate new tumors in immunocompromised mice that recapitulate the original tumor and can be passaged serially [20]. Importantly, ALDH$^+$ cells having CD44$^+$CD24$^-$ESA$^+$ phenotype possess highest level of tumor initiation ability [46]. Neuropilin-2 (NRP2), a transmembrane glycoprotein that functions as co-receptor for semaphorins [48] and vascular endothelial growth factor (VEGF) [49] has also been reported to be a marker of breast CSCs [50].

Hypoxia

Hypoxia is a condition of reduced oxygen pressure and is a common feature of most solid tumors. Hypoxia renders tumor cells more aggressive, metastatic, and resistant to radio- and chemotherapy [51–55]. Tumor hypoxia results from inadequate angiogenesis (formation of new blood vessels from pre-existing vessels) in rapidly growing tumors [56]. Importantly, however, breast cancer cells that survive in hypoxic environments often display CSC properties such as loss of estrogen receptor-α [55] and increased resistance to anoikis [57], radiotherapy, and chemotherapy [58, 59]. Thus, hypoxia can be a powerful tool to enrich for CSCs. Indeed, tumor cells isolated from the MMTV-Wnt1 mouse tumor model, cultured on reconstituted ECM under low oxygen pressure (3 % O$_2$) exhibited 100 fold more tumor forming efficiency compared to cells maintained in normoxia [60]. Moreover, breast cancer cell lines cultured in hypoxia have elevated levels of ALDH$^+$ [61] and CD44$^+$/CD24$^{-/low}$ cells [62].

Origin of Breast CSCs

Although the presence of stem cells in the normal mammary gland epithelium was anticipated before the isolation of breast CSCs based on the analysis of X-chromosome inactivation patterns [63], nothing was known about their molecular identity. The nature of mammary epithelial stem cells was established by the finding that a single mouse mammary epithelial cell with $CD29^{hi}CD24^{+}Lin^{-}$ phenotype could regenerate a full mammary gland when transplanted in the cleared mammary fat pad of a recipient mouse [64] [65]. These $CD29^{hi}CD24^{+}Lin^{-}$ cells possess self-renewal ability and can differentiate into other mammary epithelial subpopulations [65]. In the human mammary gland, epithelial cells with a $CD49f^{hi}ESA^{-}$ phenotype were shown to possess stem cell characteristics [66].

The fact that mammary stem cells and breast CSCs exhibit differences in their molecular identity based on surface markers raises the important issue of the relationship between these two populations of cells. Are breast CSCs normal mammary stem cells that possess de-regulated self-renewal ability caused by oncogenic mutations? This possibility is attractive because normal stem cells are slow cycling and have a long lifespan, which make them more vulnerable to accumulating mutations. This model also implies that tumors originate from normal SCs because they are the primary target of oncogenic mutation. To date, however, there is no definitive evidence that breast CSCs arise from normal mammary stem cells. An alternative hypothesis is that progenitor or differentiated cells are the initial targets of oncogenic transformation and that cells transformed by this mechanism acquire self-renewal ability through sequential mutations over period of time. This hypothesis infers that the CSC is not the cell of origin in breast cancer and that the major function of CSCs is to maintain the tumor, contribute to tumor dormancy and potentially metastasis.

One mechanism to account for how differentiated cells acquire stem cell properties is that an epithelial-mesenchymal transition (EMT) occurs in response to signals from the microenvironment and that the EMT has a causal role in the genesis of CSCs. The EMT is a biological process by which polarized epithelial cells undergo biochemical changes that enable them to acquire a mesenchymal phenotype that confers enhanced migratory ability, invasiveness, increased resistance to apoptosis and increased production of extracellular matrix proteins [67]. The process of EMT was first observed during embryonic development where it plays crucial roles in critical morphogenetic steps such as gastrulation and neural crest formation [68]. The activation of the EMT program has been linked to the acquisition of stem cell characteristics by both normal and neoplastic cells. Mani et al. [69] demonstrated that induction of EMT by ectopic expression of EMT-inducing transcription factors SNAI1, TWIST, and TGFβ in non-tumorigenic immortalized human mammary epithelial cells (HMLE) resulted in a mesenchymal morphology with an increase in the $CD44^{+}CD24^{-}$ population and self-renewal ability [69]. These mesenchymal cells generated 30 fold more mammospheres than did control HMLE cells [69]. Subsequent to these initial studies, numerous studies have linked the EMT to the genesis of breast CSCs [70, 71].

Some studies have challenged the EMT hypothesis for the genesis of CSCs and argued that the EMT and stemness are not linked causally, and that cells with tumor initiating potential are actually epithelial in nature [72]. This hypothesis is consistent with the fact that embryonic stem cells are epithelial [73]. Clearly, these disparate hypotheses need to be reconciled, a task that will require more insight into the characterization of *bona fide* breast CSCs. An interesting development in this context is the report that breast CSCs transit between epithelial and mesenchymal states [74]. This plasticity, which may be influenced by the tumor microenvironment, could enable these CSCs to mediate distinct functions in tumor in a spatially regulated manner. A related finding is that the $CD44^+/CD24^-$ population, which is enriched for breast CSCs, is actually comprised of distinct epithelial and mesenchymal populations that differ markedly in their tumor initiating potential [75].

Breast CSCs and Tumor Sub-Types

Gene expression profiling of breast tumors have revealed distinct tumor subtypes that include luminal A&B, basal-like, HER2, claudin low and normal-like, [76]. The relevant issues that arise from this observation are whether these subtypes differ in their content of CSCs and whether different types of CSCs contribute to their behavior. Existing evidence indicates that more aggressive subtypes of breast cancer contain a higher frequency of CSCs and that these CSCs may be responsible for their aggressive behavior. Specifically, poorly differentiated tumors, which are frequently associated with the basal-like subtype, contain a higher proportion of CSCs than more differentiated tumors [77]. Also, triple-negative breast cancers (TNBCs), which are associated with a basal-like phenotype, harbor a higher percentage of $CD44^+CD24^{-/low}$ population compared to other subtypes [78]. TNBCs are characterized by the lack of expression of estrogen receptor (ER-α), progesterone receptor (PR) and human EGF receptor 2 (Her-2) [79]. Majority of basal-like breast cancers, which express basal cytokeratins (KRT5, KRT14), p63 and alpha smooth muscle actin (α-SMA) are triple-negative and majority of TNBCs are basal-like [80–82]. In a small set of breast cancer specimens, it was observed that $CD44^+CD24^{-/low}$ cells were present in 60 % of TNBCs whereas only 26 % non-TNBCs were positive for these cells [78]. $ALDH1^+$ cells were also found to be more frequent in TNBCs compare to other subtypes [83, 84]. Moreover, a significant association was observed between human embryonic stem cells and basal-like breast cancers in their gene expression pattern [85], which justifies the fact that basal-like breast cancers harbor more stem-like cells.

The issue of whether distinct populations of CSCs contribute to the behavior of the different molecular subtypes of breast cancer has not been resolved fully but the available data do not support this possibility. The finding that luminal progenitor cells are the cells of origin for basal-like breast cancers [86, 87] strengthens the hypothesis that plasticity exists in CSCs and suggests that luminal and basal tumors, for example, may share a common CSC. This possibility is supported by the observation that breast CSCs across molecular subtypes share a common gene expression profile [50].

Clinical Importance of Breast CSCs

Breast CSCs hold enormous potential as therapeutic target for several reasons. First and foremost, their relative resistance to radio- and chemotherapy coupled with their ability to initiate new tumors infers that they are responsible for tumor recurrence, the principal cause of cancer-related mortality. This inference is supported, for example, by the observation that the frequency of $CD44^+CD24^{-/low}$ cells increases significantly after neoadjuvant chemotherapy and lapatinib (an EGFR inhibitor) treatment in patients with $HER2^+$ breast cancer [88]. Given that breast tumors can recur many years after the initial diagnosis and treatment, CSCs likely contribute to tumor dormancy, especially because they are slow cycling [89] and able to remain quiescent in the absence of appropriate stimuli from the microenvironment. Increasing evidence indicates that breast CSCs also have a significant role in metastasis [20, 90, 91]. For example, the proportion of $CD44^+CD24^-$ cells isolated from the bone marrow of breast cancer patients is much higher than in the primary site [92]. In a study on inflammatory breast cancer, an aggressive form of breast cancer, breast CSCs isolated as $ALDH^+$ cells were shown to mediate metastasis [46]. The potential contribution of CSCs to breast cancer metastasis is complicated by the fact that most metastases are epithelial in contrast to the mesenchymal phenotype of breast CSCs that has been observed in many studies. For this reason, the possibilities that breast CSCs transit between epithelial and mesenchymal states [74] or that other populations of cells interact with CSCs to facilitate metastasis are worth studying.

The challenge here is to design therapeutic approaches that can target breast CSCs specifically and effectively. A distinguishing property of CSCs is their self-renewal ability implying that targeting pathways that regulate self-renewal could be very effective. BMI1, a polycomb group transcriptional repressor has been shown to regulate self-renewal ability of breast and other CSCs [50]. Interestingly, study on colorectal cancer demonstrated that a small molecule inhibitor of BMI-1 was able to inhibit self-renewal and tumorigenic potential [93]. Clearly, this approach merits investigation in breast cancer. A related approach is based on the hypothesis that autocrine growth factor signaling sustains the self-renewal of breast CSCs [94]. A salient example of this phenomenon involves VEGF. Compelling data support the hypothesis that autocrine VEGF signaling in breast CSCs [50], as well as other CSCs [95], is essential for their self-renewal and tumor initiation. In fact, autocrine VEGF signaling mediated by NRP2 sustains BMI-1 expression in breast CSCs [50]. It should be noted that autocrine VEGF signaling in tumor cells is distinct from the role of VEGF in tumor angiogenesis. VEGF signaling that promotes angiogenesis is mediated by VEGF tyrosine kinase receptors, especially VEGFR2. Interestingly, the anti-VEGF drug bevacizumab does not block the interaction of VEGF with NRP2. This finding is important because bevacizumab and sunitinib, an inhibitor of VEGF receptor tyrosine kinases, offered only marginally improved disease free survival (DFS) and overall survival (OS) in breast cancer patients with metastatic disease [96]. Moreover, preclinical studies revealed that anti-angiogenic therapy actually increases the aggressiveness and metastatic potential of breast cancer cells [54, 97], presumably because such treatment increases tumor hypoxia, which results in an enhancement of CSCs [61]. For these reason, targeting CSCs directly could be a much better therapeutic approach. In this direction, targeting NRP2 could be an effective strategy for inhibiting the function of breast CSCs, especially given that function-blocking NRP2 antibodies exist [98].

Signaling pathways involved in embryonic development can also regulate self-renewal including the Wnt, Notch, and Hedgehog pathways [99–101]. Interestingly, perturbation of each of these pathways in the mammary gland results in tumors in transgenic mice [102–105] indicating that they are potential targets for therapy aimed at inhibiting self-renewal and CSC function. In fact, these pathways have been implicated in maintaining the function of breast CSCs, and effective inhibitors have been developed and are being tested in clinical trials. For example, salinomycin was identified in a high throughput screen designed to identify selective inhibitors of CSCs and shown to inhibit Wnt signaling [106]. Other potential approaches for targeting CSCs include inhibiting their expansion. For example, CSCs can increase in number by undergoing symmetrical cell division [16]. In HER-2 over-expressing breast cancers, restoration of p53 (a tumor suppressor protein usually mutated in majority of cancers) function results in the induction of asymmetrical cell division with reduced tumor onset [107].

Conclusions

The evidence is compelling that breast cancers harbor a relatively small population of cells that has the ability to self-renew and initiate new tumors, properties that merit their designation as CSCs. Much remains to be learned about the genesis of CSCs, mechanisms that regulate their function and their interactions with other cells in tumors. Nonetheless, there is little doubt that CSCs have a critical role in the aggressive behavior of breast cancers and that they contribute to tumor dormancy and recurrence. The challenge ahead is to develop effective therapeutic approaches for targeting CSCs, a challenge that will require a much deeper understanding of their genesis and biology.

Acknowledgments   Work in the authors' laboratory is supported by NIH Grant CA168464.

References

1. Heppner GH. Tumor heterogeneity. Cancer Res. 1984;44:2259–65.
2. Dick JE. Stem cell concepts renew cancer research. Blood. 2008;112:4793–807.
3. Meacham CE, Morrison SJ. Tumour heterogeneity and cancer cell plasticity. Nature. 2013;501:328–37.

4. Bruce WR, Van Der Gaag H. A quantitative assay for the number of murine lymphoma cells capable of proliferation in vivo. Nature. 1963;199:79–80.

5. Hewitt HB. Studies of the dissemination and quantitative transplantation of a lymphocytic leukaemia of CBA mice. Br J Cancer. 1958;12:378–401.

6. Nowell PC. The clonal evolution of tumor cell populations. Science. 1976;194:23–8.

7. Ichim CV, Wells RA. First among equals: the cancer cell hierarchy. Leuk Lymphoma. 2006;47:2017–27.

8. Reya T, Morrison SJ, Clarke MF, Weissman IL. Stem cells, cancer, and cancer stem cells. Nature. 2001;414:105–11.

9. Wicha MS, Liu S, Dontu G. Cancer stem cells: an old idea–a paradigm shift. Cancer Res. 2006; 66:1883–1890; discussion 1895–1886.

10. Kreso A, Dick JE. Evolution of the cancer stem cell model. Cell Stem Cell. 2014;14:275–91.

11. Barabe F, Kennedy JA, Hope KJ, Dick JE. Modeling the initiation and progression of human acute leukemia in mice. Science. 2007;316:600–4.

12. Bonnet D, Dick JE. Human acute myeloid leukemia is organized as a hierarchy that originates from a primitive hematopoietic cell. Nat Med. 1997;3:730–7.

13. Dalerba P, Cho RW, Clarke MF. Cancer stem cells: models and concepts. Annu Rev Med. 2007;58:267–84.

14. Clarke MF, Dick JE, Dirks PB, Eaves CJ, Jamieson CH, Jones DL, Visvader J, Weissman IL, Wahl GM. Cancer stem cells–perspectives on current status and future directions: AACR workshop on cancer stem cells. Cancer Res. 2006;66:9339–44.

15. He S, Nakada D, Morrison SJ. Mechanisms of stem cell self-renewal. Annu Rev Cell Dev Biol. 2009;25:377–406.

16. Morrison SJ, Kimble J. Asymmetric and symmetric stem-cell divisions in development and cancer. Nature. 2006;441:1068–74.

17. Hedrick SM. T cell development: bottoms-up. Immunity. 2002;16:619–22.

18. Ohneda K, Yamamoto M. Roles of hematopoietic transcription factors GATA-1 and GATA-2 in the development of red blood cell lineage. Acta Haematol. 2002;108:237–45.

19. Lapidot T, Sirard C, Vormoor J, Murdoch B, Hoang T, Caceres-Cortes J, Minden M, Paterson B, Caligiuri MA, Dick JE. A cell initiating human acute myeloid leukaemia after transplantation into SCID mice. Nature. 1994;367:645–8.

20. Al-Hajj M, Wicha MS, Benito-Hernandez A, Morrison SJ, Clarke MF. Prospective identification of tumorigenic breast cancer cells. Proc Natl Acad Sci USA. 2003;100:3983–8.

21. Kim JB, O'Hare MJ, Stein R. Models of breast cancer: is merging human and animal models the future? Breast Cancer Res BCR. 2004;6:22–30.

22. Dontu G, Abdallah WM, Foley JM, Jackson KW, Clarke MF, Kawamura MJ, Wicha MS. In vitro propagation and transcriptional profiling of human mammary stem/progenitor cells. Genes Dev. 2003;17:1253–70.

23. Grimshaw MJ, Cooper L, Papazisis K, Coleman JA, Bohnenkamp HR, Chiapero-Stanke L, Taylor-Papadimitriou J, Burchell JM. Mammosphere culture of metastatic breast cancer cells enriches for tumorigenic breast cancer cells. Breast Cancer Res BCR. 2008;10:R52.

24. Huang M, Li Y, Zhang H, Nan F. Breast cancer stromal fibroblasts promote the generation of CD44 + CD24- cells through SDF-1/CXCR4 interaction. J Exp Clin Cancer Res CR. 2010;29:80.

25. Pastrana E, Cheng LC, Doetsch F. Simultaneous prospective purification of adult subventricular zone neural stem cells and their progeny. Proc Natl Acad Sci USA. 2009;106:6387–92.

26. Reynolds BA, Rietze RL. Neural stem cells and neurospheres–re-evaluating the relationship. Nat Methods. 2005;2:333–6.

27. Bunting KD. ABC transporters as phenotypic markers and functional regulators of stem cells. Stem Cells. 2002;20:11–20.

28. Arndt-Jovin DJ, Jovin TM. Fluorescence labeling and microscopy of DNA. Methods Cell Biol. 1989;30:417–48.

29. Portugal J, Waring MJ. Assignment of DNA binding sites for 4′,6-diamidine-2-phenylindole and bisbenzimide (Hoechst 33258). A comparative footprinting study. Biochim Biophys Acta. 1988;949:158–68.
30. Golebiewska A, Brons NH, Bjerkvig R, Niclou SP. Critical appraisal of the side population assay in stem cell and cancer stem cell research. Cell Stem Cell. 2011;8:136–47.
31. Goodell MA, Brose K, Paradis G, Conner AS, Mulligan RC. Isolation and functional properties of murine hematopoietic stem cells that are replicating in vivo. J Exp Med. 1996;183:1797–806.
32. Alvi AJ, Clayton H, Joshi C, Enver T, Ashworth A, Vivanco M, Dale TC, Smalley MJ. Functional and molecular characterisation of mammary side population cells. Breast Cancer Res BCR. 2003;5:R1–8.
33. Bleau AM, Hambardzumyan D, Ozawa T, Fomchenko EI, Huse JT, Brennan CW, Holland EC. PTEN/PI3 K/Akt pathway regulates the side population phenotype and ABCG2 activity in glioma tumor stem-like cells. Cell Stem Cell. 2009;4:226–35.
34. Chiba T, Kita K, Zheng YW, Yokosuka O, Saisho H, Iwama A, Nakauchi H, Taniguchi H. Side population purified from hepatocellular carcinoma cells harbors cancer stem cell-like properties. Hepatology. 2006;44:240–51.
35. Haraguchi N, Utsunomiya T, Inoue H, Tanaka F, Mimori K, Barnard GF, Mori M. Characterization of a side population of cancer cells from human gastrointestinal system. Stem Cells. 2006;24:506–13.
36. Ho MM, Ng AV, Lam S, Hung JY. Side population in human lung cancer cell lines and tumors is enriched with stem-like cancer cells. Cancer Res. 2007;67:4827–33.
37. Patrawala L, Calhoun T, Schneider-Broussard R, Zhou J, Claypool K, Tang DG. Side population is enriched in tumorigenic, stem-like cancer cells, whereas ABCG2 + and ABCG2- cancer cells are similarly tumorigenic. Cancer Res. 2005;65:6207–19.
38. Wu C, Alman BA. Side population cells in human cancers. Cancer Lett. 2008;268:1–9.
39. Nakanishi T, Chumsri S, Khakpour N, Brodie AH, Leyland-Jones B, Hamburger AW, Ross DD, Burger AM. Side-population cells in luminal-type breast cancer have tumour-initiating cell properties, and are regulated by HER2 expression and signalling. Br J Cancer. 2010;102:815–26.
40. Marchitti SA, Brocker C, Stagos D, Vasiliou V. Non-P450 aldehyde oxidizing enzymes: the aldehyde dehydrogenase superfamily. Expert Opin Drug Metab Toxicol. 2008;4:697–720.
41. Ginestier C, Wicinski J, Cervera N, Monville F, Finetti P, Bertucci F, Wicha MS, Birnbaum D, Charafe-Jauffret E. Retinoid signaling regulates breast cancer stem cell differentiation. Cell Cycle. 2009;8:3297–302.
42. Armstrong L, Stojkovic M, Dimmick I, Ahmad S, Stojkovic P, Hole N, Lako M. Phenotypic characterization of murine primitive hematopoietic progenitor cells isolated on basis of aldehyde dehydrogenase activity. Stem Cells. 2004;22:1142–51.
43. Hess DA, Meyerrose TE, Wirthlin L, Craft TP, Herrbrich PE, Creer MH, Nolta JA. Functional characterization of highly purified human hematopoietic repopulating cells isolated according to aldehyde dehydrogenase activity. Blood. 2004;104:1648–55.
44. Corti S, Locatelli F, Papadimitriou D, Donadoni C, Salani S, Del Bo R, Strazzer S, Bresolin N, Comi GP. Identification of a primitive brain-derived neural stem cell population based on aldehyde dehydrogenase activity. Stem Cells. 2006;24:975–85.
45. Cheung AM, Wan TS, Leung JC, Chan LY, Huang H, Kwong YL, Liang R, Leung AY. Aldehyde dehydrogenase activity in leukemic blasts defines a subgroup of acute myeloid leukemia with adverse prognosis and superior NOD/SCID engrafting potential. Leukemia. 2007;21:1423–30.
46. Ginestier C, Hur MH, Charafe-Jauffret E, Monville F, Dutcher J, Brown M, Jacquemier J, Viens P, Kleer CG, Liu S, et al. ALDH1 is a marker of normal and malignant human mammary stem cells and a predictor of poor clinical outcome. Cell Stem Cell. 2007;1:555–67.
47. Charafe-Jauffret E, Ginestier C, Iovino F, Tarpin C, Diebel M, Esterni B, Houvenaeghel G, Extra JM, Bertucci F, Jacquemier J, et al. Aldehyde dehydrogenase 1-positive cancer

stem cells mediate metastasis and poor clinical outcome in inflammatory breast cancer. Clin Cancer Res (an official journal of the American Association for Cancer Research). 2010;16:45–55.

48. Uniewicz KA, Fernig DG. Neuropilins: a versatile partner of extracellular molecules that regulate development and disease. Front Biosci J Virtual Libr. 2008;13:4339–60.

49. Soker S, Takashima S, Miao HQ, Neufeld G, Klagsbrun M. Neuropilin-1 is expressed by endothelial and tumor cells as an isoform-specific receptor for vascular endothelial growth factor. Cell. 1998;92:735–45.

50. Goel HL, Pursell B, Chang C, Shaw LM, Mao J, Simin K, Kumar P, Vander Kooi CW, Shultz LD, Greiner DL, et al. GLI1 regulates a novel neuropilin-2/alpha6beta1 integrin based autocrine pathway that contributes to breast cancer initiation. EMBO Mol Med. 2013;5:488–508.

51. Zhong H, De Marzo AM, Laughner E, Lim M, Hilton DA, Zagzag D, Buechler P, Isaacs WB, Semenza GL, Simons JW. Overexpression of hypoxia-inducible factor 1alpha in common human cancers and their metastases. Cancer Res. 1999;59:5830–5.

52. Jubb AM, Buffa FM, Harris AL. Assessment of tumour hypoxia for prediction of response to therapy and cancer prognosis. J Cell Mol Med. 2010;14:18–29.

53. Dai Y, Bae K, Siemann DW. Impact of hypoxia on the metastatic potential of human prostate cancer cells. Int J Radiat Oncol Biol Phys. 2011;81:521–8.

54. Paez-Ribes M, Allen E, Hudock J, Takeda T, Okuyama H, Vinals F, Inoue M, Bergers G, Hanahan D, Casanovas O. Antiangiogenic therapy elicits malignant progression of tumors to increased local invasion and distant metastasis. Cancer Cell. 2009;15:220–31.

55. Axelson H, Fredlund E, Ovenberger M, Landberg G, Pahlman S. Hypoxia-induced dedifferentiation of tumor cells–a mechanism behind heterogeneity and aggressiveness of solid tumors. Semin Cell Dev Biol. 2005;16:554–63.

56. Hockel M, Vaupel P. Tumor hypoxia: definitions and current clinical, biologic, and molecular aspects. J Natl Cancer Inst. 2001;93:266–76.

57. Rohwer N, Welzel M, Daskalow K, Pfander D, Wiedenmann B, Detjen K, Cramer T. Hypoxia-inducible factor 1alpha mediates anoikis resistance via suppression of alpha5 integrin. Cancer Res. 2008;68:10113–20.

58. Generali D, Berruti A, Brizzi MP, Campo L, Bonardi S, Wigfield S, Bersiga A, Allevi G, Milani M, Aguggini S, et al. Hypoxia-inducible factor-1alpha expression predicts a poor response to primary chemoendocrine therapy and disease-free survival in primary human breast cancer. Clin Cancer Res (an official journal of the American Association for Cancer Research). 2006;12:4562–8.

59. Koukourakis MI, Bentzen SM, Giatromanolaki A, Wilson GD, Daley FM, Saunders MI, Dische S, Sivridis E, Harris AL. Endogenous markers of two separate hypoxia response pathways (hypoxia inducible factor 2 alpha and carbonic anhydrase 9) are associated with radiotherapy failure in head and neck cancer patients recruited in the CHART randomized trial. J Clin Oncol (official journal of the American Society of Clinical Oncology). 2006;24:727–35.

60. Castro DJ, Maurer J, Hebbard L, Oshima RG. ROCK1 inhibition promotes the self-renewal of a novel mouse mammary cancer stem cell. Stem Cells. 2013;31:12–22.

61. Conley SJ, Gheordunescu E, Kakarala P, Newman B, Korkaya H, Heath AN, Clouthier SG, Wicha MS. Antiangiogenic agents increase breast cancer stem cells via the generation of tumor hypoxia. Proc Natl Acad Sci USA. 2012;109:2784–9.

62. Louie E, Nik S, Chen JS, Schmidt M, Song B, Pacson C, Chen XF, Park S, Ju J, Chen EI. Identification of a stem-like cell population by exposing metastatic breast cancer cell lines to repetitive cycles of hypoxia and reoxygenation. Breast Cancer Res BCR. 2010;12:R94.

63. Tsai YC, Lu Y, Nichols PW, Zlotnikov G, Jones PA, Smith HS. Contiguous patches of normal human mammary epithelium derived from a single stem cell: implications for breast carcinogenesis. Cancer Res. 1996;56:402–4.

64. Kordon EC, Smith GH. An entire functional mammary gland may comprise the progeny from a single cell. Development. 1998;125:1921–30.

65. Shackleton M, Vaillant F, Simpson KJ, Stingl J, Smyth GK, Asselin-Labat ML, Wu L, Lindeman GJ, Visvader JE. Generation of a functional mammary gland from a single stem cell. Nature. 2006;439:84–8.

66. Eirew P, Stingl J, Raouf A, Turashvili G, Aparicio S, Emerman JT, Eaves CJ. A method for quantifying normal human mammary epithelial stem cells with in vivo regenerative ability. Nat Med. 2008;14:1384–9.

67. Kalluri R, Neilson EG. Epithelial-mesenchymal transition and its implications for fibrosis. J Clin Investig. 2003;112:1776–84.

68. Shook D, Keller R. Mechanisms, mechanics and function of epithelial-mesenchymal transitions in early development. Mech Dev. 2003;120:1351–83.

69. Mani SA, Guo W, Liao MJ, Eaton EN, Ayyanan A, Zhou AY, Brooks M, Reinhard F, Zhang CC, Shipitsin M, et al. The epithelial-mesenchymal transition generates cells with properties of stem cells. Cell. 2008;133:704–15.

70. Morel AP, Lievre M, Thomas C, Hinkal G, Ansieau S, Puisieux A. Generation of breast cancer stem cells through epithelial-mesenchymal transition. PLoS ONE. 2008;3:e2888.

71. May CD, Sphyris N, Evans KW, Werden SJ, Guo W, Mani SA. Epithelial-mesenchymal transition and cancer stem cells: a dangerously dynamic duo in breast cancer progression. Breast Cancer Res BCR. 2011;13:202.

72. Ocana OH, Corcoles R, Fabra A, Moreno-Bueno G, Acloque H, Vega S, Barrallo-Gimeno A, Cano A, Nieto MA. Metastatic colonization requires the repression of the epithelial-mesenchymal transition inducer Prrx1. Cancer Cell. 2012;22:709–24.

73. Baum B, Settleman J, Quinlan MP. Transitions between epithelial and mesenchymal states in development and disease. Semin Cell Dev Biol. 2008;19:294–308.

74. Liu S, Cong Y, Wang D, Sun Y, Deng L, Liu Y, Martin-Trevino R, Shang L, McDermott SP, Landis MD, et al. Breast cancer stem cells transition between epithelial and mesenchymal states reflective of their normal counterparts. Stem Cell Rep. 2014;2:78–91.

75. Goel HL, Gritsko T, Pursell B, Chang C, Shultz LD, Greiner DL, Norum JH, Toftgard R, Shaw LM, Mercurio AM. Regulated splicing of the alpha6 integrin cytoplasmic domain determines the fate of breast cancer stem cells. Cell Rep. 2014;7:747–61.

76. Cancer Genome Atlas N. Comprehensive molecular portraits of human breast tumours. Nature. 2012;490:61–70.

77. Pece S, Tosoni D, Confalonieri S, Mazzarol G, Vecchi M, Ronzoni S, Bernard L, Viale G, Pelicci PG, Di Fiore PP. Biological and molecular heterogeneity of breast cancers correlates with their cancer stem cell content. Cell. 2010;140:62–73.

78. Idowu MO, Kmieciak M, Dumur C, Burton RS, Grimes MM, Powers CN, Manjili MH. CD44(+)/CD24(-/low) cancer stem/progenitor cells are more abundant in triple-negative invasive breast carcinoma phenotype and are associated with poor outcome. Hum Pathol. 2012;43:364–73.

79. Hudis CA, Gianni L. Triple-negative breast cancer: an unmet medical need. Oncologist. 2011;16(1):1–11.

80. Banerjee S, Reis-Filho JS, Ashley S, Steele D, Ashworth A, Lakhani SR, Smith IE. Basal-like breast carcinomas: clinical outcome and response to chemotherapy. J Clin Pathol. 2006;59:729–35.

81. Rakha EA, Tan DS, Foulkes WD, Ellis IO, Tutt A, Nielsen TO, Reis-Filho JS. Are triple-negative tumours and basal-like breast cancer synonymous? Breast Cancer Res BCR. 2007;9:404; author reply 405.

82. Bertucci F, Finetti P, Cervera N, Esterni B, Hermitte F, Viens P, Birnbaum D. How basal are triple-negative breast cancers? International journal of cancer. J Int cancer. 2008;123:236–40.

83. Ohi Y, Umekita Y, Yoshioka T, Souda M, Rai Y, Sagara Y, Sagara Y, Sagara Y, Tanimoto A. Aldehyde dehydrogenase 1 expression predicts poor prognosis in triple-negative breast cancer. Histopathology. 2011;59:776–80.

84. Khoury T, Ademuyiwa FO, Chandrasekhar R, Jabbour M, Deleo A, Ferrone S, Wang Y, Wang X. Aldehyde dehydrogenase 1A1 expression in breast cancer is associated with stage, triple negativity, and outcome to neoadjuvant chemotherapy. Mod Pathol (an official journal of the United States and Canadian Academy of Pathology, Inc). 2012;25:388–397.
85. Ben-Porath I, Thomson MW, Carey VJ, Ge R, Bell GW, Regev A, Weinberg RA. An embryonic stem cell-like gene expression signature in poorly differentiated aggressive human tumors. Nat Genet. 2008;40:499–507.
86. Proia TA, Keller PJ, Gupta PB, Klebba I, Jones AD, Sedic M, Gilmore H, Tung N, Naber SP, Schnitt S, et al. Genetic predisposition directs breast cancer phenotype by dictating progenitor cell fate. Cell Stem Cell. 2011;8:149–63.
87. Molyneux G, Geyer FC, Magnay FA, McCarthy A, Kendrick H, Natrajan R, Mackay A, Grigoriadis A, Tutt A, Ashworth A, et al. BRCA1 basal-like breast cancers originate from luminal epithelial progenitors and not from basal stem cells. Cell Stem Cell. 2010;7:403–17.
88. Li X, Lewis MT, Huang J, Gutierrez C, Osborne CK, Wu MF, Hilsenbeck SG, Pavlick A, Zhang X, Chamness GC, et al. Intrinsic resistance of tumorigenic breast cancer cells to chemotherapy. J Natl Cancer Inst. 2008;100:672–9.
89. Moore N, Lyle S. Quiescent, slow-cycling stem cell populations in cancer: a review of the evidence and discussion of significance. J Oncol. 2011;2011:11.
90. Liu R, Wang X, Chen GY, Dalerba P, Gurney A, Hoey T, Sherlock G, Lewicki J, Shedden K, Clarke MF. The prognostic role of a gene signature from tumorigenic breast-cancer cells. N Engl J Med. 2007;356:217–26.
91. Weiss L. Metastatic inefficiency. Adv Cancer Res. 1990;54:159–211.
92. Giordano A, Gao H, Cohen EN, Anfossi S, Khoury J, Hess K, Krishnamurthy S, Tin S, Cristofanilli M, Hortobagyi GN, et al. Clinical relevance of cancer stem cells in bone marrow of early breast cancer patients. Ann Oncol (official journal of the European Society for Medical Oncology/ESMO). 2013;24:2515–21.
93. Kreso A, van Galen P, Pedley NM, Lima-Fernandes E, Frelin C, Davis T, Cao L, Baiazitov R, Du W, Sydorenko N, et al. Self-renewal as a therapeutic target in human colorectal cancer. Nat Med. 2014;20:29–36.
94. Scheel C, Eaton EN, Li SH, Chaffer CL, Reinhardt F, Kah KJ, Bell G, Guo W, Rubin J, Richardson AL, et al. Paracrine and autocrine signals induce and maintain mesenchymal and stem cell states in the breast. Cell. 2011;145:926–40.
95. Hamerlik P, Lathia JD, Rasmussen R, Wu Q, Bartkova J, Lee M, Moudry P, Bartek J Jr, Fischer W, Lukas J, et al. Autocrine VEGF-VEGFR2-Neuropilin-1 signaling promotes glioma stem-like cell viability and tumor growth. J Exp Med. 2012;209:507–20.
96. Bergers G, Hanahan D. Modes of resistance to anti-angiogenic therapy. Nat Rev Cancer. 2008;8:592–603.
97. Ebos JM, Lee CR, Cruz-Munoz W, Bjarnason GA, Christensen JG, Kerbel RS. Accelerated metastasis after short-term treatment with a potent inhibitor of tumor angiogenesis. Cancer Cell. 2009;15:232–9.
98. Caunt M, Mak J, Liang WC, Stawicki S, Pan Q, Tong RK, Kowalski J, Ho C, Reslan HB, Ross J, et al. Blocking neuropilin-2 function inhibits tumor cell metastasis. Cancer Cell. 2008;13:331–42.
99. Gu B, Watanabe K, Sun P, Fallahi M, Dai X. Chromatin effector Pygo2 mediates Wnt-notch crosstalk to suppress luminal/alveolar potential of mammary stem and basal cells. Cell Stem Cell. 2013;13:48–61.
100. Meier-Abt F, Milani E, Roloff T, Brinkhaus H, Duss S, Meyer DS, Klebba I, Balwierz PJ, van Nimwegen E, Bentires-Alj M. Parity induces differentiation and reduces Wnt/Notch signaling ratio and proliferation potential of basal stem/progenitor cells isolated from mouse mammary epithelium. Breast Cancer Res BCR. 2013;15:R36.
101. Sale S, Lafkas D, Artavanis-Tsakonas S. Notch2 genetic fate mapping reveals two previously unrecognized mammary epithelial lineages. Nat Cell Biol. 2013;15:451–60.

102. Simmons MJ, Serra R, Hermance N, Kelliher MA. NOTCH1 inhibition in vivo results in mammary tumor regression and reduced mammary tumorsphere-forming activity in vitro. Breast Cancer Res BCR. 2012;14:R126.
103. Vorechovsky I, Benediktsson KP, Toftgard R. The patched/hedgehog/smoothened signalling pathway in human breast cancer: no evidence for H133Y SHH, PTCH and SMO mutations. Eur J Cancer. 1999;35:711–3.
104. Kelly OG, Pinson KI, Skarnes WC. The Wnt co-receptors Lrp5 and Lrp6 are essential for gastrulation in mice. Development. 2004;131:2803–15.
105. Soriano JV, Uyttendaele H, Kitajewski J, Montesano R. Expression of an activated Notch4(int-3) oncoprotein disrupts morphogenesis and induces an invasive phenotype in mammary epithelial cells in vitro. International journal of cancer. J Int Cancer. 2000;86:652–9.
106. Gupta PB, Onder TT, Jiang G, Tao K, Kuperwasser C, Weinberg RA, Lander ES. Identification of selective inhibitors of cancer stem cells by high-throughput screening. Cell. 2009;138:645–59.
107. Cicalese A, Bonizzi G, Pasi CE, Faretta M, Ronzoni S, Giulini B, Brisken C, Minucci S, Di Fiore PP, Pelicci PG. The tumor suppressor p53 regulates polarity of self-renewing divisions in mammary stem cells. Cell. 2009;138:1083–95.

Chapter 6
Molecular Pathology of Pre-Invasive Ductal Carcinoma

Yuna Gong, Dina Kandil and Ashraf Khan

Introduction

Ductal carcinoma in situ (DCIS) of the breast consists of a group of heterogeneous and pre-invasive proliferation of neoplastic epithelial cells with the ductal phenotype. DCIS is one of the most frequently diagnosed pathologic entities of the breast, comprising approximately 25 % of all newly discovered breast carcinoma cases [1]. The incidence of DCIS in United States has increased from 1.87 per 100,000 in 1973–1975 to 32.5 in 2004 [2], reflecting in part the success of the widely adopted mammographic screening programs. With increased detection of DCIS, however, questions regarding appropriate risk assessment and therapeutic interventions have been raised, as only limited information on the natural biologic progression of untreated tumors exists.

Few long-term follow-up studies available on untreated low-grade (LG) DCIS show the risk of developing invasive breast carcinoma ranges from 14 to 60 % [3–5] after 10 years. Similar studies on high-grade (HG) DCIS are virtually nonexistent as most were excised at time of diagnosis, but it is reasonable to extrapolate that untreated HG-DCIS will be associated with even higher risks of invasive disease. Considering DCIS generally has an excellent prognosis after lumpectomy or mastectomy with 10-year breast cancer mortality rate at <2 % [6], the rationale for continuing the current standard of treatment certainly holds water. However, these statistics also demonstrate that not all DCIS invariably progress to invasive disease

Y. Gong · D. Kandil · A. Khan (✉)
Department of Pathology, University of Massachusetts Medical School,
UMassMemorial Medical Center, Three Biotech, One Innovation Drive,
Worcester, MA 01605, USA
e-mail: Ashraf.Khan@umassmemorial.org

D. Kandil
e-mail: dina.kandil@umassmemorial.org

© Springer Science+Business Media New York 2015
A. Khan et al. (eds.), *Precision Molecular Pathology of Breast Cancer*,
Molecular Pathology Library 10, DOI 10.1007/978-1-4939-2886-6_6

and as of yet, our current systems of risk stratification are inadequate in identifying those that may benefit from less or more aggressive forms of intervention.

Concerns about unnecessary anxiety experienced by the patients and possible over-treatment of DCIS have precipitated a search for improved diagnostic and prognostic parameters, and has even led to proposals for reclassification of these tumors with less ominous terminology such as "intraepithelial neoplasia" [7–10]. Recent developments in our understanding of the pathogenesis of invasive breast carcinoma has led to newly defined molecular subtypes with varying prognoses and has opened the door to more targeted therapies [11]. Although the literature on DCIS is not as extensive, emerging data suggests a similar molecular classification system may be applicable to the in situ lesions as well. In this chapter, we review the current understanding of DCIS with emphasis on its molecular pathogenesis.

Diagnosis, Classification, and Prognosis of DCIS

Diagnosis

Diagnosis of DCIS relies on several clinical and pathologic findings. Historically, DCIS was usually discovered when a tissue biopsy was performed for findings such as a palpable mass, skin retraction, or nipple discharge. Now, with the advent of the screening programs, the vast majority of DCIS are diagnosed with the mammographic discovery of clinically occult microcalcifications (76 %), soft-tissue densities (11 %), or both (13 %) [12]. Once diagnosed, the radiologically identified regions are excised with breast conserving surgery and the specimen is evaluated for extent of disease, concurrent invasive carcinoma, margins and hormone receptor status.

Microscopically, the diagnosis of DCIS is predicated on identification of clonal population of ductal epithelial cells confined within the boundary delineated by the myoepithelial cells and the basement membrane. Important diagnostic considerations for the pathologist include ruling out invasive breast carcinoma and differentiating DCIS from benign epithelial proliferations and other pre-malignant entities such as lobular carcinoma in situ (LCIS).

Compared to more benign lesions such as usual ductal hyperplasia (UDH), DCIS is comprised of a single, uniform epithelial population without the intermingling of spindled myoepithelial cells. Breast lesions with morphologic features suggestive of, but not diagnostic of DCIS are classified as atypical ductal hyperplasia (ADH). ADH essentially shares the cytologic features of DCIS, but importantly, lacks HG nuclear features and should not exceed 2 duct spaces or 2 mm. It is generally recognized that ADH and DCIS are both neoplastic proliferations with shared evolutionary pathway and the distinction between them can be quite subjective.

Classification

Several classification schemes to accurately stratify DCIS have been proposed over the years. Historically, DCIS was divided into architectural subtypes such as solid, cribriform, papillary, micropapillary, and clinging. These architectural features are still recognized and noted in pathologic reports; however, evidence has shown architectural subtyping to be of little clinical import and subject to considerable interobservor variability. Because of the insufficiencies of the architectural system, revised schemes (e.g., Holland classification [13]) focusing primarily on the cytonuclear features of the tumor cells were introduced, and found to be superior in reproducibility [14]. Van Nuys classification on the other hand, is a simplified system that categorizes DCIS based on the presence or absence of comedonecrosis and low- or HG nuclear features. Van Nuys, like the Holland classification, has demonstrated reproducibility [14] and has also been shown to be predictive of local recurrence rates and disease-free survival [15, 16]. The newly introduced concept of "ductal intraepithelial neoplasia," proposed to alleviate patient anxiety and possibly reduce over zealous treatments, has yet to gain traction in general practice. Currently, most pathologists rely on a combination of features including nuclear grade, presence of comedonecrosis, and architectural pattern to evaluate and classify DCIS. Features characteristic of each histologic grade is summarized in Fig. 6.1.

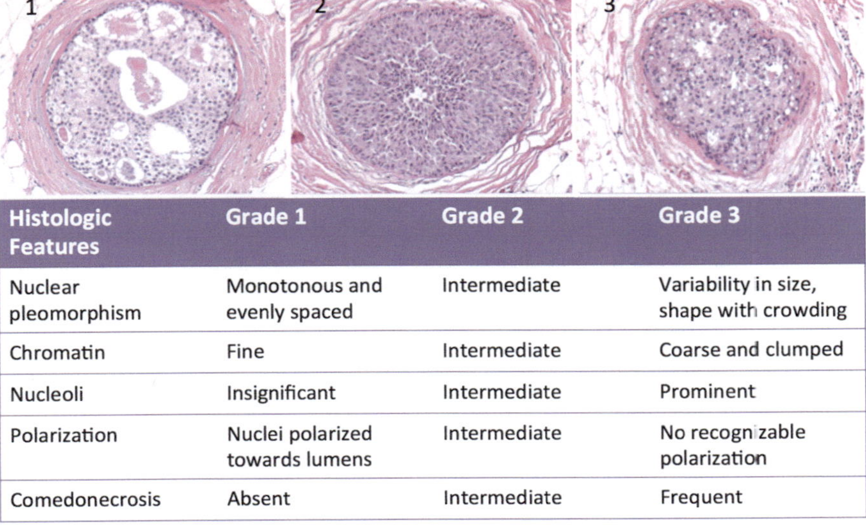

Histologic Features	Grade 1	Grade 2	Grade 3
Nuclear pleomorphism	Monotonous and evenly spaced	Intermediate	Variability in size, shape with crowding
Chromatin	Fine	Intermediate	Coarse and clumped
Nucleoli	Insignificant	Intermediate	Prominent
Polarization	Nuclei polarized towards lumens	Intermediate	No recognizable polarization
Comedonecrosis	Absent	Intermediate	Frequent

Fig. 6.1 Histologic grading of ductal carcinoma in situ (*DCIS*)

It should be noted that while interobservor variability in the classification of DCIS has improved significantly since the adoption of the newer systems, it is far from being completely eradicated. Nuclear grading is still a subjective interpretation and even the exact definition of comedonecrosis is under debate.

Prognosis

Despite the lack of extensive data on the natural progression of untreated DCIS, several large randomized clinical trials and cohort studies have identified few independent clinical and pathologic features associated with risk of disease recurrence or progression. Some of the factors associated with higher rates of local recurrence were younger age (≤ 40 years old), older age group (≥ 50 years old), symptomatic detection of DCIS, higher nuclear grade, solid or cribriform growth pattern, comedonecrosis, uncertain or involved margins or treatment with local excision alone [17–19].

Treatment modality has been shown to have significant influence on the recurrence rate, if not the overall survival. Until recently, mastectomy was the conventional treatment of DCIS [20]; however, with the success of breast conserving surgery/lumpectomy in invasive cancer, this conservative approach has been extended to DCIS as well. No randomized clinical studies comparing the efficacy of these two surgical options are currently available. On the other hand, radiotherapy (RT) has been shown to significantly decrease the rate of disease recurrence in clinical trials [17, 18, 21–26]. After lumpectomy alone, the risk of contralateral or ipsilateral disease recurrence ranges from 14 to 32 %, which is reduced by 40–50 % when paired with RT [17, 18, 21–26]. However, because RT does not seem to influence the overall survival rate, there is still a lack of consensus on the appropriate use of adjunct RT.

The use of improved DCIS classification, along with the identification of these risk factors has led to the development of prognostic systems such as the Van Nuys prognostic index (VNPI). The updated USC/VNPI stratifies DCIS patients according to age, size of the lesion, nuclear grade, and margin status and suggests differential treatment options according to the VPNI score [27, 28]. Although VPNI has been shown to be useful in a number of retrospective studies, it is yet to be validated in a prospective trial.

The current treatment protocol according to NCCN guidelines suggests lumpectomy ± radiation or mastectomy ± sentinel node biopsy. It was revised in 2008 to include lumpectomy alone as an option for those individuals with "low" risk, but does not specifically define that subset of patients. The guideline also recommends post-surgical treatment with tamoxifen in ER-positive DCIS, but does recognize that tamoxifen, like RT, reduces the risk of recurrence without improvement in overall survival rate [21, 25, 29]. The current guidelines demonstrate that despite the identification of several risk factors that are associated with higher disease recurrence, no systematically applied differential treatment protocols are currently in place for DCIS subtypes.

Tumorigenesis of DCIS

Several tumorigenesis pathways for DCIS have been proposed over the years. One model, first described by Wellings and colleagues in the 1970s, suggested flat epithelial atypia (FEA), ADH and DCIS as non-obligate precursor lesions to invasive ductal tumors [30–32]. Wellings further proposed that these ductal lesions, as well as lobular pre-malignant lesions, share a common progenitor in the terminal duct-lobular units (TDLUs) of the breast. Epidemiological, morphological, immunohistochemical and now molecular studies support this theory of evolutionary continuum between FEA, ADH, DCIS, and invasive ductal carcinoma (IDC)s, which is further detailed in the following section.

An alternative theory integrated benign epithelial proliferations such as UDH into this scheme, proposing progressive de-differentiation of UDH into malignancy [33]. Recent immunohistochemical and molecular studies however, have failed to demonstrate a clear relationship between UDH and other premalignant lesions. Rather, UDH appears to be more closely related to normal, non-proliferative breast epithelium and likely represents a distinct clinical entity unrelated to the pre-malignant lesions of the breast [34, 35].

The prevailing model of breast cancer progression has further refined Wellings' original theory and now recognizes divergent pathways for low-and HG DCIS. First discovered in IDCs, it is now recognized that the same recurrent but differential molecular changes are largely recapitulated in the in situ lesions as well. For example, loss of 16q, the hallmark chromosomal abnormality of low-grade invasive carcinoma, is also observed in greater than 70 % of LG DCIS. In contrast, 16q loss is observed in only 30 % of HG DCIS. In addition, it has been recognized that low-grade DCIS are largely ER positive, whereas only a subset of the HG lesions express the hormone receptor. Furthermore, those HG DCIS that are ER positive tend to harbor the same chromosomal abnormalities typically associated with low-grade lesions. These findings, among others, suggest that while at least two distinct carcinogenetic pathways may exist, a subset of HG DCIS may indeed represent low-grade lesions that have progressively de-differentiated and possible points of intersection can be observed among the several breast cancer pathways (Fig. 6.2).

ER Estrogen receptor; *PR* progesterone receptor; *LG* low-grade; *IG* intermediate grade; *HG* high-grade; *FEA* flat epithelial atypia; *ADH* atypical ductal hyperplasia; *TN* triple negative; *MGA* microglandular adenosis; *DCIS* ductal carcinoma in situ; *IDC* invasive ductal carcinoma

FEA and ADH, in keeping with the theory of a common evolutionary pathway, share many of the immunohistochemical and molecular signatures of low-grade DCIS. Like the low-grade DCIS, FEA and ADH are generally positive for ER and

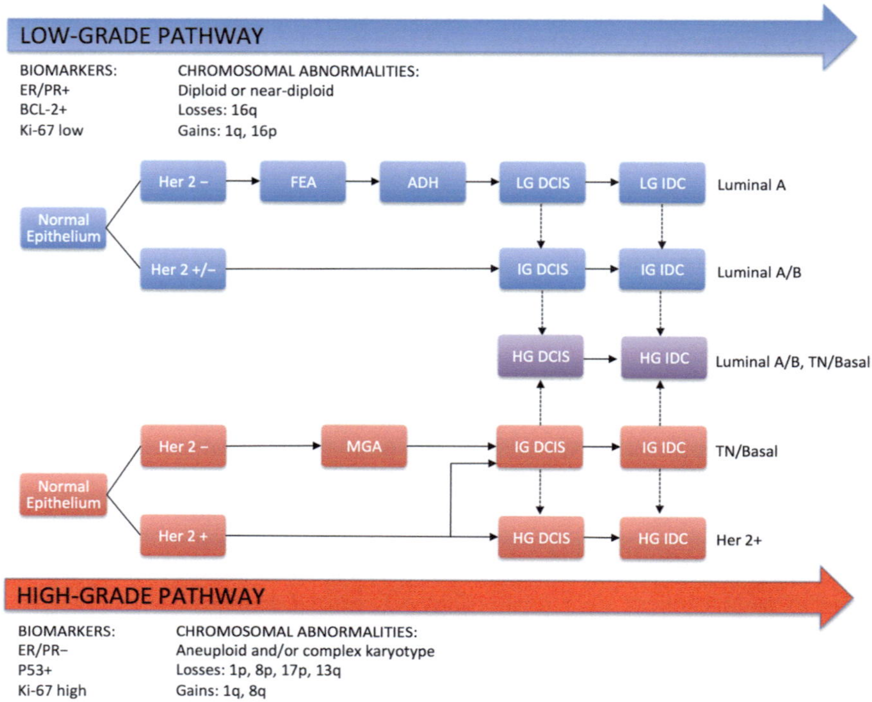

Fig. 6.2 Divergent pathways of low and high-grade breast cancer. LG pathway is characterized by positivity for ER/PR, Bcl-2 and low Ki-67 index. Chromosomes tend to be diploid or near-diploid with recurrent changes such as loss of 16q or gains of 1q or 16p. FEA and ADH are thought to be precursor lesions of the low-grade pathway and share similar expression of biomarkers and chromosomal abnormalities. Luminal A DCIS is the predominant molecular subtype seen in the low-grade pathway. HG pathway is characterized by negativity for ER/PR, positivity for p53 and high Ki-67 index, producing tumors with TN/basal-like or HER 2+ phenotype. These tumors also are frequently aneuploid and/or exhibit complex karyotype. MGA has been proposed as a possible precursor lesion for high-grade lesions with TN/basal-like phenotype. Overlap also exists between the LG and HG pathways. Some IG and HG DCIS show molecular features of both low and high-grade lesions, and may represent de-differentiated lesions of the LG pathway. (Figure adapted with permission from [36])

PR but negative for HER 2 and basal cell markers. They have also been shown to share many of the recurrent genetic imbalances (e.g., loss of 16q) and are often found in coexistence with low-grade DCIS and invasive carcinomas. These immunophenotypic, molecular, and epidemiologic evidence demonstrates the close developmental relationship among these low-grade lesions and provide strong evidence that FEA and ADH are non-obligate, neoplastic precursors of the low-grade cancerous lesions of the breast.

It is yet unclear, however, what the precursor lesion of HG DCIS may be. The complex karyotype of HG DCIS intimates both the inherent genetic volatility of these lesions and the heterogeneity of its origin. A minority of the HG DCIS that harbor a similar genomic profile to the low-grade DCIS may represent de-differentiated lesions, while others may have arisen de novo. There exists, however, recent but limited evidence showing that a subset of microglandular adenosis (MGA) may be a precursor to triple negative (ER, PR, and HER2 negative) HG DCIS [36, 37]. MGA is a rare breast lesion composed of cytologically bland glands with an infiltrative growth pattern, largely considered to be a benign process. Its rarity however, in comparison to the incidence of HG DCIS, makes it an unlikely candidate as a common progenitor for HG lesions of the breast.

Chromosomal Aberrations of Low-and High-Grade DCIS

Low and HG DCIS, like their invasive counterparts, are characterized by distinct set of chromosomal aberrations. One of the hallmark chromosomal abnormalities seen in low-grade DCIS, as mentioned before, is the loss of 16q (70 %), as evidenced by multiple comparative genomic hybridization (CGH) and loss of heterozygosity (LOH) studies [38–40]. Other recurrent abnormalities associated with low-grade DCIS include loss of 17p and gain of 1q (>70 %) and 16p (>40 %). In addition, low-grade DCIS is characterized by diploid or near-diploid chromosome number and on average, have fewer total chromosomal abnormalities.

In contrast, HG lesions exhibit greater tendencies for aneuploidy, more complex karyotype and generally harbor multiple amplifications. Some of the specific and more frequently observed chromosomal abnormalities of HG DCIS include gains of 1q, 5p, 8q and losses of 8p, 11q, 13q, and 14q. The genomic profile of intermediate-grade DCIS, much like the nuclear and cytologic features that currently define the DCIS grading system, straddle the boundaries of the low-and HG lesions. Although intermediate-grade DCIS shared some of the distinct genetic signatures with the low-grade lesions, one study also found they had on average, higher number of genetic imbalances (5.5 vs. 2.5) compared to low-grade DCIS [38]. Table 6.1 is a detailed list of the recurrent genomic changes seen in low- and HG DCIS, as well as other proliferative breast lesions.

Immunophenotype of Low-and High-Grade DCIS

Immunohistochemical (IHC) studies of the transcriptomic profiles of DCIS also support the theory of divergent tumorigenesis. DCIS, like their invasive counterpart, can be divided into broad categories based on estrogen receptor (ER) positivity. ER is one of the most valuable and extensively studied biomarkers in the breast and is expressed in approximately 70 % of DCIS overall [41]. ER expression is strongly associated with low-grade in situ and invasive ductal lesions, with nearly 100 % of the low-grade DCIS expressing the hormone receptor. Molecular studies of IDC have also shown ER-positive and ER-negative tumors

Table 6.1 Chromosomal aberrations of proliferative breast lesions

Lesion	Method	Losses	Gains	References
UDH	LOH	3p, 9p, 11p, 13q, 16q, 17q	–	[56]
	LOH	13q, 14p, 16q, 17p, 17q	–	[57]
	LOH	9p, 11q, 11p, 13q, 14q, 17p, 17q	–	[39]
	CGH	13q, 16q	12q, 16p, 20q	[58]
	CGH	None	None	[59]
	CGH	1q	16q, 17p, 21p	[60]
	CGH	13q	–	[61]
FEA	LOH	3p, 11q, 16q, 17q	–	[62]
	LOH	1p, 3p, 5q, 9p, 9q, 10q, 17p, 17q, 22q	–	[63]
	CGH	11q, 12q, 16q, 17p, 18p, 21, 22	7q, 11q, 15q, 16p, 17q, 19q	[64]
ADH	LOH	16q, 17p	–	[65]
	LOH	11p, 13q, 16q, 17p, 17q	–	[39]
	LOH	8p, 16q, 17q	–	[66]
	LOH	1q, 3p, 11p, 11q, 16q, 17p	–	[67]
	CGH	16q, 17p, 20p	1q, 16q, 11q	[60]
	CGH	13q, 16q	3p, 8q, 15q, 16p, 20q, 22q	[58]
	CGH	8p, 9p, 11q, 13q, 14q, 16q, 21q, Xp	1p, 1q, 2q, 8q, 10p, 17q, 20q, 20q, 22q, Xp	[40]
LG-DCIS	LOH	2p, 6q, 8p, 9p, 11p, 11q, 13q, 14q, 16q, 17p, 17q	–	[39]
	CGH	11p, 14q, 16q, 17p	NA	[40]
	CGH	4q, 13q	16p, 20q, 22q	[58]
	CGH	9p, 13q, 14q, 16q	1q, 17q	[38]
IG-DCIS	CGH	2q, 5q, 8p, 9q, 11q, 16q, 17p	1q, 8q, 17q	[38]
HG-DCIS	LOH	2q, 6q, 8p, 9p, 11p, 11q, 13q, 14q, 16q, 17p, 17q	–	[39]
	CGH	8p, 13q, 14q	1q, 8p, 9q, 16q, 17q, 19q	[40]
	CGH	4q, 5q, 9p, 11q, 13q	1q, 6p, 6q, 7q, 8q, 10q, 12q, 14q, 15q, 16p, 17q, 19q, 20q, 21q, 22q	[58]
	CGH	1p, 12q, 16q, 17q, 22q	1p, 1q, 2q	[61]
	CGH	2q, 5q, 6q, 8p, 9p, 11q, 13q, 14q, 16q, 17p	1q, 5p, 8q, 17q	[38]

Adapted with permission from [77]
LGDCIS low grade ductal carcinoma in situ; *HGDCIS* high grade ductal carcinoma in situ; *UDH* usual ductal hyperplasia; *FEA* flat epithelial atypia; *ADH* atypical ductal hyperplasia; *LOH* loss of heterozygosity; *CGH* comparative genomic hybridization

are intrinsically distinct entities with divergent pathologic and clinical features. ER expression, along with the presence of HER2 upregulation, is the major determinant in molecular classification of IDC.

Table 6.2   Expression of biomarkers in ductal carcinoma in situ (DCIS)

Biomarkers	Histologic grade of DCIS			
	Low	Intermediate	High	Overall
ER	94–100 % [44, 68–70]	81–100 % [44, 68–70]	30–48 % [44, 68–70]	55–77 % [44, 69]
PR	69–100 % [68, 69]	65–91 % [68, 69]	23–32 % [68, 69]	43–62 % [68, 69]
AR	36 % [44]	51 % [44]	26 % [44]	37 % [44]
Her2	0–8 % [44, 68–70]	0–26 % [44, 68–70]	55–72 % [44, 68–70]	28–47 % [44, 68–70]
Bcl-2	92 % [44]	84 % [44]	36 % [44]	64 % [44]
p53	0–8 % [44, 68, 69]	13–14 % [44, 68, 69]	28–49 % [44, 68, 69]	25–40 % [44, 69, 71]
EGFR	0 % [44, 69]	0–7 % [44, 69]	0–52 % [44, 59]	0–36 % [44, 69]
CK5/6	0 % [44]	0 % [44]	4 % [44]	2 % [44]

DCIS Ductal carcinoma in situ

Other biomarkers preferentially expressed in low-grade DCIS also include progesterone receptor (PR) and Bcl-2. PR, like ER, is a hormone receptor that is prognostic as well as predictive of response to hormone therapy [41]. Bcl-2 is an anti-apoptotic protein whose de-regulation has been associated with pathogenesis of breast cancer. The expressions of both proteins are positively associated with ER, and help define the immunoprofile of the low-grade ductal lesions of the breast.

Conversely, higher-grade lesions are negatively associated with ER, positively associated with [42–44] HER2 expression, p53 expression, and basal markers (CK5/6, EGFR) and display higher Ki-67 index. Somewhat paradoxically, HER2 amplification, which is typically associated with worse clinical outcome in invasive tumors, is seen with higher frequency in the in situ lesions (15–25 vs. 55–70 %). The reason for this disparity remains unclear, however. Some of the proposed mechanisms include: loss of HER2 expression as HER2-positive DCIS progresses to IDC; higher rates of disease progression in HER2-negative DCIS; and mammographic detection bias for HER2-positive DCIS due to their association with comedo necrosis and calcification, which may be more easily identified by imaging. Table 6.2 summarizes the expression rate of various biomarkers stratified by DCIS histologic grades.

Molecular Subtyping of DCIS

Microarray profiling of invasive breast carcinomas in the early 2000s introduced a novel classification method into at least four major intrinsic molecular subtypes with variable clinical outcomes: luminal A, luminal B, human epidermal growth factor receptor-2 (HER2) overexpressing and TN/basal-like (Table 6.3) [45].

Table 6.3 Molecular subtypes defined as: Luminal A (ER+, HER2−), Luminal B (ER+, HER2+), HER2 (ER−, HER2+), TN/Basal-like (ER−, HER2−, EGFR, and/or cytokeratin 5/6 +)

Lesion	Molecular subtypes of DCIS				
	Luminal A (%)	Luminal B (%)	HER2 (%)	TN/Basal-like (%)	References
DCIS	62.5	13.2	13.6	NA/7.7	[47][a]
	61	9	16	6/8	[48][a]
	48.8	8.7	17.4	7.1	[50]
	38.3	6.9	14.9	7.5	[72][a]
IDC	58–75	5–16	3–6	11–20	[47, 73–76]

DCIS Ductal carcinoma in situ; *IDC* invasive ductal carcinoma

[a]3, 6, and 35 % of tumors were unclassified, respectively (negative for all four defining markers or missing information)

Studies have shown the intrinsic molecular subtypes can be approximated with a panel of immunohistochemical markers, most commonly including ER, PR, HER2, CK5/6, and EGFR [46]. Similar categorization of DCIS has been explored in several studies [47–50], which were largely successful in recapitulating the molecular subtypes found in invasive tumors.

Several differences in the prevalence of the distinct molecular phenotypes between the in situ and invasive ductal lesions were noted in these studies. HER2 subtype was consistently shown to be more prevalent in DCIS (14–17 %) compared to IDC (3–6 %), as previously discussed. On the other hand, luminal type A was generally less common in DCIS (38–63 %) compared to IDC (58–75 %). Overall, no statistically significant difference was noted between the prevalence of luminal type B and TN/basal phenotypes, although the TN/basal phenotype was generally less common in DCIS.

Although the limited number of studies should preclude premature generalizations of the DCIS molecular subtypes, one study showed TN/basal-like phenotype to be associated with elevated risk of disease recurrence at 10 years [50], as well as being associated with other unfavorable prognostic variables such as high-grade nuclei, p53 expression, and elevated Ki-67 index [47, 48].

Molecular Features of DCIS Versus IDC

DCIS is generally recognized as a non-obligate precursor lesion to IDC due to a multitude of indirect but convincing evidence. Tissue resections of IDC nearly invariably show concurrent DCIS, usually of similar nuclear grade, helping demonstrate a close relationship between the two lesions and suggestive of a shared evolutionary pathway. However, contrary to expectations, global gene expression studies have shown no significant differences in molecular changes between invasive and in situ carcinomas [38], suggesting that the potential for invasiveness already resides in the mutations that first gave rise to the in situ neoplastic proliferations.

In light of this failure to find the specific genetic signatures that define invasiveness, several other mechanisms have been proposed. One theory suggests that epigenetic alterations regulating the expression of various genes may be contributory. Few studies have demonstrated stage-specific methylation of tumor suppressor genes in the tumor cells [51, 52], suggesting a possible role in the disease progression. On the other hand, others have shown that the changes in the microenvironment of the tumor may also be instrumental. Studies have shown that similar to the epithelial tumor cells that exhibit differential epigenetic gene regulation, the surrounding stromal cells and myoepithelial cells also show significant changes in gene expression during the transition from in situ to invasive carcinoma [53]. It has been suggested that these phenotypically aberrant stromal and myoepithelial cells, having lost their normal function, may facilitate invasion by creating a more permissive environment for the tumor cells.

It is likely that the progression of the in situ to IDC involves a complex set of changes including the intrinsic genetic abnormalities of the tumor, epigenetic deregulation of the tumor/stromal/myoepithelial cells' gene expression and other as-of-yet undefined deviations from the norm.

Future of Molecular Testing in DCIS

Recent advancements in molecular methodologies have allowed the emergence of multiple RNA-and DNA-based commercial tests to categorize breast carcinomas into prognostically significant subgroups. Tests such as Oncotype Dx® and Mammaprint® are RNA-or DNA-based assays used to evaluate the expression of key genes involved in cell proliferation, invasion, hormone receptors, HER-2, and other house keeping genes. Oncotype DX for example, is an assay performed using quantitative RT-PCR on formalin-fixed, paraffin-embedded samples to generate Recurrence Score® (RS) to categorize the tumors into three prognostic categories. For early stage invasive tumors, these molecular assays have become widely accepted as ancillary tests to help identify those patients that may benefit from adjuvant chemotherapy.

More recently in 2011, a validation study using ECOG E5194 dataset showed these assays might also be applicable to in situ tumors as well [54, 55]. Oncotype DX assays on DCIS showed that similar to invasive tumors, the risk of ipslateral breast event (IBE) was significantly increased in those with higher RS. Low, intermediate, and high-risk groups within this study had 10-year risk of IBE of 10.6, 26.7, and 25.9 % respectively, and 3.7, 12.3, and 19.2 % risk of invasive IBE (both log rank $P \leq 0.006$) [55]. These results indicate that DCIS can be stratified into meaningful prognostic subgroups using this tool and we may be one step closer to identifying those patients in the "low-risk" category mentioned, but not specified, in the NCCN guidelines. Oncotype Dx® in DCIS has, however, not been universally accepted as is the case in invasive carcinoma and additional larger studies with long term follow-up may be needed to clearly define its role in planning adjuvant RT in DCIS. With accurate identification of risk groups, we can better individualize treatment for women with DCIS and reduce the incidence of morbidity that can often accompany aggressive therapy.

Key Points

- DCIS is a heterogeneous group of breast lesions hitherto categorized into three grades based primarily on nuclear and cytologic features.
- The prevailing model of breast cancer progression now recognizes divergent pathways for low-and high-grade DCIS.
- FEA, ADH, and low-grade DCIS are now considered to be non-obligate precursors of low-grade invasive ductal breast carcinoma; the precursor lesions of HG DCIS and invasive carcinoma are yet unknown.
- Low-grade DCIS, like its invasive counterpart, is characterized by loss of 16q and ER/PR positivity. HG DCIS is characterized by aneuploidy, p53 positivity, and HER2 amplification.
- Molecular studies of DCIS have shown categorization of the in situ lesions into at least four intrinsic molecular subtypes is possible, albeit with some differences from their invasive counterpart (e.g., higher incidence of HER2 type).
- Progression from in situ to invasive ductal lesions may be facilitated by epigenetic changes in the tumors' gene expression, as well as changes in their microenvironment.
- Commercial molecular testing for DCIS is now available and may play a role in directing adjuvant therapy for some patients. Caution should still be exercised in interpreting the results of these tests however, as the data supporting the validity of molecular testing for DCIS is not yet extensive.

References

1. Brinton LA, et al. Recent trends in breast cancer among younger women in the United States. J Natl Cancer Inst. 2008;100(22):1643–8.
2. Virnig BA, et al. Ductal carcinoma in situ of the breast: a systematic review of incidence, treatment, and outcomes. J Natl Cancer Inst. 2010;102(3):170–8.
3. Betsill WL Jr, et al. Intraductal carcinoma. long-term follow-up after treatment by biopsy alone. JAMA. 1978;239(18):1863–7.
4. Eusebi V, et al. Long-term follow-up of in situ carcinoma of the breast. Semin Diagn Pathol. 1994;11(3):223–35.
5. Page DL, et al. Continued local recurrence of carcinoma 15-25 years after a diagnosis of low grade ductal carcinoma in situ of the breast treated only by biopsy. Cancer. 1995;76(7):1197–200.
6. Ernster VL, et al. Mortality among women with ductal carcinoma in situ of the breast in the population-based surveillance, epidemiology and end results program. Arch Intern Med. 2000;160(7):953–8.

7. Tavassoli FA. Ductal carcinoma in situ: introduction of the concept of ductal intraepithelial neoplasia. Mod Pathol. 1998;11(2):140–54.

8. Tavassoli FA. Breast pathology: rationale for adopting the ductal intraepithelial neoplasia (DIN) classification. Nat Clin Pract Oncol. 2005;2(3):116–7.

9. Veronesi U, et al. Rethinking TNM: breast cancer TNM classification for treatment decision-making and research. Breast. 2006;15(1):3–8.

10. Veronesi U, et al. Breast cancer classification: time for a change. J Clin Oncol. 2009;27(15):2427–8.

11. Prat A, Perou CM. Deconstructing the molecular portraits of breast cancer. Mol Oncol. 2011;5(1):5–23.

12. Stomper PC, et al. Clinically occult ductal carcinoma in situ detected with mammography: analysis of 100 cases with radiologic-pathologic correlation. Radiology. 1989;172(1):235–41.

13. Holland R, et al. Ductal carcinoma in situ: a proposal for a new classification. Semin Diagn Pathol. 1994;11(3):167–80.

14. Bethwaite P, et al. Reproducibility of new classification schemes for the pathology of ductal carcinoma in situ of the breast. J Clin Pathol. 1998;51(6):450–4.

15. Silverstein MJ, et al. Prognostic classification of breast ductal carcinoma-in-situ. Lancet. 1995;345(8958):1154–7.

16. Poller DN, et al. Ideas in pathology. Ductal carcinoma in situ of the breast: a proposal for a new simplified histological classification association between cellular proliferation and c-erbB-2 protein expression. Mod Pathol. 1994;7(2):257–62.

17. Bijker N, et al. Risk factors for recurrence and metastasis after breast-conserving therapy for ductal carcinoma-in-situ: analysis of european organization for research and treatment of cancer trial 10853. J Clin Oncol. 2001;19(8):2263–71.

18. Fisher ER, et al. Pathologic findings from the National Surgical Adjuvant Breast Project (NSABP) Protocol B-17. Intraductal carcinoma (ductal carcinoma in situ). The national surgical adjuvant breast and bowel project collaborating investigators. Cancer. 1995;75(6):1310–9.

19. Kerlikowske K, et al. Characteristics associated with recurrence among women with ductal carcinoma in situ treated by lumpectomy. J Natl Cancer Inst. 2003;95(22):1692–702.

20. Fonseca R, et al. Ductal carcinoma in situ of the breast. Ann Intern Med. 1997;127(11):1013–22.

21. Houghton J, et al. Radiotherapy and tamoxifen in women with completely excised ductal carcinoma in situ of the breast in the UK, Australia, and New Zealand: randomised controlled trial. Lancet. 2003;362(9378):95–102.

22. Julien JP, et al. Radiotherapy in breast-conserving treatment for ductal carcinoma in situ: first results of the EORTC randomised phase III trial 10853. EORTC breast cancer cooperative group and EORTC radiotherapy group. Lancet. 2000;355(9203):528–33.

23. Fisher B, et al. Lumpectomy compared with lumpectomy and radiation therapy for the treatment of intraductal breast cancer. N Engl J Med. 1993;328(22):1581–6.

24. Fisher B, et al. Lumpectomy and radiation therapy for the treatment of intraductal breast cancer: findings from national surgical adjuvant breast and bowel project B-17. J Clin Oncol. 1998;16(2):441–52.

25. Fisher B, et al. Prevention of invasive breast cancer in women with ductal carcinoma in situ: an update of the national surgical adjuvant breast and bowel project experience. Semin Oncol. 2001;28(4):400–18.

26. Fisher ER, et al. Pathologic findings from the national surgical adjuvant breast project (NSABP) eight-year update of protocol B-17: intraductal carcinoma. Cancer. 1999;86(3):429–38.

27. Silverstein MJ. The university of Southern California/Van Nuys prognostic index for ductal carcinoma in situ of the breast. Am J Surg. 2003;186(4):337–43.

28. Silverstein MJ, Buchanan C. Ductal carcinoma in situ: USC/Van Nuys prognostic index and the impact of margin status. Breast. 2003;12(6):457–71.

29. Fisher B, et al. Tamoxifen in treatment of intraductal breast cancer: national surgical adjuvant breast and bowel project B-24 randomised controlled trial. Lancet. 1999;353(9169):1993–2000.
30. Wellings SR, Jensen HM, Marcum RG. An atlas of subgross pathology of the human breast with special reference to possible precancerous lesions. J Natl Cancer Inst. 1975;55(2):231–73.
31. Wellings SR, Jensen HM. On the origin and progression of ductal carcinoma in the human breast. J Natl Cancer Inst. 1973;50(5):1111–8.
32. Lerwill MF. Flat epithelial atypia of the breast. Arch Pathol Lab Med. 2008;132(4):615–21.
33. Xu S, et al. Evidence of chromosomal alterations in pure usual ductal hyperplasia as a breast carcinoma precursor. Oncol Rep. 2008;19(6):1469–75.
34. Boecker W, et al. Usual ductal hyperplasia of the breast is a committed stem (progenitor) cell lesion distinct from atypical ductal hyperplasia and ductal carcinoma in situ. J Pathol. 2002;198(4):458–67.
35. Otterbach F, et al. Cytokeratin 5/6 immunohistochemistry assists the differential diagnosis of atypical proliferations of the breast. Histopathology. 2000;37(3):232–40.
36. Bombonati A, Sgroi DC. The molecular pathology of breast cancer progression. J Pathol. 2011;223(2):307–17.
37. Shin SJ, et al. Molecular evidence for progression of microglandular adenosis (MGA) to invasive carcinoma. Am J Surg Pathol. 2009;33(4):496–504.
38. Buerger H, et al. Comparative genomic hybridization of ductal carcinoma in situ of the breast-evidence of multiple genetic pathways. J Pathol. 1999;187(4):396–402.
39. O'Connell P, et al. Analysis of loss of heterozygosity in 399 premalignant breast lesions at 15 genetic loci. J Natl Cancer Inst. 1998;90(9):697–703.
40. Gao Y, et al. Genetic changes at specific stages of breast cancer progression detected by comparative genomic hybridization. J Mol Med (Berl). 2009;87(2):145–52.
41. Lari SA, Kuerer HM. Biological markers in DCIS and risk of breast recurrence: a systematic review. J Cancer. 2011;2:232–61.
42. Claus EB, et al. Pathobiologic findings in DCIS of the breast: morphologic features, angiogenesis, HER-2/neu and hormone receptors. Exp Mol Pathol. 2001;70(3):303–16.
43. Lebrecht A, et al. Histological category and expression of hormone receptors in ductal carcinoma in situ of the breast. Anticancer Res. 2002;22(3):1909–11.
44. Meijnen P, et al. Immunohistochemical categorisation of ductal carcinoma in situ of the breast. Br J Cancer. 2008;98(1):137–42.
45. Perou CM, et al. Molecular portraits of human breast tumours. Nature. 2000;406(6797):747–52.
46. Cheang MC, et al. Basal-like breast cancer defined by five biomarkers has superior prognostic value than triple-negative phenotype. Clin Cancer Res. 2008;14(5):1368–76.
47. Tamimi RM, et al. Comparison of molecular phenotypes of ductal carcinoma in situ and invasive breast cancer. Breast Cancer Res. 2008;10(4):R67.
48. Livasy CA, et al. Identification of a basal-like subtype of breast ductal carcinoma in situ. Hum Pathol. 2007;38(2):197–204.
49. Dabbs DJ, et al. Basal phenotype of ductal carcinoma in situ: recognition and immunohistologic profile. Mod Pathol. 2006;19(11):1506–11.
50. Zhou W, et al. Molecular subtypes in ductal carcinoma in situ of the breast and their relation to prognosis: a population-based cohort study. BMC Cancer. 2013;13:512.
51. Pasquali L, et al. Quantification of CpG island methylation in progressive breast lesions from normal to invasive carcinoma. Cancer Lett. 2007;257(1):136–44.
52. Ai L, et al. Epigenetic silencing of the tumor suppressor cystatin M occurs during breast cancer progression. Cancer Res. 2006;66(16):7899–909.
53. Hu M, et al. Distinct epigenetic changes in the stromal cells of breast cancers. Nat Genet. 2005;37(8):899–905.
54. Duggal S, Julian TB. A multigene expression assay to predict local recurrence risk for ductal carcinoma in situ. J Natl Cancer Inst. 2013;105(10):681–3.

55. Solin LJ, et al. A multigene expression assay to predict local recurrence risk for ductal carcinoma in situ of the breast. J Natl Cancer Inst. 2013;105(10):701–10.
56. Washington C, et al. Loss of heterozygosity in fibrocystic change of the breast: genetic relationship between benign proliferative lesions and associated carcinomas. Am J Pathol. 2000;157(1):323–9.
57. Lakhani SR, et al. Detection of allelic imbalance indicates that a proportion of mammary hyperplasia of usual type are clonal, neoplastic proliferations. Lab Invest. 1996;74(1):129–35.
58. Aubele MM, et al. Accumulation of chromosomal imbalances from intraductal proliferative lesions to adjacent in situ and invasive ductal breast cancer. Diagn Mol Pathol. 2000;9(1):14–9.
59. Boecker W, et al. Ductal epithelial proliferations of the breast: a biological continuum? Comparative genomic hybridization and high-molecular-weight cytokeratin expression patterns. J Pathol. 2001;195(4):415–21.
60. Gong G, et al. Genetic changes in paired atypical and usual ductal hyperplasia of the breast by comparative genomic hybridization. Clin Cancer Res. 2001;7(8):2410–4.
61. Jones C, et al. Molecular cytogenetic comparison of apocrine hyperplasia and apocrine carcinoma of the breast. Am J Pathol. 2001;158(1):207–14.
62. Moinfar F, et al. Genetic abnormalities in mammary ductal intraepithelial neoplasia-flat type ("clinging ductal carcinoma in situ"): a simulator of normal mammary epithelium. Cancer. 2000;88(9):2072–81.
63. Dabbs DJ, et al. Molecular alterations in columnar cell lesions of the breast. Mod Pathol. 2006;19(3):344–9.
64. Simpson PT, et al. Columnar cell lesions of the breast: the missing link in breast cancer progression? A morphological and molecular analysis. Am J Surg Pathol. 2005;29(6):734–46.
65. Lakhani SR, et al. Atypical ductal hyperplasia of the breast: clonal proliferation with loss of heterozygosity on chromosomes 16q and 17p. J Clin Pathol. 1995;48(7):611–5.
66. Amari M, et al. LOH analyses of premalignant and malignant lesions of human breast: frequent LOH in 8p, 16q, and 17q in atypical ductal hyperplasia. Oncol Rep. 1999;6(6):1277–80.
67. Larson PS, et al. Quantitative analysis of allele imbalance supports atypical ductal hyperplasia lesions as direct breast cancer precursors. J Pathol. 2006;209(3):307–16.
68. Bijker N, et al. Histological type and marker expression of the primary tumour compared with its local recurrence after breast-conserving therapy for ductal carcinoma in situ. Br J Cancer. 2001;84(4):539–44.
69. Lebeau A, et al. EGFR, HER-2/neu, cyclin D1, p21 and p53 in correlation to cell proliferation and steroid hormone receptor status in ductal carcinoma in situ of the breast. Breast Cancer Res Treat. 2003;79(2):187–98.
70. Collins LC, Schnitt SJ. HER2 protein overexpression in estrogen receptor-positive ductal carcinoma in situ of the breast: frequency and implications for tamoxifen therapy. Mod Pathol. 2005;18(5):615–20.
71. Warnberg F, et al. Tumour markers in breast carcinoma correlate with grade rather than with invasiveness. Br J Cancer. 2001;85(6):869–74.
72. Clark SE, et al. Molecular subtyping of DCIS: heterogeneity of breast cancer reflected in pre-invasive disease. Br J Cancer. 2011;104(1):120–7.
73. Carey LA, et al. Race, breast cancer subtypes, and survival in the carolina breast cancer study. JAMA. 2006;295(21):2492–502.
74. Kurebayashi J, et al. The prevalence of intrinsic subtypes and prognosis in breast cancer patients of different races. Breast. 2007;16(Suppl 2):S72–7.
75. Rakha EA, et al. Prognostic markers in triple-negative breast cancer. Cancer. 2007;109(1):25–32.
76. Kwan ML, et al. Epidemiology of breast cancer subtypes in two prospective cohort studies of breast cancer survivors. Breast Cancer Res. 2009;11(3):R31.
77. Lopez-Garcia MAl, Geyer FC, Lacroix-Triki M, Marchió C, Reis-Filho JS. Breast cancer precursors revisited: molecular features and progression pathways. Histopathology. 2010;57:171–92.

Chapter 7
Molecular Pathology of Lobular Carcinoma

Ali Sakhdari, Lloyd Hutchinson and Ediz F. Cosar

Background

Lobular neoplasia (LN), a term that was introduced more than 30 years ago encompasses atypical lobular hyperplasia (ALH) and lobular carcinoma in situ (LCIS) [1, 2]. LN was initially thought to be only a risk indicator of subsequent development of breast cancer and not a true precursor [3, 4]. More recently, studies have shown that the molecular and epidemiologic profiles of ALH and LCIS are similar and share common features with invasive lobular carcinoma (ILC) [5–9].

ILC is a type of breast cancer with distinct clinical, morphological and molecular features. ILC is the second most common type of invasive breast carcinoma and accounts for 5-15 % of invasive lesions of the breast [10–12]. The incidence of lobular carcinoma has been rising at a faster rate than ductal carcinoma and has been mainly attributed to postmenopausal hormone therapy [13, 14]. Some ILC have a mammographic or gross appearance identical to that of invasive ductal carcinomas (IDC), however in many cases no mass lesion is evident. In such instances, the excised breast issue may only show slight abnormalities such as a slightly rubbery consistency, or may even appear normal [15, 16]. Consequently, the true size of the ILC may be substantially underestimated in clinical, mammographic or gross examinations compared with the microscopic finding [16]. Histologically, ILC shows distinct cytological features and patterns of tumor cell infiltration of the stroma [15, 17]. The classical form, which is the most common type, is characterized by small, relatively uniform cells that insidiously infiltrate

A. Sakhdari · L. Hutchinson · E.F. Cosar (✉)
Department of Pathology, University of Massachusetts Medical School, UMassMemorial
Medical Center, Three Biotech, One Innovation Drive, Worcester, MA 01605, USA
e-mail: Ediz.Cosar@umassmemorial.org

© Springer Science+Business Media New York 2015
A. Khan et al. (eds.), *Precision Molecular Pathology of Breast Cancer*,
Molecular Pathology Library 10, DOI 10.1007/978-1-4939-2886-6_7

the breast stroma and adipose tissue in a single-file pattern. This pattern of invasion may invoke no or minimal stromal fibrous reaction with no significant disruption in the background breast tissue architecture [18]. Often times, a targetoid growth pattern is seen around normal breast ducts, which gives the tumor a combination of linear strands and concentric pattern. In the classic form of ILC, the nuclei are usually small, with little variation in size or shape and are often eccentric. Some cells contain intracytoplasmic lumina with or without eosinophilic globules which may give them a signet ring cell appearance. Mitotic activity is insignificant [12, 16, 17].

Histological Subtypes

In addition to the classical type, which accounts for the majority of ILC, there are a number of histologic variants including pleomorphic, alveolar, tubulolobular, solid, histiocytoid and signet ring cell. They differ from the classical type in regard to architectural and/or cytological features [18–21]. The pleomorphic variant displays the growth pattern of the classical ILC, but the tumor cells exhibit a higher degree of cellular atypia, pleomorphism and mitotic activity. ILC may also show mixed morphologies, such as combinations of classical type or pleomorphic type with other less common variants. Mixed morphologies represent the most common presentation after the classical type [22–26]. To date, most of the molecular studies have focused on the classical and pleomorphic variants, and future studies are needed to assess whether the other histological subtypes have distinct molecular signatures. All of these subtypes lack cell-to-cell adhesion, which is a universal characteristic of lobular breast lesions which has been attributed to loss of E-cadherin [18–21].

Role of E-Cadherin in Lobular Carcinoma

The cells in LN and lobular carcinoma are characteristically dishesive. This is best visualized in ILC as individually dispersed cells in the stroma. This feature represents the first molecular abnormality identified in LN and is attributed to the loss of E-cadherin expression, an essential intercellular adhesion molecule on the cell surface [7, 27–30]. E-cadherin (Cadherin-1, Uvomorulin, CD324 or CAM120/80) is a transmembrane glycoprotein, which along with catenins, vinculin and actinins plays an indispensable role in the cell-to-cell adhesion of epithelial cells [27, 31].

E-cadherin is an essential component of zonula adherens type of cell-cell junction and forms homodimers in a calcium-dependent manner with other E-cadherin molecules on adjacent cells. The E-cadherin molecule comprises of extracellular, juxtamembrane and intracellular domains. The intracellular domain interacts with β-, α-, δ-catenins along with vinculin and establishes a complex of proteins with close interaction with cytoskeleton [32, 33].

An interesting interaction exists between E-cadherin and δ-catenin (P120 catenin) molecules. In normal breast epithelium P120 catenin is expressed on the cell membrane. If E-cadherin is lost, as in LN, P120 catenin is upregulated and accumulates in the cytoplasm and is no longer detectable at the cell membrane by immunohistochemistry (IHC) methods [34–36]. These cells, therefore, show cytoplasmic rather than membrane localization of P120 protein [37].

Loss of expression of E-cadherin, encoded by the *CDH1* gene, is seen in most cases of LCIS and ILC, but not in ductal carcinoma in situ (DCSI) or IDC [27]. The main mechanisms responsible for the loss of E-cadherin expression in LN are; (a) nonsense or stop codon mutation in the *CDH1* gene resulting in the truncation of the E-cadherin protein (b) silencing of the *CDH1* gene through promoter methylation and (c) loss of heterozygosity (LOH) involving the *CDH1* gene [8, 38–44]. LOH of the *CDH1* gene at 16q22.1 occurs in approximately 65 % whereas *CDH1* gene mutations occur in approximately 35 % of LN [45, 46].

Loss of E-cadherin expression may be detected by IHC and is characterized by lack of tumor cell staining in a background of non-neoplastic cells showing membranous staining. However, up to 10-12 % of ILC show some E-cadherin membrane staining, but this is usually patchy and weak. Occasionally there is diffuse or dot-like cytoplasmic expression. In some instances a *CDH1* mutation may inactivate the E-cadherin protein, yet preserve the antibody binding epitope. Another explanation is the gradual loss of E-cadherin expression during clonal evolution with some residual preservation in tumors early in development. Indeed in almost all of these cases the E-cadherin protein is nonfunctional and not associated with the catenin complex [47]. Consequently, it is possible to have an ILC with typical morphology, and a *CDH1* mutation that still retains E-cadherin membrane staining by IHC [47–50].

Classification of Lobular Neoplasia Using Transcriptional Profiling

Variation in messenger RNA (mRNA) expression patterns, mainly assessed by complementary DNA (cDNA) microarrays, has been used in the past decade to classify breast tumors through hierarchical clustering analysis into distinct molecular taxonomies [51–53]. Based on these classifications, breast carcinomas have been successfully categorized into at least five distinct groups, namely Luminal A, Luminal B, HER2-enriched, normal breast-like and basal-like [51, 53]. The genomic complexity, the specific genetic changes and the clinical outcomes are significantly different among different subtypes of breast cancers [53–55].

Briefly, the preferential expression of the genes normally expressed by luminal epithelium resulted in the names of the luminal subtypes. The luminal tumors express cytokeratin (CK) 8/18, GATA3, and ER-related genes [51–53, 56, 57].

Estrogen receptor (ER) is highly expressed in Luminal A tumors that have low levels of proliferation-related genes and usually results in a low grade histology and excellent prognosis. Luminal B tumors express lower levels of ER relative to Luminal A tumors. Luminal B tumors also express higher levels of proliferation-related genes, often resulting in a higher histological grade and a significantly worse prognosis [51, 58–60]. Tumors in HER2-enriched group are characterized by *HER2* gene amplification on chromosome 17q12 [56]. These tumors often demonstrate strong HER2 protein expression (3+ IHC staining) and are completely negative for ER and progesterone receptor (PgR) [61]. The HER2-enriched subtype tends to have a more aggressive clinical course [60]. In the basal-like subtype, the tumors frequently express basal/myoepithelial cell genes, such as CK5, CK14, CK17, caveolins 1/2 and EGFR [56, 62–64]. Interestingly, the basal-like tumors are usually triple negative for ER, PR and HER2 expression [65]. This subtype also shows an aggressive clinical behavior with high histological grade and high proliferative index [66, 67].

Gene expression profiling studies have demonstrated that ILCs are most frequently classified as Luminal A type cancers. However, a small portion of ILCs may show molecular signatures of normal breast-like, luminal B, HER2-enriched and rarely basal-like cancers [68]. Classical ILCs almost invariably express ER and PgR and rarely show HER2 overexpression or *HER2* gene amplification [69–71]. In contrast, a lower percentage of the pleomorphic variant of ILC shows ER/PgR expression [72]. The pleomorphic variant may also show HER2 protein overexpression and *HER2* gene amplification [26, 28]. Notably, the gene expression profiling data indicate that ILCs differ from grade-matched and molecular subtype-matched IDC in the expression of genes associated with cell adhesion (*ITGB1, LAMA3, LAMC, ADAM10, ADAM9*), actin cytoskeleton signaling (e.g. *ROCK1, ROCK2*) and cell-to-cell signaling. Particularly, ILCs have reduced expression of E-cadherin and of genes that are involved in cytoskeleton remodeling, cell adhesion, TGF-β signaling, DNA repair and ubiquitination. In addition, increased expression of prostaglandin biosynthesis genes, transcription factor and cell migration associated genes is observed [73–76].

Chromosomal Abnormalities

The most common abnormalities identified in ILC are loss of chromosome 16q and gain of chromosomes 1q and 16p [28, 77–79]. There are other genomic alterations that are less common and more heterogeneous across different types of lobular carcinoma. These alterations are not specific to lobular breast cancers. Genomic changes, such as gains (8q, 6q), amplifications (1q32, 8p, 11q) and losses (8p, 11q, 13q, 6q, 17p) are identified in the classical type of ILC [80, 81]. Similar genomic alterations can commonly be detected in pleomorphic variant of ILC, but in addition, other changes such as amplifications at loci of 8q24, 17q12 and 20q13, which are typically more characteristic of high grade invasive carcinoma can be also seen [28, 45, 80].

Molecular analysis of LN and synchronous ILC has demonstrated that the LN is a clonal neoplastic proliferation and a precursor for ILC [79]. LOH at 11q13, 16q, 17p and 17q, which are commonly seen in ILC, has been observed in LN as well. Other frequently observed alterations are losses of 16p, 16q, 17p, 22q and gain of 6q [81–83].

LCIS is morphologically classified into classical (CLCIS) and pleomorphic (PLCIS) types [84–86]. Some studies have suggested that more complex molecular alterations observed in the apocrine type of PLCIS may be associated with more aggressive behavior for this subtype [86]. PLCIS harbors greater genomic instability with increased copy number alterations, including 8p, 16p, 17q and amplification of loci such as 8q24 and 17q12. Compared with CLCIS, PLCIS showed significantly higher Ki67 index, lower ER and PgR expression, and occasionally *HER2* gene amplification. The accumulation of genomic changes in PLCIS has greater similarities to those of high grade DCIS, reflecting the more aggressive nature of PLCIS compared with CLCIS [85, 87, 88].

Genomic Alterations at the Gene Level

Different studies have found heterogeneous, but reproducible alterations in different genes [74, 89]. These changes include, but are not limited to, mutations, deletions and amplifications [46]. Comprehensive sequence analysis including mutations and translocations revealed highly altered genes among different subtypes of breast carcinomas. Inactivation of E-cadherin (*CDH1, 16q22.1*), the most commonly identified genetic alteration in LN and ILC, occurs as an early event in oncogenesis [8]. Single nucleotide mutational changes can be commonly seen in low or intermediate grade lobular carcinoma and accumulation of additional genetic alterations can occur with disease progression [90]. Genes commonly altered in ductal and/or lobular breast cancers include *TP53 (17p13.1)*, *PIK3CA (3q26.32)*, *AKT1 (14q32.32)*, *GATA3 (10p15)*, *MAP3K1 (5q11.2)*, *CBFB (16q22.1)*, *RUNX1 (21q22.3)* and *CDH1 (16q22.1)* (Table 7.1)[91–98]. Other less frequently altered genes are *CCND1 (11q13)*, *ERBB2 (17q12)*, *FGFR1 (8p11)*, *MCL1 (1q21)*, *KRAS (12p12.1)*, *NF1 (17q11.2)*, *MEN1 (11q13)*, *ATM (11q22–q23)*, *CCNF (16p13.3)*, *RB1 (13q14.2)* and *BRCA2 (13q12.3)* [52, 91, 98–103].

Recent studies in The Cancer Genome Atlas Research Network (TCGA) shed more light on the gene deletions, mutations and amplifications commonly seen in ILC [46, 104]. Comprehensive genomic and transcriptomic analysis of breast cancers show that the major differences between ILC and IDC are mutations in *TP53, PIK3CA, GATA3, MYC, MAP3K1/MAP2K4*, which are more common in IDC versus *PIK3CA, FOXA1, HER2* and *PTEN* which are more common in ILC. It is important to emphasize that the rate of *HER2* gene mutation is much higher in ILC (10 % vs. <1 %), whereas *HER2* gene amplification is more common in IDC (15 % vs. <5 %) [46]. The biologic significance and clinical utility of some of these alterations will need to be elucidated with further comprehensive molecular studies.

Table 7.1 Genes frequently mutated in lobular breast carcinoma

Gene	Name	Location	Function
TP53	Tumor protein 53	17p13.1	Tumor suppressor
PIK3CA	phosphatidylinositol-4,5-bisphosphate 3-kinase	3q26.32	Cell growth, division and survival
AKT1	v-akt murine thymoma viral oncogene homolog 1	14q32.32	Cell growth, division and survival
GATA3	GATA binding protein 3	10p15	Transcription factors important in T cell and endothelial development
MAP3K1	mitogen-activated protein kinase kinase kinase 1	5q11.2	Protein kinase activating ERK and JNK kinase pathways
CBFB	core-binding factor, β subunit	16q22.1	Master regulator of RUNX genes
RUNX1	runt-related transcription factor 1	21q22.3	Part of core-binding factor complex
CDH1	cadherin 1 (E-cadherin)	16q22.1	Cell adhesion

There is little known about the hereditary genetics of lobular cancer. Current evidence suggests that there is a significant overlap between genetic predisposition to IDC and ILC. However, newer studies have identified novel nucleotide polymorphisms at locus 7q34 conferring a predisposition that is specific to lobular breast cancer [105].

Molecular characterization of lobular carcinomas in the literature is relatively limited. With the advent of more advanced and readily available technologies additional molecular findings will likely emerge.

Key Points

- Lobular breast carcinoma (ILC) is the second most common type of breast carcinoma.
- The incidence of lobular carcinoma is rising that is due to better diagnosis and use of postmenopausal hormone therapy.
- Morphologically, ILC comprises of small, dyshesive and relatively uniform cells that insidiously infiltrate the breast stroma in a single-file pattern without significant stromal reaction.
- There are different subtype of ILC, with classical and pleomorphic subtypes are two most prevalent.
- Loss of E-cadherin is the characteristic molecular feature of the ILC.
- Underlying alteration in *CDH1* gene in the form of mutation or splicing or loss of heterozygosity is seen in almost all of the ILC.
- Most ILC, particularly the classical subtype, belong to luminal A molecular type of breast carcinomas.
- Although there are several other chromosomal abnormalities in ILC, loss of chromosome 16q and gain of chromosomes 1q and 16p are most common changes.
- Apart from changes in *CDH1* gene, alterations in *TP53*, *PIK3CA* and *GATA3* are also commonly seen in ILC.

References

1. Foote FW, Stewart FW. Lobular carcinoma in situ: a rare form of mammary cancer. Am J Pathol. 1941;17(4):491–6.
2. Haagensen CD, et al. Lobular neoplasia (so-called lobular carcinoma in situ) of the breast. Cancer. 1978;42(2):737–69.
3. Wheeler JE, et al. Lobular carcinoma in situ of the breast: long-term followup. Cancer. 1974;34(3):554–63.
4. Andersen JA. Lobular carcinoma in situ: a long-term follow-up in 52 cases. Acta Pathol Microbiol Scand A. 1974;82(4):519–33.
5. Brogi E, Murray MP, Corben AD. Lobular carcinoma, not only a classic. Breast J. 2010;16(Suppl 1):S10–4.
6. Mastracci TL, et al. E-cadherin alterations in atypical lobular hyperplasia and lobular carcinoma in situ of the breast. Mod Pathol. 2005;18(6):741–51.
7. De Leeuw WJ, et al. Simultaneous loss of E-cadherin and catenins in invasive lobular breast cancer and lobular carcinoma in situ. J Pathol. 1997;183(4):404–11.
8. Vos CB, et al. E-cadherin inactivation in lobular carcinoma in situ of the breast: an early event in tumorigenesis. Br J Cancer. 1997;76(9):1131–3.
9. Arpino G, Laucirica R, Elledge RM. Premalignant and in situ breast disease: biology and clinical implications. Ann Intern Med. 2005;143(6):446–57.
10. Rakha EA, Ellis IO. Lobular breast carcinoma and its variants. Semin Diagn Pathol. 2010;27(1):49–61.
11. Simpson PT, et al. The diagnosis and management of pre-invasive breast disease: pathology of atypical lobular hyperplasia and lobular carcinoma in situ. Breast Cancer Res. 2003;5(5):258–62.
12. Lakhani SRE, Simpson PT. Invasive lobular carcinoma. In: Lakhani SEI, Schnitt SJ, Tan P-H, van de Vijver MJ, editors. WHO classification of tumors of the breast. Lyon: IARC; 2012.
13. Daling JR, et al. Relation of regimens of combined hormone replacement therapy to lobular, ductal, and other histologic types of breast carcinoma. Cancer. 2002;95(12):2455–64.
14. Chen CL, et al. Hormone replacement therapy in relation to breast cancer. JAMA. 2002;287(6):734–41.
15. Shetty MR. Infiltrating lobular carcinoma: is it different from infiltrating duct carcinoma? Cancer. 1994;74(3):986–7.
16. Silverstein MJ, et al. Infiltrating lobular carcinoma: is it different from infiltrating duct carcinoma? Cancer. 1994;73(6):1673–7.
17. Wheeler JE, Enterline HT. Lobular carcinoma of the breast in situ and infiltrating. Pathol Annu. 1976;11:161–88.
18. Martinez V, Azzopardi JG. Invasive lobular carcinoma of the breast: incidence and variants. Histopathology. 1979;3(6):467–88.
19. Fechner RE. Histologic variants of infiltrating lobular carcinoma of the breast. Hum Pathol. 1975;6(3):373–8.
20. Shousha S, et al. Alveolar variant of invasive lobular carcinoma of the breast: a tumor rich in estrogen receptors. Am J Clin Pathol. 1986;85(1):1–5.
21. Van Bogaert LJ, Maldague P. Infiltrating lobular carcinoma of the female breast: deviations from the usual histopathologic appearance. Cancer. 1980;45(5):979–84.
22. Bentz JS, Yassa N, Clayton F. Pleomorphic lobular carcinoma of the breast: clinicopathologic features of 12 cases. Mod Pathol. 1998;11(9):814–22.
23. Weidner N, Semple JP. Pleomorphic variant of invasive lobular carcinoma of the breast. Hum Pathol. 1992;23(10):1167–71.
24. Eusebi V, Magalhaes F, Azzopardi JG. Pleomorphic lobular carcinoma of the breast: an aggressive tumor showing apocrine differentiation. Hum Pathol. 1992;23(6):655–62.

25. Silver SA, Tavassoli FA. Pleomorphic carcinoma of the breast: clinicopathological analysis of 26 cases of an unusual high-grade phenotype of ductal carcinoma. Histopathology. 2000;36(6):505–14.
26. Middleton LP, et al. Pleomorphic lobular carcinoma: morphology, immunohistochemistry, and molecular analysis. Am J Surg Pathol. 2000;24(12):1650–6.
27. Gamallo C, et al. Correlation of E-cadherin expression with differentiation grade and histological type in breast carcinoma. Am J Pathol. 1993;142(4):987–93.
28. Simpson PT, et al. Molecular profiling pleomorphic lobular carcinomas of the breast: evidence for a common molecular genetic pathway with classic lobular carcinomas. J Pathol. 2008;215(3):231–44.
29. Rasbridge SA, et al. Epithelial (E-) and placental (P-)cadherin cell adhesion molecule expression in breast carcinoma. J Pathol. 1993;169(2):245–50.
30. Moll R, et al. Differential loss of E-cadherin expression in infiltrating ductal and lobular breast carcinomas. Am J Pathol. 1993;143(6):1731–42.
31. Takeichi M. Cadherin cell adhesion receptors as a morphogenetic regulator. Science. 1991;251(5000):1451–5.
32. Golenhofen N, Drenckhahn D. The catenin, p120ctn, is a common membrane-associated protein in various epithelial and non-epithelial cells and tissues. Histochem Cell Biol. 2000;114(2):147–55.
33. Hatzfeld M. The p120 family of cell adhesion molecules. Eur J Cell Biol. 2005;84(2–3):205–14.
34. Davis MA, Ireton RC, Reynolds AB. A core function for p120-catenin in cadherin turnover. J Cell Biol. 2003;163(3):525–34.
35. Peifer M, Yap AS. Traffic control: p120-catenin acts as a gatekeeper to control the fate of classical cadherins in mammalian cells. J Cell Biol. 2003;163(3):437–40.
36. Sarrio D, et al. Cytoplasmic localization of p120ctn and E-cadherin loss characterize lobular breast carcinoma from preinvasive to metastatic lesions. Oncogene. 2004;23(19):3272–83.
37. Shibata T, et al. Cytoplasmic p120ctn regulates the invasive phenotypes of E-cadherin-deficient breast cancer. Am J Pathol. 2004;164(6):2269–78.
38. Kanai Y, et al. Point mutation of the E-cadherin gene in invasive lobular carcinoma of the breast. Jpn J Cancer Res. 1994;85(10):1035–9.
39. Droufakou S, et al. Multiple ways of silencing E-cadherin gene expression in lobular carcinoma of the breast. Int J Cancer. 2001;92(3):404–8.
40. Berx G, et al. E-cadherin is a tumour/invasion suppressor gene mutated in human lobular breast cancers. EMBO J. 1995;14(24):6107–15.
41. Graff JR, et al. E-cadherin expression is silenced by DNA hypermethylation in human breast and prostate carcinomas. Cancer Res. 1995;55(22):5195–9.
42. Yoshiura K, et al. Silencing of the E-cadherin invasion-suppressor gene by CpG methylation in human carcinomas. Proc Natl Acad Sci USA. 1995;92(16):7416–9.
43. Yonemura Y, et al. Decreased E-cadherin expression correlates with poor survival in patients with gastric cancer. Anal Cell Pathol. 1995;8(2):177–90.
44. Berx G, et al. E-cadherin is inactivated in a majority of invasive human lobular breast cancers by truncation mutations throughout its extracellular domain. Oncogene. 1996;13(9):1919–25.
45. Mohsin SK, et al. Biomarker profile and genetic abnormalities in lobular carcinoma in situ. Breast Cancer Res Treat. 2005;90(3):249–56.
46. Cancer Genome Atlas Network. Comprehensive molecular portraits of human breast tumours. Nature. 2012;490(7418):61–70.
47. Da Silva L, et al. Aberrant expression of E-cadherin in lobular carcinomas of the breast. Am J Surg Pathol. 2008;32(5):773–83.
48. Zhao L, et al. Diagnostic role of immunohistochemistry in the evaluation of breast pathology specimens. Arch Pathol Lab Med. 2014;138(1):16–24.
49. Rakha EA, et al. Clinical and biological significance of E-cadherin protein expression in invasive lobular carcinoma of the breast. Am J Surg Pathol. 2010;34(10):1472–9.

50. Lopez-Garcia MA, et al. Breast cancer precursors revisited: molecular features and progression pathways. Histopathology. 2010;57(2):171–92.
51. Sorlie T, et al. Repeated observation of breast tumor subtypes in independent gene expression data sets. Proc Natl Acad Sci USA. 2003;100(14):8418–23.
52. Perou CM, et al. Molecular portraits of human breast tumours. Nature. 2000;406(6797):747–52.
53. Sorlie T, et al. Gene expression patterns of breast carcinomas distinguish tumor subclasses with clinical implications. Proc Natl Acad Sci USA. 2001;98(19):10869–74.
54. Gatza ML, et al. A pathway-based classification of human breast cancer. Proc Natl Acad Sci USA. 2010;107(15):6994–9.
55. Stephens PJ, et al. Complex landscapes of somatic rearrangement in human breast cancer genomes. Nature. 2009;462(7276):1005–10.
56. Andre F, Pusztai L. Molecular classification of breast cancer: implications for selection of adjuvant chemotherapy. Nat Clin Pract Oncol. 2006;3(11):621–32.
57. Reis-Filho JS, Westbury C, Pierga JY. The impact of expression profiling on prognostic and predictive testing in breast cancer. J Clin Pathol. 2006;59(3):225–31.
58. Geyer FC, et al. Genetic characterization of breast cancer and implications for clinical management. J Cell Mol Med. 2009;13(10):4090–103.
59. Geyer FC, Reis-Filho JS. Microarray-based gene expression profiling as a clinical tool for breast cancer management: are we there yet? Int J Surg Pathol. 2009;17(4):285–302.
60. Weigelt B, Baehner FL, Reis-Filho JS. The contribution of gene expression profiling to breast cancer classification, prognostication and prediction: a retrospective of the last decade. J Pathol. 2010;220(2):263–80.
61. Rouzier R, et al. Breast cancer molecular subtypes respond differently to preoperative chemotherapy. Clin Cancer Res. 2005;11(16):5678–85.
62. Livasy CA, et al. Phenotypic evaluation of the basal-like subtype of invasive breast carcinoma. Mod Pathol. 2006;19(2):264–71.
63. Nielsen TO, et al. Immunohistochemical and clinical characterization of the basal-like subtype of invasive breast carcinoma. Clin Cancer Res. 2004;10(16):5367–74.
64. Cheang MC, et al. Basal-like breast cancer defined by five biomarkers has superior prognostic value than triple-negative phenotype. Clin Cancer Res. 2008;14(5):1368–76.
65. Bhargava R, Dabbs DJ. Use of immunohistochemistry in diagnosis of breast epithelial lesions. Adv Anat Pathol. 2007;14(2):93–107.
66. Turner NC, Reis-Filho JS. Basal-like breast cancer and the BRCA1 phenotype. Oncogene. 2006;25(43):5846–53.
67. Foulkes WD, et al. The prognostic implication of the basal-like (cyclin E high/p27 low/p53+/glomeruloid-microvascular-proliferation+) phenotype of BRCA1-related breast cancer. Cancer Res. 2004;64(3):830–5.
68. Weigelt B, et al. Refinement of breast cancer classification by molecular characterization of histological special types. J Pathol. 2008;216(2):141–50.
69. Soomro S, et al. c-erbB-2 expression in different histological types of invasive breast carcinoma. J Clin Pathol. 1991;44(3):211–4.
70. Rakha EA, et al. Invasive lobular carcinoma of the breast: response to hormonal therapy and outcomes. Eur J Cancer. 2008;44(1):73–83.
71. Arpino G, et al. Infiltrating lobular carcinoma of the breast: tumor characteristics and clinical outcome. Breast Cancer Res. 2004;6(3):R149–56.
72. Radhi JM. Immunohistochemical analysis of pleomorphic lobular carcinoma: higher expression of p53 and chromogranin and lower expression of ER and PgR. Histopathology. 2000;36(2):156–60.
73. Zhao H, et al. Different gene expression patterns in invasive lobular and ductal carcinomas of the breast. Mol Biol Cell. 2004;15(6):2523–36.
74. Weigelt B, et al. The molecular underpinning of lobular histological growth pattern: a genome-wide transcriptomic analysis of invasive lobular carcinomas and grade- and molecular subtype-matched invasive ductal carcinomas of no special type. J Pathol. 2010;220(1):45–57.

75. Turashvili G, et al. Novel markers for differentiation of lobular and ductal invasive breast carcinomas by laser microdissection and microarray analysis. BMC Cancer. 2007;7:55.
76. Korkola JE, et al. Differentiation of lobular versus ductal breast carcinomas by expression microarray analysis. Cancer Res. 2003;63(21):7167–75.
77. Nishizaki T, et al. Genetic alterations in lobular breast cancer by comparative genomic hybridization. Int J Cancer. 1997;74(5):513–7.
78. Loo LW, et al. Array comparative genomic hybridization analysis of genomic alterations in breast cancer subtypes. Cancer Res. 2004;64(23):8541–9.
79. Hwang ES, et al. Clonality of lobular carcinoma in situ and synchronous invasive lobular carcinoma. Cancer. 2004;100(12):2562–72.
80. Masuda S. Breast cancer pathology: the impact of molecular taxonomy on morphological taxonomy. Pathol Int. 2012;62(5):295–302.
81. Lu YJ, et al. Comparative genomic hybridization analysis of lobular carcinoma in situ and atypical lobular hyperplasia and potential roles for gains and losses of genetic material in breast neoplasia. Cancer Res. 1998;58(20):4721–7.
82. Lakhani SR, et al. Loss of heterozygosity in lobular carcinoma in situ of the breast. Clin Mol Pathol. 1995;48(2):M74–8.
83. Nayar R, et al. Loss of heterozygosity on chromosome 11q13 in lobular lesions of the breast using tissue microdissection and polymerase chain reaction. Hum Pathol. 1997;28(3):277–82.
84. Shin SJ, et al. Florid lobular carcinoma in situ: molecular profiling and comparison to classic lobular carcinoma in situ and pleomorphic lobular carcinoma in situ. Hum Pathol. 2013;44(10):1998–2009.
85. Mastracci TL, et al. Genomic alterations in lobular neoplasia: a microarray comparative genomic hybridization signature for early neoplastic proliferation in the breast. Genes Chromosomes Cancer. 2006;45(11):1007–17.
86. Chen YY, et al. Genetic and phenotypic characteristics of pleomorphic lobular carcinoma in situ of the breast. Am J Surg Pathol. 2009;33(11):1683–94.
87. Boldt V, et al. Positioning of necrotic lobular intraepithelial neoplasias (LIN, grade 3) within the sequence of breast carcinoma progression. Genes Chromosom Cancer. 2010;49(5):463–70.
88. Reis-Filho JS, et al. Pleomorphic lobular carcinoma of the breast: role of comprehensive molecular pathology in characterization of an entity. J Pathol. 2005;207(1):1–13.
89. Ross JS, et al. Relapsed classic E-cadherin (CDH1)-mutated invasive lobular breast cancer shows a high frequency of HER2 (ERBB2) gene mutations. Clin Cancer Res. 2013;19(10):2668–76.
90. Green AR, et al. Loss of expression of chromosome 16q genes DPEP1 and CTCF in lobular carcinoma in situ of the breast. Breast Cancer Res Treat. 2009;113(1):59–66.
91. Banerji S, et al. Sequence analysis of mutations and translocations across breast cancer subtypes. Nature. 2012;486(7403):405–9.
92. Sjoblom T, et al. The consensus coding sequences of human breast and colorectal cancers. Science. 2006;314(5797):268–74.
93. Samuels Y, et al. High frequency of mutations of the PIK3CA gene in human cancers. Science. 2004;304(5670):554.
94. Carpten JD, et al. A transforming mutation in the pleckstrin homology domain of AKT1 in cancer. Nature. 2007;448(7152):439–44.
95. Usary J, et al. Mutation of GATA3 in human breast tumors. Oncogene. 2004;23(46):7669–78.
96. Kan Z, et al. Diverse somatic mutation patterns and pathway alterations in human cancers. Nature. 2010;466(7308):869–73.
97. Derksen PW, et al. Mammary-specific inactivation of E-cadherin and p53 impairs functional gland development and leads to pleomorphic invasive lobular carcinoma in mice. Dis Model Mech. 2011;4(3):347–58.

98. Dabbs DJ, et al. Lobular neoplasia of the breast revisited with emphasis on the role of E-cadherin immunohistochemistry. Am J Surg Pathol. 2013;37(7):e1–11.
99. Shah SP, et al. Mutational evolution in a lobular breast tumour profiled at single nucleotide resolution. Nature. 2009;461(7265):809–13.
100. Wilkerson PM, Reis-Filho JS. The 11q13–q14 amplicon: clinicopathological correlations and potential drivers. Genes Chromosom Cancer. 2013;52(4):333–55.
101. Natrajan R, et al. An integrative genomic and transcriptomic analysis reveals molecular pathways and networks regulated by copy number aberrations in basal-like, HER2 and luminal cancers. Breast Cancer Res Treat. 2010;121(3):575–89.
102. Weigelt B, Reis-Filho JS. Histological and molecular types of breast cancer: is there a unifying taxonomy? Nat Rev Clin Oncol. 2009;6(12):718–30.
103. Stephens PJ, et al. The landscape of cancer genes and mutational processes in breast cancer. Nature. 2012;486(7403):400–4.
104. Gatza M. Genomic characterization of invasive lobular breast carcinoma. 2014. Available from: http://www.genome.gov/multimedia/slides/tcga3/21_gatza.pdf.
105. Sawyer E, et al. Genetic predisposition to in situ and invasive lobular carcinoma of the breast. PLoS Genet. 2014;10(4):e1004285.

Chapter 8
Molecular Pathology of Hormone Regulation in Breast Cancer: Hormone Receptor Evaluation and Therapeutic Implications

Emad A. Rakha

Introduction

Steroids hormone receptor together with growth factors drive the development, growth and differentiation of hormone responsive tissue including breast epithelial tissue following activation of the nuclear estrogen (ER) and progesterone receptor (PR) [1–3]. ER and PR are expressed in breast cancer respectively in 70–90 % and 55–65 % of cases. Hormone receptor activation—mainly through paracrine signaling—triggers diverse gene networks to activate metabolic and cell regulatory pathways involved in the initiation and progression of hormone receptor positive breast cancer [4]. ER is activated by the hormone estrogen (17β-estradiol) and once activated, the ER is able to translocate into the nucleus and bind to DNA to regulate the activity of different genes functioning as a DNA-binding transcription factor. There are two different forms of the estrogen receptor, usually referred to as α and β. In this article ER refers to ERα. PR is encoded by a single *PR* gene residing on chromosome 11q22 and its protein product is activated by the steroid hormone progesterone. After progesterone binds to the receptor, PR enters the nucleus and binds to DNA.

The expression of ER and PR is predictive for endocrine response and prognostic for breast cancer outcome but to a different extend for each receptor. Women with an ER-positive breast cancer not receiving endocrine therapy have a better outcome than women with an ER-negative tumour [5, 6]. This outcome difference is further enhanced with endocrine therapy as ER expression predicts response to

E.A. Rakha (✉)
Department of Histopathology, Division of Cancer and Stem Cells,
School of Medicine, Nottingham University Hospitals NHS Trust,
Nottingham City Hospital, The University of Nottingham, Nottingham, NG5 1PB, UK
e-mail: Emad.Rakha@nottingham.ac.uk

© Springer Science+Business Media New York 2015
A. Khan et al. (eds.), *Precision Molecular Pathology of Breast Cancer*,
Molecular Pathology Library 10, DOI 10.1007/978-1-4939-2886-6_8

anti-oestrogen therapeutic strategies [7, 8] including inhibition of hormone production through oophorectomy or administration of drugs that inhibit hormone synthesis in other organs of origin such as aromatase inhibitors in post-menopausal women. The other approach of endocrine therapy includes the use of hormone receptor antagonists that bind to the normal hormone receptor and prevent its activation. Selective estrogen receptor modulators (SERM) are an important class of estrogen receptor antagonist that are used primarily for the treatment and chemoprevention of breast cancer. Tamoxifen, which is currently first-line treatment for nearly all pre-menopausal women with hormone receptor-positive breast cancer is an example of SERM that has partial agonist function in some tissues, such as the endometrium. The use of Tamoxifen for 5-years after surgery reduces the risk of recurrence by 47 % and of death by 26 % [9]. Example of SERM that has little or no agonist function is Fulvestrant are used for treatment of metastatic BC.

Although ER predicts response to endocrine therapy, its predictive power appears to decreases over time indicating that it is a time-dependent factor [10]. The PR-positivity increases the predictive power of ER but on its own does not predict response [11, 12]. Some studies have demonstrated prognostic value for PR but did not identify significant effect on the response to endocrine therapy [13, 14]. However, other authors have demonstrated that high PR expression is associated with clinical outcomes and effect of hormone therapy in ER positive premenopausal patients [15, 16]. Compared to ER+/PR+ cases, ER+/PR− tumours constitute a more aggressive breast cancer phenotype more often seen in the so called luminal B breast cancers [13, 14, 17]. ER+/PR− tumours tend to have a lower nuclear ER-activity, a greater genomic instability, a higher proliferation rate, HER2 positivity, carry frequently PI3K mutations and showing more crosstalk between ER and growth factors [18]. It was also demonstrated that the presence of PR in ER-negative tumours is associated with an enhanced chance of response [19] but may mostly indicate a false-negative ER assay rather than a biologic phenomenon [20]. Therefore several authors have concluded that ER and PR should be reported in combination with the HER-2 status, since these clinical phenotypes, available for every patient in daily routine, possess discriminative prognostic information comparable to gene expression profiling [21, 22].

Assessment and Reporting Hormone Receptor

The substantial survival benefit from hormone therapy has made treatment with one of these well-tolerated agents mandatory in ER-positive breast cancer; therefore, ER assessment of ER status has been rendered essential for all invasive primary breast carcinomas [23]. Therefore a test that can assess ER status with a high degree of accuracy, reliability, precision and reproducibility is of crucial importance. Measurement and characterization of ER was first reported by Jensen et al. [24] in 1960s. Until about 1990, ER was quantified using a variety of biochemical ligand-binding assays (LBAs) that depended on homogenization of fresh-frozen portion of breast cancer tissue. This assay depended on homogenization of a portion of fresh-frozen breast cancer tissue and preparation of cytosol by centrifugation for the performance of a LBA involving incubation with radioactively labeled estradiol. Separation of receptor-bound estradiol from the unbound fraction was most frequently achieved with a suspension of dextran-coated charcoal (DCC). Initially LBA techniques were used extensively to quantify ER concentrations in breast cancer tissue. LBA remained the most widely used service assay until the early 1990s. Although the results of ER measurement was quantitative most clinical trials used 10 fmol/mg protein as a cutoff [7]. The availability of monoclonal antibodies to ER led to the development of an enzyme immunoassay (EIA) as a more precise and less labour intensive alternative to the LBA/DCC. Excellent linear correlations were reported between the two methodologies [25]. Retrospective analyses have shown that semi-quantitative analysis of ER-expression by immunohistochemistry (IHC) is superior to biochemical assays for both prognostic and predictive purposes [26–29]. IHC application of monoclonal anti-ER antibodies was initially successful only on frozen sections, but the introduction of antigen retrieval methods and the development of new antibodies allowed application on routinely fixed tissues. IHC approach has soon become widespread because of the ease of the assays, low cost, use of minimal amounts of tissue, and applicability to routine histopathological samples. IHC is also safe and usable for evaluating cytology, fresh frozen tissue and formalin-fixed paraffin-embedded specimens. Additionally, IHC offers the advantage of morphology, allowing pathologists to discriminate between malignant and benign hormone receptor positive cells. This led laboratories around the world to abandon LBA in favour of IHC, which is currently the standard routine practice [30, 31].

However, lack of standardized protocols in the pre-analytical phase including type of fixative and time of fixation and specimen type, in the analytical phase including primary antibody, antigen retrieval and detection system and post analytical phase including scoring method and definition of positivity remained critical issues and were a likely reason for discordant results in different laboratories [32, 33]. This is in addition the availability of several antibodies that recognise different epitopes and may vary in their sensitivity. Previous studies have demonstrated that the sensitivity of detection of ER expression is related to the quality of fixation and antigen retrieval methods and the clone of antibody used in addition to other analytical variables [34]. Therefore guideline recommendation that aimed at improving assays reproducibility, accuracy and precision have been published [23, 35]. Quality control programs have also been implemented in the UK and elsewhere to guarantee reproducibility and comparability between different centres [36]. Indeed, false negative but also false positive results for ER do exist, with error rates reported in some centres as high as 20 % [30, 33].

Newer molecular technologies such as Real Time quantitative Reverse Transcription Polymerase Chain Reaction (qRT-PCR) and gene-expression microarrays are expected to further refine the assessment of hormone receptor expression. For example, the pre-treatment Oncotype DX®Recurrence Score uses RT-PCR ER gene information together with information obtained from 20 other genes and is not only a highly significant predictor of recurrence (prognostic), but it is also being tested as a predictive tool to estimate the benefit of adjuvant chemotherapy as well [37]. Future studies will need to further assess and validate both the prognostic and predictive qualities of RT-PCR compared with IHC. Although the techniques assess ER/PR totally different, the concordance among local IHC, central IHC, and central RT-PCR by the proprietary gene assay for ER and PR status is high [37].

The main points recognised as a source of IHC ER assay variation include the followings: *Choice of specimen and fixation*: Hormone receptor studies are most optimally performed on the preoperative needle core biopsies. Recent studies show near 100 % concordance between needle core and resection specimens [38]. However, to reduce any possibility of false negative cases, repeat testing of ER-negative cases on resection specimens is recommended. Bilateral carcinomas, histologically distinct ipsilateral carcinomas or widely separated carcinomas considered to be separate synchronous primary tumours should each be assessed if the core biopsy is ER negative. It is deemed reasonable not to assess multiple ipsilateral tumours if they are histologically similar and the core biopsy was ER positive. Currently there is no consensus on testing residual invasive tumour following neoadjuvant therapy, although some recommend this approach. Cases negative on resection specimens but show true positivity on needle core biopsy may be a reflection of poor fixation of the resection specimen. Good fixation of specimens used for hormone receptor testing should be ensured and the cold ischaemic time (time from removal from the patient to placing in fixative (cold ischaemic time) should be as short as possible, certainly less than 1 h [39]. Tumours samples should be fixed in buffered formalin and embedded in paraffin wax. Other methods of tissue fixation may adversely affect antigen reactivity. At least 6 h fixation is recommended for core biopsies. Surgical specimens should be incised as soon as possible through the carcinoma to allow initial penetration of fixative and then sliced into 5–10 mm slices to ensure rapid penetration and even fixation. Tissue should be placed in an adequate volume (ideally 10:1; fixative:tissue) of fixative for at least 24 h and not more than 72 h Centres using rapid fixation and processing must validate their methodology for HER2 assessment (http://www.ukneqasicc.ucl.ac.uk/neqasicc.shtml) [26]. Inadequate fixation of specimens increases the risk of false-negative ER status. Given the lack of control some laboratories have over the fixation duration, and given the liability of the ER antigen, it is still advisable to look for 'built-in' positive controls in the form of non-neoplastic breast epithelium when identifying an ER-negative case.

Choice of antibody: Although a number of anti-ER antibodies are available, the ideal antibody is one that is both robust and has been clinically validated; to date, there are few such antibodies including the mouse monoclonal antibodies 1D5 and 6F11 and the rabbit monoclonal antibodies SP1 and EP1 clones, which have been demonstrated to produce results that correlate with clinical outcome and have also been demonstrated to be equal or superior to LBA [34].

Threshold for positivity: The use of reproducible clinically validated, and standardized scoring system and cutoffs for determining positive results is critical.

Several different IHC semi-quantitative scoring systems for reporting hormone receptors have been developed over time. Amongst the first was McCarthy's "H" score, calculated by multiplying the percentage of positive cells by a factor representing the intensity of immunoreactivity (1 for weak, 2 for moderate and 3 for strong), giving a minimum score of 0 and a maximum score of 300 (3+). Originally, a score of <50 was considered negative (−) and a score of 50–100 was considered weakly positive (1+). Another score still in use is the immunoreactive Remmele score [27], described in 1987 and also called IRS which is the product of o proportion score and an intensity score with a ranger of 0–12. The "Allred" or "modified quick" score which is a nine-point, semiquantitative (ranging from 0 to 8) score that combine percent of positive tumour cells stratified into 6 groups (0 no; 1 less than 1 %; 2 between 1 and 10 %; 3 between 11 and 33 %; 4 between 34 and 66 % and 5 between 67 and 100 % of the cells staining) and intensity of staining (0–3) was introduced and used frequently in clinical trials [28]. The Allred score was the only clinically validated scoring system and most widely used hormone receptor scoring system [28]. Although there was a strong direct association between the level of ER expression and response to hormonal therapy, studies have revealed that a score of 3 or more that corresponds to as few as 1 % of cells showing staining define ER positivity. When <1 % of the tumor cells stain (proportion score = 1), the tumour is per definition receptor-negative, regardless of the intensity score [23]. However, ER percent alone was used for assessment of hormone receptor in many laboratories and a wide range of arbitrary cutoffs (e.g. 5, 10 and 20 % of tumour cells) were employed by different laboratories to define positivity. In 2010, a consensus ASCO/CAP meeting of expert panelists have set the consensus threshold for reporting ER as positive at 1 % staining [23]. This cutoff has also been endorsed in the UK and elsewhere. It is our practice to assess and report percent, H-score and Allred score and define ER positivity based on a 1 % cutoff. However, it is important to be aware that cases expressing ER staining in 1–9 % of tumour cells on needle core biopsy should be repeated on resection specimens and the proportions of false positive and false negative results are the highest among those cases [29]. Discordances between H-score and Allred score for defining ER-positivity and the resulting benefit from anti-estrogen therapy also occur when 1–10 % of cells stain [31].

Evaluation and quality: For assessment of hormone receptor training and experience in interpretation of histological characteristics of breast tissue is essential. Hormone receptor should only be determined on the invasive portion of the tumour. Image analysis systems may provide alternatives to manual scoring for hormone receptor. The inclusion of controls, ideally including on slide control(s), and their detailed scrutiny are essential to ensure test accuracy. Tissue-based controls, from breast cancers, should also be used. Control material should be similarly fixed and processed to the test tissue. Control sections should be ideally cut at the same time as the test material. Long-term storage of pre-cut control sections is strongly discouraged. There is no evidence that storage of blocks leads to deterioration of signal. Crushing and edge artefact, particularly affect core biopsies may make interpretation difficult. A repeat staining may be prudent in these cases.

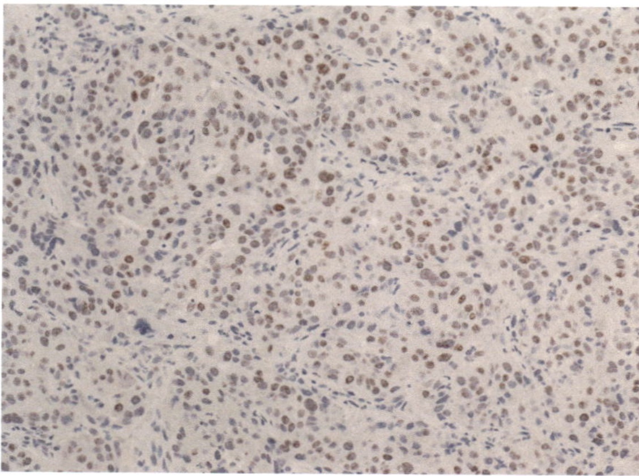

Fig. 8.1 Immunohistochemical staining of estrogen receptor showing granular/punctate brown nuclear staining in consistent with false positive pattern [55]

The potential gradient effects of suboptimal fixation, particularly in larger surgical specimens, should also be considered in interpretation of staining. New batches of antibody should also be tested before commencing routine application. Use of standardized operating procedures, including routine use of control materials, is recommended. In the UK, participation and satisfactory performance in the UK NEQAS IHC modules is a requirement (www.ukneqasicc.ucl.ac.uk). If a commercial kit/assay is utilised, it is recommended that laboratories adhere strictly to the kit/assay protocol.

False positive ER staining: Although 6F11 is widely used and has been validated in several studies, we and other have experienced some difficulties with the interpretation of staining patterns, and in some instances, we observed weak granular/punctate nuclear staining on core biopsy that gave false-positive results. We have identified some cases with this staining pattern in our routine practice and repeated the ER assessment by using different antibodies on resection specimens that yielded negative results (Fig. 8.1), which suggested that the pattern observed with 6F11 is likely to constitute a false-positive staining [29].

Predictive Value of Hormone Receptor Expression in Breast Cancer

A factor is predictive if it predicts the likelihood of responding to specific types of therapies both in the adjuvant and metastatic neoadjuvant setting. Hormone receptor expression in breast cancer is predictive of response to endocrine therapy that has been proven to be highly effective and appropriate for nearly all women with hormone receptor positive breast cancer, making such treatment the most widely prescribed therapy for patients with cancer in the world. For many years, tamoxifen taken for 5 years was the standard endocrine therapy for breast cancer. In a systematic review of randomised trials of adjuvant tamoxifen among women with early breast cancer (55 trials including 37,000 women) [40], it was demonstrated that in women with ER negative tumours ($n = 8000$) the overall effects of tamoxifen appeared to be small. In ER positive women ($n = 30,000$), adjuvant tamoxifen reduced the proportional recurrence during about 10 years of follow-up by 21, 29, and 47 %, for 1-year, 2-years and 5-years of treatment respectively. The corresponding proportional mortality reductions were 12, 17, and 26 %. The proportional mortality reductions were similar for women with node-positive and node-negative disease, but the absolute mortality reductions were greater in node-positive women [40]. More recently, patients who are postmenopausal also have been offered the option of taking an aromatase inhibitor (AI) as an alternative to tamoxifen or in sequence after tamoxifen [41].

Despite its advantages, the fact that patients who do not express ER do not benefit from hormone therapy added to an approximate 40 % of ER-positive BC patients who also do not respond to hormone therapy [42] provides important clinical context for researchers to explore more signalling pathways which may provide alternatives for novel targeted therapies. The understanding of the molecular biology and behaviour of breast cancer and a more robust classification of its different molecular subtypes is crucial in identifying newer therapeutic strategies. Using cDNA microarray, Jansen et al. [43] determined 81 genes for tamoxifen response among 46 ER-positive tumours from women with advanced ER-positive breast cancer after tamoxifen treatment. The genes were then shortlisted to 44 and validated on 66 tumours where they could predict tamoxifen response in 27 out of 35 cases. In another study, a new gene signature comprising 78 genes was identified using a set of 69 independent tumours from patients treated with tamoxifen [44]. The resistance to tamoxifen was also correctly predicted in 78 % of patients with relapse using a molecular signature of 36 genes, many of them were related to DNA proliferation and replication such as TK1 and CDC2 [45].

In patients with ER-positive disease, it is a major concern for oncologists as whether to add chemotherapy to the treatment plan or not. It has been reported that tumours which are ER positive are relatively resistant to chemotherapy compared to ER-negative ones with the absolute benefit from adjuvant chemotherapy significantly worse (7 % of ER-positive tumours vs. 22.8 % of ER-negative tumours) survived to 5 year disease free when receiving adjuvant chemotherapy [46, 47]. Tumours with high levels of both ER and PR are highly sensitive to endocrine therapy and the benefit of adjuvant chemotherapy is small in these cases, irrespective of menopausal status [48]. It remains unclear whether the lack of benefit from chemotherapy in these patients is due to an excellent outcome or due to genuine lack of biological effect. Recent data indicate that response to chemotherapy in ER positive breast cancer can be predicted using the commercially available Oncotype DX gene signature which is composed of a set of 16 genes with 5 reference genes using a polymerase chain reaction-type array [49].

Currently, the use of hormonal therapy in breast cancer is restricted to patients with tumours expressing ER and is prescribed in one of the following two clinical contexts: (1) in limited disease, it is either used in the adjuvant setting, i.e. after surgery to halt the growth of the metastatic cancer cells or as part of the neoadjuvant protocol to help shrink the tumour prior to surgery, OR (2) in the metastatic setting where surgical eradication of the disease in unlikely.

Although there is a gradient of increasing response to endocrine agents with increasing levels of ER, the gradient is skewed such that tumours expressing even very low numbers of positive cells (e.g. 1–10 %) show a significant benefit far above that of ER negative tumours, which are essentially unresponsive. The predictive value of quantitative PR expression for response to tamoxifen is less clear. Some authors showed that the benefit of endocrine adjuvant therapy is not affected by quantitative PR expression in ER positive breast cancer [50] while others have reported that the benefit of tamoxifen seems to be restricted to ER-positive breast cancers with a strong expression of PR (>75 %) [15]. Although some trials reported benefit of tamoxifen in ER negative breast cancer when PR is positive cases this may represent ER false negative assays [20, 29]. Tumours expressing both hormone receptor and HER2 pathways may be resistant to one or both targeted treatments due to interplay between these pathways and combination therapy may be more beneficial. The significance of the effect of adjuvant trastuzumab in ER-positive breast cancers is dependent on PR's presence in HERA [51].

In menopausal women with ER positive breast cancer, there is a linear relationship between the quantitative expression of ER and the chance of responding to endocrine therapy, both for tamoxifen and oral AIs [52, 53]. Metastatic post-menopausal breast cancer patients diagnosed with ER positive breast cancer have an estimated clinical benefit from first line tamoxifen or AIs of 38–59 % [54].

In an update of guideline recommendations on adjuvant endocrine therapy for women with ER positive breast cancer by ASCO/CAP [41], it was recommended that:

1. Pre- or perimenopausal women should be offered adjuvant endocrine therapy with Tamoxifen for an initial duration of 5 years. Additional therapy after 5 years should be based on menopausal status as follows:

    A. If women are pre- or perimenopausal, or if menopausal status is unknown or cannot be determined, they should be offered continued tamoxifen for a total duration of 10 years
    B. If women have become definitively postmenopausal, they should be offered continued tamoxifen for a total duration of 10 years or switching to up to 5 years of AIs, for a total duration of up to 10 years of adjuvant endocrine therapy.

2. Women diagnosed with ER positive breast cancer who are postmenopausal should be offered adjuvant endocrine therapy with Tamoxifen for a duration of 10 years OR AIs for a duration of 5 years OR Tamoxifen for an initial duration of 5 years, then switching to an AI for up to 5 years, for a total duration of up to 10 years of adjuvant endocrine therapy OR Tamoxifen for a duration of 2–3 years and switching to an AI for up to 5 years, for a total duration of up to 7–8 years of adjuvant endocrine therapy.

3. Women who are postmenopausal and are intolerant of either tamoxifen or an AI should be offered the alternative type of adjuvant endocrine therapy.
   If women have received an AI but discontinued treatment at less than 5 years, they may be offered tamoxifen for a total of 5 years.
   If women have received tamoxifen for 2–3 years, they should be offered switching to an AI for up to 5 years, for a total duration of up to 7–8 years of adjuvant endocrine therapy.
4. Women who have received 5 years of tamoxifen as adjuvant endocrine therapy should be offered additional adjuvant endocrine treatment.

If women are postmenopausal, they should be offered continued tamoxifen for a total duration of 10 years or switching to up to 5 years AI, for a total duration of up to 10 years of adjuvant endocrine therapy.

If women are pre- or perimenopausal, or menopausal status cannot be ascertained, they should be offered 5 additional years of tamoxifen, for a total duration of 10 years of adjuvant endocrine therapy.

Conclusion

Hormone receptor is a strong predictor of endocrine therapy and should be assessed in all breast cancers including primary and recurrent. Hormone therapy is offered to all patients with ER positive breast cancer. Guideline recommendations for assessment of hormone receptor expression in breast cancer have been published. Adoption of these guidelines and implementation of various quality assurance methods should be encouraged to ensure high level of accuracy, precision and reproducibility of hormone receptor assays performance

References

1. Hankinson SE, Colditz GA, Willett WC. Towards an integrated model for breast cancer etiology: the lifelong interplay of genes, lifestyle, and hormones. Breast Cancer Res. 2004;6(5):213–8.
2. Anderson E, Clarke RB. Steroid receptors and cell cycle in normal mammary epithelium. J Mammary Gland Biol Neoplasia. 2004;9(1):3–13.
3. Asselin-Labat ML, et al. Control of mammary stem cell function by steroid hormone signalling. Nature. 2010;465(7299):798–802.
4. Frasor J, et al. Profiling of estrogen up- and down-regulated gene expression in human breast cancer cells: insights into gene networks and pathways underlying estrogenic control of proliferation and cell phenotype. Endocrinology. 2003;144(10):4562–74.
5. Knight WA, et al. Estrogen receptor as an independent prognostic factor for early recurrence in breast cancer. Cancer Res. 1977;37(12):4669–71.
6. Blamey RW, et al. Reading the prognosis of the individual with breast cancer. Eur J Cancer. 2007;43(10):1545–7.
7. Effects of chemotherapy and hormonal therapy for early breast cancer on recurrence and 15-year survival: an overview of the randomised trials. Lancet, 2005;365(9472):1687–1717.

8. Bartlett JM, et al. Estrogen receptor and progesterone receptor as predictive biomarkers of response to endocrine therapy: a prospectively powered pathology study in the Tamoxifen and Exemestane Adjuvant Multinational trial. J Clin Oncol. 2011;29(12):1531–8.

9. Al-Mubarak M, et al. Extended adjuvant tamoxifen for early breast cancer: a meta-analysis. PLoS one. 2014;9(2):e88238.

10. Hilsenbeck SG, et al. Time-dependence of hazard ratios for prognostic factors in primary breast cancer. Breast Cancer Res Treat. 1998;52(1–3):227–37.

11. Mohsin SK, et al. Progesterone receptor by immunohistochemistry and clinical outcome in breast cancer: a validation study. Mod Pathol. 2004;17(12):1545–54.

12. Bardou VJ, et al. Progesterone receptor status significantly improves outcome prediction over estrogen receptor status alone for adjuvant endocrine therapy in two large breast cancer databases. J Clin Oncol. 2003;21(10):1973.

13. Rakha EA, et al. Biologic and clinical characteristics of breast cancer with single hormone receptor positive phenotype. J Clin Oncol. 2007;25(30):4772–8.

14. Arpino G, et al. Estrogen receptor-positive, progesterone receptor-negative breast cancer: association with growth factor receptor expression and tamoxifen resistance. J Natl Cancer Inst. 2005;97(17):1254–61.

15. Stendahl M, et al. High progesterone receptor expression correlates to the effect of adjuvant tamoxifen in premenopausal breast cancer patients. Clin Cancer Res. 2006;12(15):4614–8.

16. Liu S, et al. Progesterone receptor is a significant factor associated with clinical outcomes and effect of adjuvant tamoxifen therapy in breast cancer patients. Breast Cancer Res Treat. 2010;119(1):53–61.

17. Sorlie T, et al. Repeated observation of breast tumor subtypes in independent gene expression data sets. Proc Natl Acad Sci U S A. 2003;100(14):8418–23.

18. Thakkar JP, Mehta DG. A review of an unfavorable subset of breast cancer: estrogen receptor positive progesterone receptor negative. Oncologist. 2011;16(3):276–85.

19. McGuire WL, et al. Current status of estrogen and progesterone receptors in breast cancer. Cancer. 1977;39(6 Suppl):2934–47.

20. Rakha E, et al. Oestrogen receptor negative progesterone receptor positive phenotype in breast cancer is a technical artefact. J Path. 2012;228(S1):S22.

21. Van Belle V, et al. Qualitative assessment of the progesterone receptor and HER2 improves the Nottingham Prognostic Index up to 5 years after breast cancer diagnosis. J Clin Oncol. 2010;28(27):4129–34.

22. Rakha EA, Reis-Filho JS, Ellis IO. Combinatorial biomarker expression in breast cancer. Breast Cancer Res Treat. 2010;120(2):293–308.

23. Hammond ME, et al. American Society of Clinical Oncology/College of American Pathologists guideline recommendations for immunohistochemical testing of estrogen and progesterone receptors in breast cancer. J Clin Oncol. 2010;28(16):2784–95.

24. Jensen EV, et al. Estrogen-receptor interactions in target tissues. Arch Anat Microsc Morphol Exp. 1967;56(3):547–69.

25. Thorpe SM. Monoclonal antibody technique for detection of estrogen receptors in human breast cancer: greater sensitivity and more accurate classification of receptor status than the dextran-coated charcoal method. Cancer Res. 1987;47(24 Pt 1):6572–5.

26. Bartlett JM, Rea D, Rimm DL. Quantification of hormone receptors to guide adjuvant therapy choice in early breast cancer: better methods required for improved utility. J Clin Oncol. 2011;29(27):3715–6.

27. Allred DC. Issues and updates: evaluating estrogen receptor-alpha, progesterone receptor, and HER2 in breast cancer. Mod Pathol. 2010;23(Suppl 2):S52–9.

28. Cheang MC, et al. Immunohistochemical detection using the new rabbit monoclonal antibody SP1 of estrogen receptor in breast cancer is superior to mouse monoclonal antibody 1D5 in predicting survival. J Clin Oncol. 2006;24(36):5637–44.

29. Nofech-Mozes S, et al. Cancer care Ontario guideline recommendations for hormone receptor testing in breast cancer. Clin Oncol (R Coll Radiol). 2012;24(10):684–96.

30. Leake R, et al. Immunohistochemical detection of steroid receptors in breast cancer: a working protocol. UK receptor group, UK NEQAS, The Scottish breast cancer pathology group, and the receptor and biomarker study group of the EORTC. J Clin Pathol. 2000;53(8):634–5.
31. Rhodes A, et al. Frequency of oestrogen and progesterone receptor positivity by immunohistochemical analysis in 7016 breast carcinomas: correlation with patient age, assay sensitivity, threshold value, and mammographic screening. J Clin Pathol. 2000;53(9):688–96.
32. Badve SS, et al. Estrogen- and progesterone-receptor status in ECOG 2197: comparison of immunohistochemistry by local and central laboratories and quantitative reverse transcription polymerase chain reaction by central laboratory. J Clin Oncol. 2008;26(15):2473–81.
33. Hodi Z, et al. The reliability of assessment of oestrogen receptor expression on needle core biopsy specimens of invasive carcinomas of the breast. J Clin Pathol. 2007;60(3):299–302.
34. Lee AH, et al. The effect of delay in fixation on HER2 expression in invasive carcinoma of the breast assessed with immunohistochemistry and in situ hybridisation. J Clin Pathol. 2014;67(7):573–5.
35. Rakha EA, et al. Updated UK recommendations for HER2 assessment in breast cancer. J Clin Pathol. 2015;68(2):93–9.
36. Remmele W, Stegner HE. Recommendation for uniform definition of an immunoreactive score (IRS) for immunohistochemical estrogen receptor detection (ER-ICA) in breast cancer tissue. Pathologe. 1987;8(3):138–40.
37. Harvey JM, et al. Estrogen receptor status by immunohistochemistry is superior to the ligand-binding assay for predicting response to adjuvant endocrine therapy in breast cancer. J Clin Oncol. 1999;17(5):1474–81.
38. Rakha EA, et al. Low-estrogen receptor-positive breast cancer: the impact of tissue sampling, choice of antibody, and molecular subtyping. J Clin Oncol, 2012;30(23):2929–30; author reply 2931.
39. Shousha S. Oestrogen receptor status of breast carcinoma: Allred/H score conversion table. Histopathology. 2008;53(3):346–7.
40. Tamoxifen for early breast cancer. Cochrane Database Syst Rev, 2001;1:CD000486.
41. Burstein HJ et al. Adjuvant endocrine therapy for women with hormone receptor-positive breast cancer: american society of clinical oncology clinical practice guideline focused update. J Clin Oncol, 2014;32(21):2255–69.
42. Osborne CK. Tamoxifen in the treatment of breast cancer. N Engl J Med. 1998;339(22):1609–18.
43. Jansen MPHM, et al. Molecular classification of tamoxifen-resistant breast carcinomas by gene expression profiling. J Clin Oncol. 2005;23(4):732.
44. Kok M, et al. Comparison of gene expression profiles predicting progression in breast cancer patients treated with tamoxifen. Breast Cancer Res Treat. 2009;113(2):275–83.
45. Chanrion M, et al. A gene expression signature that can predict the recurrence of tamoxifen-treated primary breast cancer. Clin Cancer Res. 2008;14(6):1744.
46. Allegra JC, et al. An association between steroid hormone receptors and response to cytotoxic chemotherapy in patients with metastatic breast cancer. Cancer Res. 1978;38(11 Pt 2):4299–304.
47. Berry DA, et al. Estrogen-receptor status and outcomes of modern chemotherapy for patients with node-positive breast cancer. JAMA. 2006;295(14):1658–67
48. Thurlimann B, et al. Is chemotherapy necessary for premenopausal women with lower-risk node-positive, endocrine responsive breast cancer? 10-year update of International Breast Cancer Study Group trial 11–93. Breast Cancer Res Treat. 2009;113(1):137–44.
49. Paik S, et al. A multigene assay to predict recurrence of tamoxifen-treated, node-negative breast cancer. N Engl J Med. 2004;351(27):2817–26.
50. Early Breast Cancer Trialists' Collaborative, G., et al., Relevance of breast cancer hormone receptors and other factors to the efficacy of adjuvant tamoxifen: patient-level meta-analysis of randomised trials. Lancet, 2011;378(9793):771–784.
51. Untch M, et al. Estimating the magnitude of trastuzumab effects within patient subgroups in the HERA trial. Ann Oncol. 2008;19(6):1090–6.

52. Colleoni M, et al. Increasing steroid hormone receptors expression defines breast cancer subtypes non responsive to preoperative chemotherapy. Breast Cancer Res Treat. 2009;116(2):359–69.
53. Ellis MJ, et al. Letrozole is more effective neoadjuvant endocrine therapy than tamoxifen for ErbB-1- and/or ErbB-2-positive, estrogen receptor-positive primary breast cancer: evidence from a phase III randomized trial. J Clin Oncol. 2001;19(18):3808–16.
54. Buzdar AU, Vergote I, Sainsbury R. The impact of hormone receptor status on the clinical efficacy of the new-generation aromatase inhibitors: a review of data from first-line metastatic disease trials in postmenopausal women. Breast J. 2004;10(3):211–7.
55. Immunocytochemistry. Improving immunocytochemistry for over 25 years. UK NEQAS ICC and ISH for Immunocytochemistry and In Situ Hybridisation 2013, Run 103/32. (http://www.ukneqasicc.ucl.ac.uk/Run_103_Journal.pdf).

Chapter 9
Molecular Pathology of HER Family of Oncogenes in Breast Cancer: HER-2 Evaluation and Role in Targeted Therapy

Ali Sakhdari, Lloyd Hutchinson and Ediz F. Cosar

Background

Currently, there are four different members in the epidermal growth factor receptor (EGFR) family. These consist of the erbB lineage of proteins and include erbB1 (EGFR), erbB2 (HER2), erbB3, and erbB4. Each of these molecules consists of an extracellular domain, a single hydrophobic transmembrane segment, an intracellular portion with a juxtamembrane segment, a protein kinase domain, and a carboxy terminal tail [1–3].

The *human epidermal growth factor receptor-2* (*HER2* or *ERBB2*) gene product is a transmembrane growth factor receptor, which is normally expressed in secretory epithelia. It is involved in the cellular signaling that regulates growth and development [3–5]. Other HER (ErbB) proteins can preferentially heterodimerize with HER2, which leads to phosphorylation of the tyrosine residues and activation of downstream effectors such as mitogen activating protein kinase (MAPK), phosphatidylinositol-3 kinase (PI3K), and signal transducer and activator of transcription (STAT). Depending on the particular signal cascades triggered, HER2 can be involved in different biological processes, including cell survival, proliferation, differentiation, invasion, adhesion, migration, and angiogenesis, as well as malignant transformation (Fig. 9.1) [6–8].

A. Sakhdari · L. Hutchinson · E.F. Cosar (✉)
Department of Pathology, University of Massachusetts Medical School,
UMassMemorial Medical Center, Three Biotech, One Innovation Drive,
Worcester, MA 01605, USA
e-mail: Ediz.Cosar@umassmemorial.org

© Springer Science+Business Media New York 2015
A. Khan et al. (eds.), *Precision Molecular Pathology of Breast Cancer*,
Molecular Pathology Library 10, DOI 10.1007/978-1-4939-2886-6_9

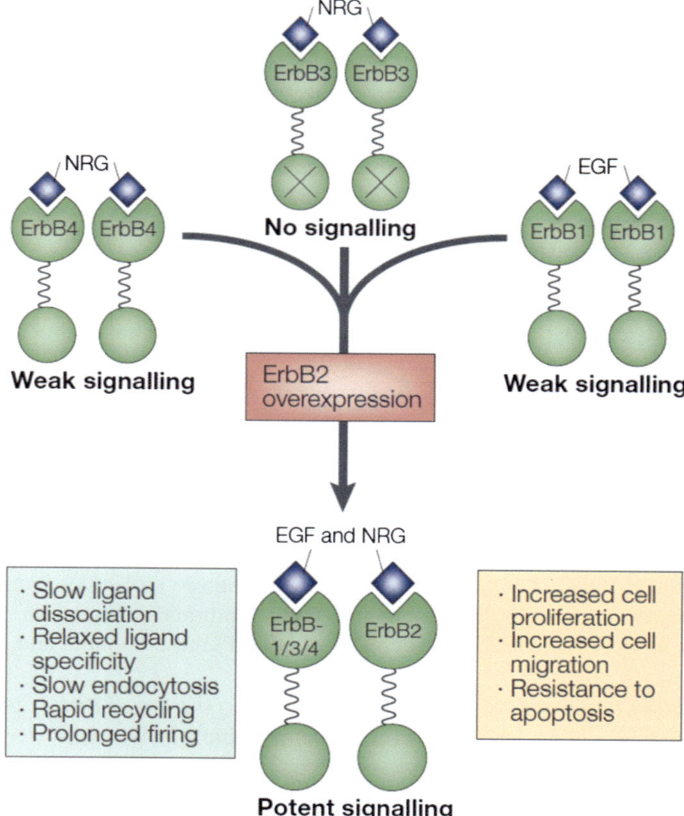

Fig. 9.1 Signaling by ErbB homodimers in comparison with ErbB2-containing heterodimers. Receptors are shown as two lobes connected by a transmembrane stretch. Binding of a ligand (EGF-like or NRG) to the extracellular lobe of ErbB1, ErbB3 (*note* inactive kinase, marked by a cross), or ErbB4 induces homodimer formation. Unlike homodimers, which are either inactive (ErbB3 homodimers) or signal only weakly, ErbB2-containing heterodimers have attributes that prolong and enhance downstream signaling (*green box*) and their outputs (*yellow box*). *NRG* Neuregulin, *EGF* Epidermal Growth Factor. With permission from [4]. Copyright Nature Publishing Group 2001

Biology of HER2

HER2 protein is expressed at low levels in normal epithelial cells [9]. *HER2* amplification and/or overexpression, however, is often observed in several cancers of epithelial origin, such as breast, colorectal, ovarian, pancreatic, and renal cell carcinomas [9, 10]. Studies using erbB2-deficient mouse models have shown lethal neural and cardiac defects during embryonic development [3, 11]. Over the past 20 years many mouse models have been developed to study the role of *HER2* gene expression in breast cancer. These studies have shown that the erbB2 receptor can have a causal role in the development of breast carcinoma [12, 13].

The erbB-receptor family plays a crucial role in cell lineage differentiation into many tissue types, including the epithelial–mesenchymal transformation in epithelial tissues [14]. Although no ligand has been identified for erbB2, the receptor is recruited into heterodimers with other erbB receptors and this process increases ligand binding affinity of other erbB-receptor family members. Among erbB-family members, HER2 is the favored receptor for heterodimerization [6, 15].

Several mechanisms have been proposed to explain the role of erbB2 in oncogenesis. For instance, overexpression of erbB2 on the cell membrane may lead to increased heterodimerization with the kinase-defective erbB3 (HER3). These heterodimers may undergo a conformational change into the ligand-active state leading to weak, but prolonged activation of the receptor. Alternatively, spontaneous erbB2 homodimers may be formed upon overexpression of the protein with subsequent activation of the receptor tyrosine kinase [4, 16–18].

HER2 in Clinical Setting

HER2 overexpression can be seen in a number of tumors, including, but not limited to, breast, gastroesophageal, endometrial, lung, ovarian, bladder, and pancreatic carcinomas [17, 19–27]. *HER2* gene amplification is the most common mechanism driving HER2 protein overexpression. This mechanism is observed in 15–20 % of breast and gastroesophageal carcinomas and at lower rates in other carcinomas [21, 24, 26]. In normal breast tissue, the ductal epithelial cells display an average of 80,000–100,000 HER2 receptors on the cell surface, whereas breast carcinoma cells can show 500,000 to 1,000,000 receptors on their surface [28–31].

Overexpression of HER2 receptor in breast cancer leads to increased homodimerization (HER2:HER2) and heterodimerization (e.g., HER2:HER3) of the receptors, which initiates a strong pro-tumorigenic signaling cascade [4].

HER2 gene amplification has been associated with a more aggressive clinical course.

In addition, *HER2* gene amplification in breast carcinoma correlates with lymph node metastasis, negative hormone receptor status, high nuclear grade, and high proliferation index, such as high Ki67 positivity or increased mitotic activity [31–37].

Current evidence suggests that HER2 receptor overexpression can serve as a negative prognostic indicator [38]. HER2 protein overexpression has consistently been shown to act as an independent marker of poor prognosis in patients with lymph node-positive disease. Interestingly, this feature is often found in concert with other poor prognostic factors, such as large tumor size, higher histologic grade, or positive nodal status [29, 32, 38, 39].

Therapies Targeting HER2

HER2 gene amplification represents the underlying molecular event for the vast majority of HER2-driven breast cancers [40–44]. Since HER2 receptor plays a role in biological and clinical behavior of breast cancers, targeting this receptor in breast carcinomas with HER2 overexpression has been an attractive therapeutic approach. HER2 was the first molecule to be targeted with a novel humanized monoclonal antibody [45].

In 1998, the U.S. Food and Drug Administration (FDA) approved trastuzumab (Genentech, Inc., San Francisco, California), a humanized monoclonal antibody that targets the extracellular portion of the HER2 receptor. Clinical trials with trastuzumab showed that this treatment improves survival, response rates, and time to progression when used alone or in combination with chemotherapy [46–49]. Although approved for use in metastatic cancer, several prospective randomized clinical trials have also shown therapeutic benefit of trastuzumab in early stage breast cancers, by reducing the mortality rate by one-third and recurrence rate by one-half [50–55]. This therapy has been shown to be effective as a single agent or in combination with more traditional chemotherapy [56–59]. However, both clinical and in vitro studies have demonstrated that trastuzumab is only active against HER2-overexpressing (HER2 positive) tumors [49, 56, 58, 60]. There are also several reports showing that patients with relatively lower expression of HER2 protein on the cell surface derive some benefit from anti-HER2 therapy [61, 62].

Lapatinib (GlaxoSmithKline, King of Prussia, Pennsylvania), a tyrosine kinase inhibitor of HER2 and EGFR was the next therapeutic agent approved by the FDA for the treatment of HER2 positive breast cancers. Lapatinib is an ATP competitor that blocks phosphorylation of the HER2/EGFR1 tyrosine kinase domains inhibiting activation of AKT/PIK3CA and MAP kinase pathways. Lapatinib provided a significant improvement in disease-free survival of breast cancer patients after progression on trastuzumab [45, 63–65].

More recently, additional monoclonal antibody therapies have been approved for the treatment of HER2 positive metastatic breast cancer. In one instance, the original trastuzumab antibody has been conjugated to the cytotoxic agent mertansine. In one study, this antibody-drug conjugate, ado-trastuzumab emtansine (T-DM1), offered a better tolerance and improved both progression-free and overall survival when compared with the standard drug combination lapatinib–capecitabine [66]. A meta-analysis indicates that this antibody-drug conjugate is effective for HER2-positive metastatic breast cancer in patients previously treated with a variety of therapeutic agents, including trastuzumab, lapatinib, and a taxane [67, 68].

Another recently approved frontline therapy for HER2 positive metastatic breast cancer is the monoclonal antibody pertuzumab (Genentech, Inc) [69–73]. This represents a new class of monoclonal antibody that targets a different site on the HER2 molecule. Unlike trastuzumab, which binds to extracellular domain IV [74], a region that does not contribute to receptor dimerization, pertuzumab binds to domain II and blocks dimerization of the HER2 receptor. In vitro studies have shown that pertuzumab is more effective than trastuzumab in disrupting the HER1–HER2 and HER3–HER2 dimers [75, 76]. Several clinical trials are currently underway to show efficacy and potential side effects of these therapeutic agents (NCT01966471, NCT01855828, NCT02003209). These new HER2-targeting agents have been tested in the adjuvant setting, including trials with single agent or dual antibody regimens without concomitant or sequential chemotherapy [72, 77–82]. So far, pertuzumab therapy is associated with increased progression-free survival and a strong trend toward improved overall survival [73]. All of these ongoing efforts point to the fact that accurate HER2 testing is now more critical than ever to ensure that the patients receive the correct treatment.

Resistance to HER2 Targeted Therapy

The fact that still a fraction of HER2 positive breast carcinomas treated with these targeted therapies ultimately relapse or develop a more progressive disease, suggests that there are some de novo or acquired intrinsic mechanisms of resistance to these drugs [83]. Resistance may be innate or develop during the course of HER2-targeted therapy. Some of these mechanisms include mutations in *HER2* gene itself, the use of compensatory signaling pathways and other resistance mutations affecting response to therapy (e.g., apoptosis). Mechanisms involving HER2 receptor alter the antibody binding site through alternative transcription and splicing. Compensatory signaling through other receptor or intracellular signaling pathways, such as insulin-like growth factor 1 receptor (IGF-1R), which widely bypass the HER2 receptor signaling, may also occur (Fig. 9.2). In addition, acquired mutations in *PIK3CA* or *PTEN* genes have been shown to confer resistance to trastuzumab. Finally, defects in cell cycle regulation or apoptosis, such as elevated levels of the apoptosis inhibitor survivin, as well as host factors that affect the immunomodulatory function of these drugs, may contribute to resistance [83–95].

Methods of HER2 Testing

Accurate determination of HER2 status is essential, given the significant therapeutic benefit derived from targeted therapy in HER2 positive tumors. This is underscored by the most recent American Society of Clinical Oncology/College of American Pathologists (ASCO/CAP) recommendations, which require HER2 testing of all newly diagnosed invasive breast cancers [95]. In addition, these therapeutic agents are not without complications or even serious side effects, necessitating the proper selection of patients who really benefit from them [96–98].

There are several methods that can be used to assess routine formalin-fixed paraffin-embedded (FFPE) clinical breast samples for HER2 status. These include

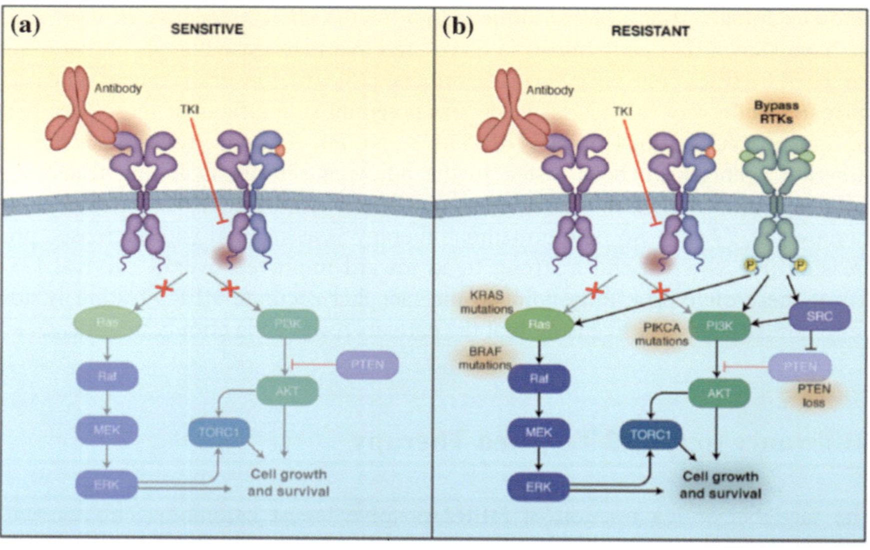

Fig. 9.2 Schematic depicting resistance to EGFR and HER2 inhibitors due to activation of bypass track signaling. **a** model of a sensitive EGFR or HER2-addicted cancer treated with an erbB small-molecule inhibitor or antibody resulting in suppression of downstream signaling. EGFR or HER2 homodimers and heterodimers are shown. **b** Model of an EGFR-mutant or *HER2*-amplified cancer with resistance due to maintenance of downstream signaling in the presence of the EGFR or HER2 inhibitors. Activation of signaling can be caused by activation of other receptor tyrosine kinases (RTKs) or mutational activation of downstream signaling. With permission from [83]. Copyright Elsevier 2014

the evaluation for HER2 protein overexpression at the tumor cell membrane by immunohistochemistry (IHC), the assessment of *HER2* gene amplification by in situ hybridization [fluorescence in situ hybridization (FISH), chromogenic in situ hybridization (CISH), silver in situ hybridization (SISH)], by multiplex ligation-dependent probe amplification or reverse transcription polymerase chain reaction (RT-PCR) [99–103].

Two of these methods, namely IHC and FISH, have been studied more thoroughly and gained popularity for assessing HER2 status in breast carcinomas in routine clinical practice. These methods offer several advantages. Both of these assays allow correlation between HER2 protein expression or *HER2* gene status and the morphologic features in tissue sections. Both methodologies have received FDA approval for HER2 evaluation [104, 105].

Assessment of HER2 Status by IHC

There are two FDA-approved antibodies, namely Herceptest (Dako, Carpinteria, California) and Pathway (Ventana, Tucson, Arizona), which may be used to assess HER2 protein status by IHC. These IHC systems have been reviewed in more detail elsewhere [95, 106]. A standardized scoring system for IHC studies has been developed and was most recently updated in 2013 (Fig. 9.3) [95, 104, 105].

Briefly, a positive HER2 IHC is defined by intense, complete circumferential membrane staining in >10 % of invasive tumor cells (score 3+). HER2 IHC result is negative if weak and incomplete pattern of staining is seen in ≤10 % of tumor cells (score 0/1+). In approximately 20 % of cases, an equivocal result is observed showing incomplete and/or weak to moderate circumferential staining in >10 % of the invasive tumor cells or complete and intense circumferential membrane staining is present in ≤10 % of the invasive tumor cells. All equivocal HER2 results should be reflexed to an alternative testing (i.e., FISH or CISH) on the same or another specimen, if available (Fig. 9.4) [95].

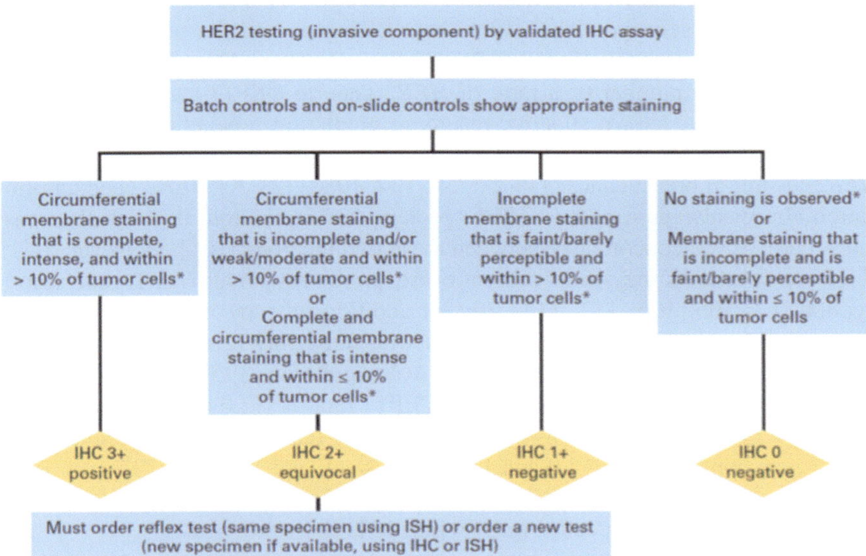

Fig. 9.3 Algorithm for evaluation of HER2 protein expression by IHC assay of the invasive component of a breast cancer specimen. *ISH* in situ hybridization. (*Asterisk*) Readily appreciated using a low-power objective and observed within a homogeneous and contiguous invasive tumor cell population. With permission from [95]. Copyright American Society of Clinical Oncology 2014

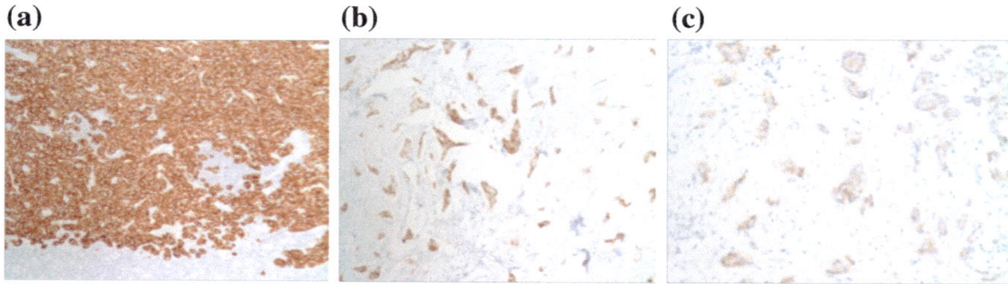

Fig. 9.4 HER2 immunohistochemistry showing 3+ (**a**); 2+ (**b**); and 1+ (**c**) staining in invasive breast carcinoma (a, b, c 100× magnification)

Assessment of HER2 Status by FISH

FISH is a molecular cytogenetic technique designed to detect specific chromosomal DNA sequences using fluorescent-labeled complementary DNA probes [106, 107]. There are three FDA-approved FISH probes manufactured by Abbott (PathVysion, Des Plaines, Illinois), Dako (HER2 FISH pharmaDx), and Ventana (INFORM, Tucson, Arizona) to assess *HER2* gene status. These FISH systems have been reviewed in more detail elsewhere [95, 106]. A standardized scoring system for FISH has been developed and was most recently updated in 2013 (Figs. 9.5 and 9.6) [95, 104, 105].

Probe sets for HER2 may include a single-color HER2 probe or dual-color probes with one sequence labeled for the *HER2* gene and the other for the centromere of chromosome 17 (CEP17). To determine amplification, an absolute *HER2* gene copy number or a ratio of *HER2* gene to CEP17 can be used. Since FISH studies have shown superior results in predicting a benefit from monoclonal antibody therapy, this approach has gained acceptance as a primary mode for *HER2* testing in breast cancer [49, 56, 59, 100, 108–112]. As *HER2* gene amplification almost always results in HER2 protein overexpression, it generally translates to 90−95 % concordance between these two methods [105]. However, 3−15 % of breast cancers may show protein overexpression without *HER2* gene amplification [63, 105, 106, 113, 114]. Recent addition of copy number to the scoring guidelines may help to identify cases with polysomy (greater than 2 copies) of chromosome 17 with HER2 protein overexpression. FISH result should be reported as positive, if dual-probe *HER2*/CEP17 ratio is ≥2.0 or an average *HER2* gene copy number ≥6.0 signals/cell. An equivocal result is defined as an average *HER2* gene copy number ≥4.0 and <6.0 signals/cell and *HER2*/CEP17 ratio <2.0. Negative result is defined as *HER2*/CEP17 ratio <2.0 and an average *HER2* gene copy number <4.0 signals/cell (Fig. 9.7) [95, 104, 108].

Although true polysomy 17 is not a common finding in breast carcinoma [115–117], in the presence of simultaneous increase in CEP17 and *HER2* gene copy number, the ratio of *HER2*/CEP17 may remain less than 2.0 and mask the true amplification of the *HER2* gene [118, 119]. In this regard, several other genes on

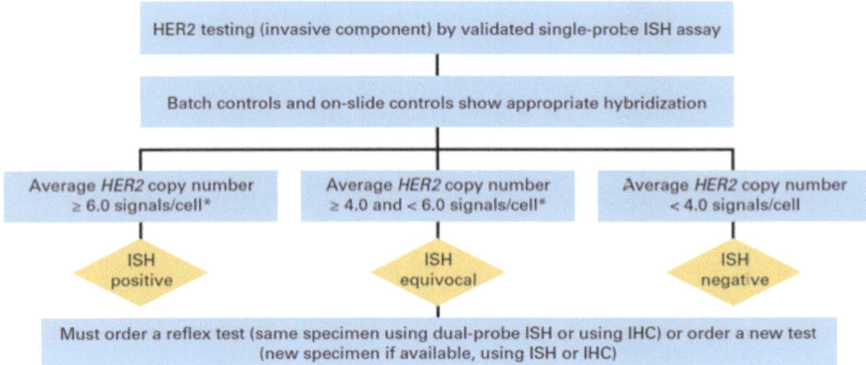

Fig. 9.5 Algorithm for evaluation of *HER2* gene amplification by ISH assay of the invasive component of a breast cancer specimen using a single-signal (*HER2* gene) assay (single-probe ISH). Amplification in a single-probe ISH assay is defined by examining the average *HER2* gene copy number. If there is a second contiguous population of cells with increased HER2 signals per cell, and this cell population consists of more than 10 % of tumor cells on the slide, a separate counting of at least 20 nonoverlapping tumor cells must also be performed within this cell population and also reported. (*Asterisk*) Observed in a homogeneous and contiguous population. With permission from [95]. Copyright American Society of Clinical Oncology 2014

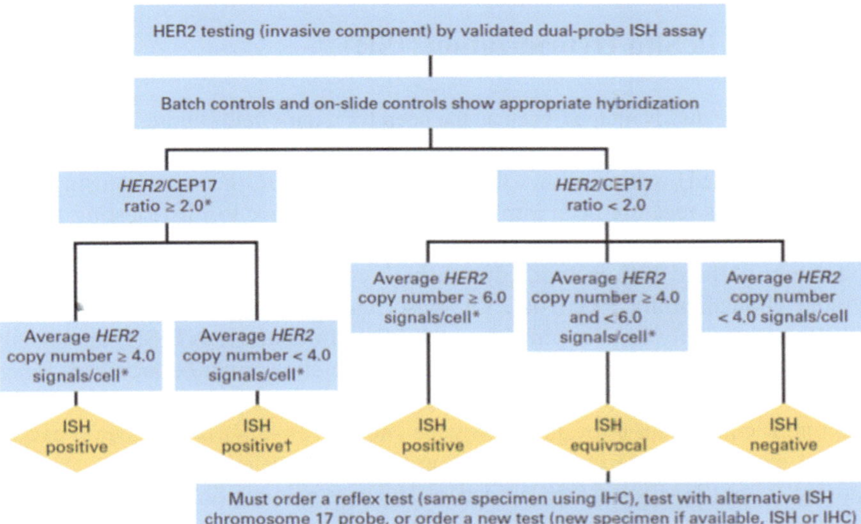

Fig. 9.6 Algorithm for evaluation of *HER2* gene amplification by ISH assay of the invasive component of a breast cancer specimen using a dual-signal (*HER2* gene) assay (dual-probe ISH). Amplification in a dual-probe ISH assay is defined by examining first the *HER2*/CEP17 ratio followed by the average *HER2* gene copy number. If there is a second contiguous population of cells with increased HER2 signals per cell, and this cell population consists of more than 10 % of tumor cells on the slide, a separate counting of at least 20 nonoverlapping tumor cells must also be performed within this cell population and also reported. CEP17, chromosome enumeration probe 17 (*Asterisk*) Observed in a homogeneous and contiguous population. With permission from [95]. Copyright American Society of Clinical Oncology 2014

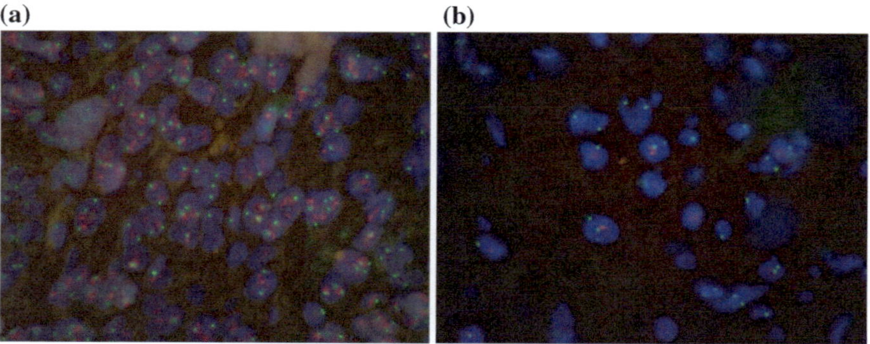

Fig. 9.7 Dual-color (*orange HER2, green* CEP17) FISH for *HER2* gene status on tissue sections from invasive breast carcinoma (a, b, 1000× magnification). **a** Tumor with *HER2* gene amplification; **b** tumor without *HER2* gene amplification

chromosome 17, such as *RARA, SMS,* or *TP53,* have been tested as alternative probes in determining the true *HER2* gene amplification and used successfully in different studies [120].

Brightfield In Situ Hybridization (ISH)

FISH has some disadvantages, such as the need for a dark field (fluorescence) microscope, which limits the ability to assess the conventional morphological details.

Brightfield ISH, which allows the user to assess *HER2* gene status using light microscopy, has recently been introduced as an alternative to FISH testing for the detection of *HER2* gene amplification. The current ASCO/CAP guidelines also endorse brightfield ISH methods due to high concordance with FISH and comparable clinical utility [95, 106]. Of these, chromogenic in situ hybridization (CISH) has recently been approved by the FDA. In contrast to FISH, the signals from these techniques do not fade. Therefore, the slides may be archived. Since CISH uses the brightfield microscopy, the viewer is able to easily locate the invasive tumor component to evaluate the gene status [121–124]. This method can be used to enumerate gene copy number (amplification, deletion) and chromosome translocation [125–128]. CISH similar to IHC uses enzyme-linked antibodies and chromogens to detect a hapten-labeled probe specific for the target DNA that can be applied to formalin-fixed paraffin-embedded (FFPE) tissues. Under the light microscopy the brown and red signals are visualized with better preservation of morphologic details. The interpretation of the signals may be difficult due to limitation in discriminating between discrete and overlapping signals on light microscopy [129]. However, the advantage of CISH over FISH in routine practice is that simultaneous verification of brightfield histology can be performed using CISH [130]. Although, CISH does not permit the actual determination of gene copy number, it has been shown to correlate with FISH [131]. Silver in situ hybridization (SISH) is a novel brightfield ISH technique [130]. It is a fully automated system which uses an enzyme-linked probe to deposit silver ions on the target site that improves the efficacy and consistency of ISH and reduces the risk of error. Automated detection of chromogenic signals also allows *HER2* and CEP17 assays to be performed on consecutive tissue slides [130], making interpretation easier and resulting in a readily identifiable signals [129, 130, 132, 133]. This strategy allows *HER2* gene status to be determined in reference to chromosome 17, so that a *HER2*/CEP17 ratio can be determined using the same reported ranges as those recommended by ASCO/CAP guidelines for FISH [129, 134]. The main disadvantage of these assays is an inherent risk of sectioning through the smaller tumors, when biopsy material is used for analysis [129, 135].

Correlation of Immunohistochemistry (IHC) with Fluorescence in Situ Hybridization (FISH)

In most studies, only cases with uniform intense circumferential membrane staining (score 3+) show a good concordance with *HER2* gene amplification detected by FISH assay. This group of patients will be the most likely to benefit from HER2 monoclonal antibody therapies [49, 56, 58, 111, 136–142]. On the contrary, when there is no HER2 membrane staining or only faint and barely perceptible incomplete staining is observed (scores 0 or 1+), gene amplification studies typically demonstrate a normal *HER2* gene status and these cases are regarded as negative [137, 138, 141, 143–145]. Cases with incomplete and/or weak to moderate circumferential membranous staining (score 2+) show poor agreement with FISH results and are considered inconclusive [66, 138, 143]. In this regard, an accurate and quantitative assessment of hormone receptor (HR) results is critical, when using IHC studies to determine therapeutic targets [95, 146, 147]. It should be emphasized that a number of pre-analytical (such as tissue handling and fixation), analytical (such as reagents, antibodies, protocols), and post-analytical (reporting, quality analysis, interpretation) factors can adversely affect immune reactivity of HER2 protein [108, 148]. These are discussed in more detail in chap. 19.

Key Points

- Currently, there are four members in EGFR family of molecules. They include erbB1 (EGFR), erbB2 (HER2), erbB3 and erbB4.
- In normal states, HER2 is expressed at low levels on the surface of epithelial cells.
- HER2 protein overexpression can be seen in a number of epithelial tumors, including breast, gastroesophageal, endometrial, ovarian and lung carcinomas.

- *HER2* gene amplification as the most common mechanism for HER2 protein overexpression is seen in 15 % to 20 % of breast carcinomas.
- HER2 protein overexpression can serve as a negative prognostic factor.
- HER2 overexpression can be determined at the protein or gene levels by IHC or ISH assays.
- HER2 overexpressing breast carcinomas can be targeted by several therapeutics, including monoclonal anti-HER2 antibodies or small molecules.
- Currently trastuzumab, pertuzumab and lapatinib have been approved by FDA as targeted therapies for breast carcinomas with HER2 protein overexpression.

References

1. Roskoski R Jr. The ErbB/HER receptor protein-tyrosine kinases and cancer. Biochem Biophys Res Commun. 2004;319(1):1–11.
2. Roskoski R Jr. ErbB/HER protein-tyrosine kinases: structures and small molecule inhibitors. Pharmacol Res. 2014;87C:42–59.
3. Burgess AW. EGFR family: structure physiology signalling and therapeutic targets. Growth Factors. 2008;26(5):263–74.
4. Yarden Y, Sliwkowski MX. Untangling the ErbB signalling network. Nat Rev Mol Cell Biol. 2001;2(2):127–37.
5. Waterman H, et al. The C-terminus of the kinase-defective neuregulin receptor ErbB-3 confers mitogenic superiority and dictates endocytic routing. EMBO J. 1999;18(12):3348–58.
6. Citri A, Skaria KB, Yarden Y. The deaf and the dumb: the biology of ErbB-2 and ErbB-3. Exp Cell Res. 2003;284(1):54–65.
7. Wallasch C, et al. Heregulin-dependent regulation of HER2/neu oncogenic signaling by heterodimerization with HER3. EMBO J. 1995;14(17):4267–75.
8. Seliger B, Kiessling R. The two sides of HER2/neu: immune escape versus surveillance. Trends Mol Med. 2013;19(11):677–84.
9. Press MF, Cordon-Cardo C, Slamon DJ. Expression of the HER-2/neu proto-oncogene in normal human adult and fetal tissues. Oncogene. 1990;5(7):953–62.
10. Seidman JD, Frisman DM, Norris HJ. Expression of the HER-2/neu proto-oncogene in serous ovarian neoplasms. Cancer. 1992;70(12):2857–60.
11. Negro A, Brar BK, Lee KF. Essential roles of Her2/erbB2 in cardiac development and function. Recent Prog Horm Res. 2004;59:1–12.
12. Suda Y, et al. Induction of a variety of tumors by c-erbB2 and clonal nature of lymphomas even with the mutated gene (Val659—Glu659). EMBO J. 1990;9(1):181–90.
13. Ursini-Siegel J, et al. Insights from transgenic mouse models of ERBB2-induced breast cancer. Nat Rev Cancer. 2007;7(5):389–97.
14. Burden S, Yarden Y. Neuregulins and their receptors: a versatile signaling module in organogenesis and oncogenesis. Neuron. 1997;18(6):847–55.
15. Citri A, Yarden Y. EGF-ERBB signalling: towards the systems level. Nat Rev Mol Cell Biol. 2006;7(7):505–16.
16. Di Fiore PP, et al. erbB-2 is a potent oncogene when overexpressed in NIH/3T3 cells. Science. 1987;237(4811):178–82.
17. Hudziak RM, Schlessinger J, Ullrich A. Increased expression of the putative growth factor receptor p185HER2 causes transformation and tumorigenesis of NIH 3T3 cells. Proc Natl Acad Sci USA. 1987;84(20):7159–63.
18. Kokai Y, et al. Synergistic interaction of p185c-neu and the EGF receptor leads to transformation of rodent fibroblasts. Cell. 1989;58(2):287–92.

19. Gonzaga IM, et al. Alterations in epidermal growth factor receptors 1 and 2 in esophageal squamous cell carcinomas. BMC Cancer. 2012;12:569.
20. Cappuzzo F, Bemis L, Varella-Garcia M. HER2 mutation and response to trastuzumab therapy in non-small-cell lung cancer. N Engl J Med. 2006;354(24):2619–21.
21. Boku N. HER2-positive gastric cancer. Gastric Cancer. 2014;17(1):1–12.
22. Boku N. Molecular target for Her2 positive gastric cancer. Nihon Shokakibyo Gakkai Zasshi. 2012;109(12):2014–20.
23. Bang YJ, et al. Trastuzumab in combination with chemotherapy versus chemotherapy alone for treatment of HER2-positive advanced gastric or gastro-oesophageal junction cancer (ToGA): a phase 3, open-label, randomised controlled trial. Lancet. 2010;376(9742):687–97.
24. Yan M, et al. HER2 aberrations in cancer: implications for therapy. Cancer Treat Rev. 2014;40(6):770–80.
25. Zhang HT, et al. New perspectives on anti-HER2/neu therapeutics. Drug News Perspect. 2000;13(6):325–9.
26. Koeppen HK, et al. Overexpression of HER2/neu in solid tumours: an immunohistochemical survey. Histopathology. 2001;38(2):96–104.
27. Chan DS, Twine CP, Lewis WG. Systematic review and meta-analysis of the influence of HER2 expression and amplification in operable oesophageal cancer. J Gastrointest Surg. 2012;16(10):1821–9.
28. Ross JS, et al. The Her-2/neu gene and protein in breast cancer 2003: biomarker and target of therapy. Oncologist. 2003;8(4):307–25.
29. Slamon DJ, et al. Human breast cancer: correlation of relapse and survival with amplification of the HER-2/neu oncogene. Science. 1987;235(4785):177–82.
30. Stefano R, et al. Expression levels and clinical-pathological correlations of HER2/neu in primary and metastatic human breast cancer. Ann NY Acad Sci. 2004;1028:463–72.
31. Yaziji H, Gown AM. Accuracy and precision in HER2/neu testing in breast cancer: are we there yet? Hum Pathol. 2004;35(2):143–6.
32. Yu D, Hung MC. Overexpression of ErbB2 in cancer and ErbB2-targeting strategies. Oncogene. 2000;19(53):6115–21.
33. Penault-Llorca F, Cayre A. Assessment of HER2 status in breast cancer. Bull Cancer. 2004;91(Suppl 4):S211–5.
34. Varga Z, et al. Assessment of HER2 status in breast cancer: overall positivity rate and accuracy by fluorescence in situ hybridization and immunohistochemistry in a single institution over 12 years: a quality control study. BMC Cancer. 2013;13:615.
35. Dowsett M, et al. Assessment of HER2 status in breast cancer: why, when and how? Eur J Cancer. 2000;36(2):170–6.
36. Yarden Y. Biology of HER2 and its importance in breast cancer. Oncology. 2001;61(Suppl 2):1–13.
37. Eccles SA. The role of c-erbB-2/HER2/neu in breast cancer progression and metastasis. J Mammary Gland Biol Neoplasia. 2001;6(4):393–406.
38. Pegram MD. Treating the HER2 pathway in early and advanced breast cancer. Hematol Oncol Clin North Am. 2013;27(4):751–65.
39. Slamon DJ, et al. Studies of the HER-2/neu proto-oncogene in human breast and ovarian cancer. Science. 1989;244(4905):707–12.
40. Gown AM. Current issues in ER and HER2 testing by IHC in breast cancer. Mod Pathol. 2008;21(Suppl 2):S8–15.
41. Garcia-Caballero T, et al. Determination of HER2 amplification in primary breast cancer using dual-colour chromogenic in situ hybridization is comparable to fluorescence in situ hybridization: a European multicentre study involving 168 specimens. Histopathology. 2010;56(4):472–80.

42. Owens MA, Horten BC, Da Silva MM. HER2 amplification ratios by fluorescence in situ hybridization and correlation with immunohistochemistry in a cohort of 6556 breast cancer tissues. Clin Breast Cancer. 2004;5(1):63–9.
43. Peintinger F, et al. Hormone receptor status and pathologic response of HER2-positive breast cancer treated with neoadjuvant chemotherapy and trastuzumab. Ann Oncol. 2008;19(12):2020–5.
44. Paik S, Kim C, Wolmark N. HER2 status and benefit from adjuvant trastuzumab in breast cancer. N Engl J Med. 2008;358(13):1409–11.
45. Robidoux A, et al. Lapatinib as a component of neoadjuvant therapy for HER2-positive operable breast cancer (NSABP protocol B-41): an open-label, randomised phase 3 trial. Lancet Oncol. 2013;14(12):1183–92.
46. Slamon D, Pegram M. Rationale for trastuzumab (Herceptin) in adjuvant breast cancer trials. Semin Oncol. 2001;28(1 Suppl 3):13–9.
47. Horton J. Trastuzumab use in breast cancer: clinical issues. Cancer Control. 2002;9(6):499–507.
48. Tan-Chiu E, Piccart M. Moving forward: herceptin in the adjuvant setting. Oncology. 2002;63(Suppl 1):57–63.
49. Vogel CL, et al. Efficacy and safety of trastuzumab as a single agent in first-line treatment of HER2-overexpressing metastatic breast cancer. J Clin Oncol. 2002;20(3):719–26.
50. Ferretti G, et al. Adjuvant trastuzumab with docetaxel or vinorelbine for HER-2-positive breast cancer. Oncologist. 2006;11(7):853–4.
51. Joensuu H, et al. Adjuvant docetaxel or vinorelbine with or without trastuzumab for breast cancer. N Engl J Med. 2006;354(8):809–20.
52. Piccart-Gebhart MJ, et al. Trastuzumab after adjuvant chemotherapy in HER2-positive breast cancer. N Engl J Med. 2005;353(16):1659–72.
53. Untch M, et al. Neoadjuvant treatment with trastuzumab in HER2-positive breast cancer: results from the GeparQuattro study. J Clin Oncol. 2010;28(12):2024–31.
54. Romond EH, et al. Trastuzumab plus adjuvant chemotherapy for operable HER2-positive breast cancer. N Engl J Med. 2005;353(16):1673–84.
55. Smith I, et al. 2-year follow-up of trastuzumab after adjuvant chemotherapy in HER2-positive breast cancer: a randomised controlled trial. Lancet. 2007;369(9555):29–36.
56. Slamon DJ, et al. Use of chemotherapy plus a monoclonal antibody against HER2 for metastatic breast cancer that overexpresses HER2. N Engl J Med. 2001;344(11):783–92.
57. Pegram MD, et al. Rational combinations of trastuzumab with chemotherapeutic drugs used in the treatment of breast cancer. J Natl Cancer Inst. 2004;96(10):739–49.
58. Tedesco KL, et al. Docetaxel combined with trastuzumab is an active regimen in HER-2 3+ overexpressing and fluorescent in situ hybridization-positive metastatic breast cancer: a multi-institutional phase II trial. J Clin Oncol. 2004;22(6):1071–7.
59. Cobleigh MA, et al. Multinational study of the efficacy and safety of humanized anti-HER2 monoclonal antibody in women who have HER2-overexpressing metastatic breast cancer that has progressed after chemotherapy for metastatic disease. J Clin Oncol. 1999;17(9):2639–48.
60. Pegram M, Slamon D. Biological rationale for HER2/neu (c-erbB2) as a target for monoclonal antibody therapy. Semin Oncol. 2000;27(5 Suppl 9):13–9.
61. Borley A, et al. Impact of HER2 copy number in IHC2+/FISH-amplified breast cancer on outcome of adjuvant trastuzumab treatment in a large UK cancer network. Br J Cancer. 2014;110(8):2139–43.
62. Dowsett M, et al. Disease-free survival according to degree of HER2 amplification for patients treated with adjuvant chemotherapy with or without 1 year of trastuzumab: the HERA Trial. J Clin Oncol. 2009;27(18):2962–9.
63. Sauter G, et al. Guidelines for human epidermal growth factor receptor 2 testing: biologic and methodologic considerations. J Clin Oncol. 2009;27(8):1323–33.
64. Inoue T, et al. Clinical evaluation of lapatinib therapy in metastatic breast cancer using the Bayes meta-analysis. Gan Kagaku Ryoho. 2014;41(3):347–52.

65. Garcia-Munoz C, et al. Lapatinib plus transtuzumab for HER-2 positiva metastatic breast cancer: experience of use. Farm Hosp. 2014;38(2):130–4.
66. Verma S, et al. Trastuzumab emtansine for HER2-positive advanced breast cancer. N Engl J Med. 2012;367(19):1783–91.
67. Krop IE, et al. Trastuzumab emtansine versus treatment of physician's choice for pretreated HER2-positive advanced breast cancer (TH3RESA): a randomised, open-label, phase 3 trial. Lancet Oncol. 2014;15(7):689–99.
68. Corrigan PA, et al. Ado-trastuzumab Emtansine: A HER2-positive targeted antibody-drug conjugate. Ann Pharmacother. 2014;48:1484–93.
69. Lynce F, Swain SM. Pertuzumab for the treatment of breast cancer. Cancer Invest. 2014;32:430–8.
70. McCormack PL. Pertuzumab: a review of its use for first-line combination treatment of HER2-positive metastatic breast cancer. Drugs. 2013;73(13):1491–502.
71. O'Sullivan CC, Connolly RM. Pertuzumab and its accelerated approval: evolving treatment paradigms and new challenges in the management of HER2-positive breast cancer. Oncology (Williston Park). 2014;28(3):186–94 196.
72. Gianni L, et al. Efficacy and safety of neoadjuvant pertuzumab and trastuzumab in women with locally advanced, inflammatory, or early HER2-positive breast cancer (NeoSphere): a randomised multicentre, open-label, phase 2 trial. Lancet Oncol. 2012;13(1):25–32.
73. Schneeweiss A, et al. Pertuzumab plus trastuzumab in combination with standard neoadjuvant anthracycline-containing and anthracycline-free chemotherapy regimens in patients with HER2-positive early breast cancer: a randomized phase II cardiac safety study (TRYPHAENA). Ann Oncol. 2013;24(9):2278–84.
74. Cho HS, et al. Structure of the extracellular region of HER2 alone and in complex with the Herceptin Fab. Nature. 2003;421(6924):756–60.
75. Jhaveri K, Esteva FJ. Pertuzumab in the treatment of HER2+ breast cancer. J Natl Compr Canc Netw. 2014;12(4):591–8.
76. Franklin MC, et al. Insights into ErbB signaling from the structure of the ErbB2-pertuzumab complex. Cancer Cell. 2004;5(4):317–28.
77. Swain SM, et al. Pertuzumab, trastuzumab, and docetaxel for HER2-positive metastatic breast cancer (CLEOPATRA study): overall survival results from a randomised, double-blind, placebo-controlled, phase 3 study. Lancet Oncol. 2013;14(6):461–71.
78. Baselga J, et al. Pertuzumab plus trastuzumab plus docetaxel for metastatic breast cancer. N Engl J Med. 2012;366(2):109–19.
79. de Azambuja E, et al. Lapatinib with trastuzumab for HER2-positive early breast cancer (NeoALTTO): survival outcomes of a randomised, open-label, multicentre, phase 3 trial and their association with pathological complete response. Lancet Oncol. 2014;15(10):1137–46.
80. Baselga J, et al. Lapatinib with trastuzumab for HER2-positive early breast cancer (NeoALTTO): a randomised, open-label, multicentre, phase 3 trial. Lancet. 2012;379(9816):633–40.
81. Baselga J, Swain SM. CLEOPATRA: a phase III evaluation of pertuzumab and trastuzumab for HER2-positive metastatic breast cancer. Clin Breast Cancer. 2010;10(6):489–91.
82. Blackwell KL, et al. Randomized study of Lapatinib alone or in combination with trastuzumab in women with ErbB2-positive, trastuzumab-refractory metastatic breast cancer. J Clin Oncol. 2010;28(7):1124–30.
83. Arteaga CL, Engelman JA. ERBB receptors: from oncogene discovery to basic science to mechanism-based cancer therapeutics. Cancer Cell. 2014;25(3):282–303.
84. Engelman JA, et al. MET amplification leads to gefitinib resistance in lung cancer by activating ERBB3 signaling. Science. 2007;316(5827):1039–43.
85. Nahta R, et al. Insulin-like growth factor-I receptor/human epidermal growth factor receptor 2 heterodimerization contributes to trastuzumab resistance of breast cancer cells. Cancer Res. 2005;65(23):11118–28.
86. Lu Y, et al. Insulin-like growth factor-I receptor signaling and resistance to trastuzumab (Herceptin). J Natl Cancer Inst. 2001;93(24):1852–7.

87. Berns K, et al. A functional genetic approach identifies the PI3K pathway as a major determinant of trastuzumab resistance in breast cancer. Cancer Cell. 2007;12(4):395–402.
88. Nagata Y, et al. PTEN activation contributes to tumor inhibition by trastuzumab, and loss of PTEN predicts trastuzumab resistance in patients. Cancer Cell. 2004;6(2):117–27.
89. Esteva FJ, et al. PTEN, PIK3CA, p-AKT, and p-p70S6 K status: association with trastuzumab response and survival in patients with HER2-positive metastatic breast cancer. Am J Pathol. 2010;177(4):1647–56.
90. Xia W, et al. A model of acquired autoresistance to a potent ErbB2 tyrosine kinase inhibitor and a therapeutic strategy to prevent its onset in breast cancer. Proc Natl Acad Sci USA. 2006;103(20):7795–800.
91. Valabrega G, et al. HER2-positive breast cancer cells resistant to trastuzumab and lapatinib lose reliance upon HER2 and are sensitive to the multitargeted kinase inhibitor sorafenib. Breast Cancer Res Treat. 2011;130(1):29–40.
92. Oliveras-Ferraros C, et al. Inhibitor of Apoptosis (IAP) survivin is indispensable for survival of HER2 gene-amplified breast cancer cells with primary resistance to HER1/2-targeted therapies. Biochem Biophys Res Commun. 2011;407(2):412–9.
93. Musolino A, et al. Immunoglobulin G fragment C receptor polymorphisms and clinical efficacy of trastuzumab-based therapy in patients with HER-2/neu-positive metastatic breast cancer. J Clin Oncol. 2008;26(11):1789–96.
94. Gennari R, et al. Pilot study of the mechanism of action of preoperative trastuzumab in patients with primary operable breast tumors overexpressing HER2. Clin Cancer Res. 2004;10(17):5650–5.
95. Wolff AC, et al. Recommendations for human epidermal growth factor receptor 2 testing in breast cancer: American Society of clinical oncology/college of American pathologists clinical practice guideline update. J Clin Oncol. 2013;31(31):3997–4013.
96. Keefe DL. Trastuzumab-associated cardiotoxicity. Cancer. 2002;95(7):1592–600.
97. Ewer SM, Ewer MS. Cardiotoxicity profile of trastuzumab. Drug Saf. 2008;31(6):459–67.
98. Babar T, et al. Anti-HER2 cancer therapy and cardiotoxicity. Curr Pharm Des. 2014;20(30):4911–9.
99. Moelans CB, et al. Current technologies for HER2 testing in breast cancer. Crit Rev Oncol Hematol. 2011;80(3):380–92.
100. Pauletti G, et al. Assessment of methods for tissue-based detection of the HER-2/neu alteration in human breast cancer: a direct comparison of fluorescence in situ hybridization and immunohistochemistry. J Clin Oncol. 2000;18(21):3651–64.
101. Xing WR, et al. FISH detection of HER-2/neu oncogene amplification in early onset breast cancer. Breast Cancer Res Treat. 1996;39(2):203–12.
102. Persons DL, et al. Fluorescence in situ hybridization (FISH) for detection of HER-2/neu amplification in breast cancer: a multicenter portability study. Ann Clin Lab Sci. 2000;30(1):41–8.
103. Susini T, et al. Preoperative assessment of HER-2/neu status in breast carcinoma: the role of quantitative real-time PCR on core-biopsy specimens. Gynecol Oncol. 2010;116(2):234–9.
104. Wolff AC, et al. Recommendations for human epidermal growth factor receptor 2 testing in breast cancer: American Society of clinical oncology/college of American pathologists clinical practice guideline update. Arch Pathol Lab Med. 2014;138(2):241–56.
105. Wolff AC, et al. American Society of clinical oncology/college of American pathologists guideline recommendations for human epidermal growth factor receptor 2 testing in breast cancer. Arch Pathol Lab Med. 2007;131(1):18–43.
106. Wolff AC, et al. American Society of clinical oncology/college of American pathologists guideline recommendations for human epidermal growth factor receptor 2 testing in breast cancer. J Clin Oncol. 2007;25(1):118–45.
107. Bartlett J, Mallon E, Cooke T. The clinical evaluation of HER-2 status: which test to use? J Pathol. 2003;199(4):411–7.
108. Cornejo KM, et al. Theranostic and molecular classification of breast cancer. Arch Pathol Lab Med. 2014;138(1):44–56.

109. Shak S. Overview of the trastuzumab (Herceptin) anti-HER2 monoclonal antibody clinical program in HER2-overexpressing metastatic breast cancer. Herceptin multinational investigator study group. Semin Oncol. 1999;26((4 Suppl 12)):71–7.

110. Ross JS, et al. HER-2/neu testing in breast cancer. Am J Clin Pathol. 2003;120(Suppl):S53–71.

111. Press MF, et al. Evaluation of HER-2/neu gene amplification and overexpression: comparison of frequently used assay methods in a molecularly characterized cohort of breast cancer specimens. J Clin Oncol. 2002;20(14):3095–105.

112. Addition of trastuzumab to chemotherapy produces 50 % increase in survival in patients selected by FISH. Oncology (Williston Park), 2001; 15(10): 1345, 1364.

113. Dyhdalo KS, et al. Laboratory compliance with the american society of clinical oncology/college of american pathologists human epidermal growth factor receptor 2 testing guidelines: a 3-year comparison of validation procedures. Arch Pathol Lab Med. 2014;138(7):876–84.

114. Grimm EE, et al. Achieving 95 % cross-methodological concordance in HER2 testing: causes and implications of discordant cases. Am J Clin Pathol. 2010;134(2):284–92.

115. Moelans CB, de Weger RA, van Diest PJ. Absence of chromosome 17 polysomy in breast cancer: analysis by CEP17 chromogenic in situ hybridization and multiplex ligation-dependent probe amplification. Breast Cancer Res Treat. 2010;120(1):1–7.

116. Yeh IT, et al. Clinical validation of an array CGH test for HER2 status in breast cancer reveals that polysomy 17 is a rare event. Mod Pathol. 2009;22(9):1169–75.

117. Viale G. Be precise! The need to consider the mechanisms for CEP17 copy number changes in breast cancer. J Pathol. 2009;219(1):1–2.

118. Vranic S, et al. Assessment of HER2 gene status in breast carcinomas with polysomy of chromosome 17. Cancer. 2011;117(1):48–53.

119. Perez EA, et al. HER2 and chromosome 17 effect on patient outcome in the N9831 adjuvant trastuzumab trial. J Clin Oncol. 2010;28(28):4307–15.

120. Tse CH, et al. Determining true HER2 gene status in breast cancers with polysomy by using alternative chromosome 17 reference genes: implications for anti-HER2 targeted therapy. J Clin Oncol. 2011;29(31):4168–74.

121. Clark BZ, Bhargava R. Bright-field microscopy for HER2 gene assessment: not just DISHful thinking? Am J Clin Pathol. 2013;139(2):137–9.

122. Bhargava R, Lal P, Chen B. Chromogenic in situ hybridization for the detection of HER-2/neu gene amplification in breast cancer with an emphasis on tumors with borderline and low-level amplification: does it measure up to fluorescence in situ hybridization? Am J Clin Pathol. 2005;123(2):237–43.

123. Isola J, et al. Interlaboratory comparison of HER-2 oncogene amplification as detected by chromogenic and fluorescence in situ hybridization. Clin Cancer Res. 2004;10(14):4793–8.

124. Mayr D, et al. Chromogenic in situ hybridization for Her-2/neu-oncogene in breast cancer: comparison of a new dual-colour chromogenic in situ hybridization with immunohistochemistry and fluorescence in situ hybridization. Histopathology. 2009;55(6):716–23.

125. Kato N, et al. Evaluation of HER2 gene amplification in invasive breast cancer using a dual-color chromogenic in situ hybridization (dual CISH). Pathol Int. 2010;60(7):510–5.

126. Todorovic-Rakovic N, et al. Prognostic value of HER2 gene amplification detected by chromogenic in situ hybridization (CISH) in metastatic breast cancer. Exp Mol Pathol. 2007;82(3):262–8.

127. Di Palma S, et al. Chromogenic in situ hybridisation (CISH) should be an accepted method in the routine diagnostic evaluation of HER2 status in breast cancer. J Clin Pathol. 2007;60(9):1067–8.

128. Arnould L, et al. Agreement between chromogenic in situ hybridisation (CISH) and FISH in the determination of HER2 status in breast cancer. Br J Cancer. 2003;88(10):1587–91.

129. Francis GD, et al. Bright-field in situ hybridization for HER2 gene amplification in breast cancer using tissue microarrays: correlation between chromogenic (CISH) and

automated silver-enhanced (SISH) methods with patient outcome. Diagn Mol Pathol. 2009;18(2):88–95.

130. Park K, et al. Silver-enhanced in situ hybridization as an alternative to fluorescence in situ hybridization for assaying HER2 amplification in clinical breast cancer. J Breast Cancer. 2011;14(4):276–82.

131. Schnitt SJ, Jacobs TW. Current status of HER2 testing: caught between a rock and a hard place. Am J Clin Pathol. 2001;116(6):806–10.

132. Bae YK, et al. HER2 status by standardized immunohistochemistry and silver-enhanced in situ hybridization in Korean breast cancer. J Breast Cancer. 2012;15(4):381–7.

133. Koh YW, et al. Dual-color silver-enhanced in situ hybridization for assessing HER2 gene amplification in breast cancer. Mod Pathol. 2011;24(6):794–800.

134. Unal B, et al. Determination of HER2 gene amplification in breast cancer using dual-color silver enhanced in situ hybridization (dc- SISH) and comparison with fluorescence ISH (FISH). Asian Pac J Cancer Prev. 2013;14(10):6131–4.

135. Jacquemier J, et al. SISH/CISH or qPCR as alternative techniques to FISH for determination of HER2 amplification status on breast tumors core needle biopsies: a multicenter experience based on 840 cases. BMC Cancer. 2013;13:351.

136. Dowsett M, et al. Correlation between immunohistochemistry (HercepTest) and fluorescence in situ hybridization (FISH) for HER-2 in 426 breast carcinomas from 37 centres. J Pathol. 2003;199(4):418–23.

137. Bilous M, et al. Current perspectives on HER2 testing: a review of national testing guidelines. Mod Pathol. 2003;16(2):173–82.

138. Ridolfi RL, Jamehdor MR, Arber JM. HER-2/neu testing in breast carcinoma: a combined immunohistochemical and fluorescence in situ hybridization approach. Mod Pathol. 2000;13(8):866–73.

139. Tubbs RR, Hicks DG. HER-2 testing in breast cancer. JAMA. 2004; 292(15): p 1817-8 (author reply 1818).

140. Lal P, et al. HER-2 testing in breast cancer using immunohistochemical analysis and fluorescence in situ hybridization: a single-institution experience of 2,279 cases and comparison of dual-color and single-color scoring. Am J Clin Pathol. 2004;121(5):631–6.

141. Yaziji H, et al. HER-2 testing in breast cancer using parallel tissue-based methods. JAMA. 2004;291(16):1972–7.

142. Elkin EB, et al. HER-2 testing and trastuzumab therapy for metastatic breast cancer: a cost-effectiveness analysis. J Clin Oncol. 2004;22(5):854–63.

143. Zhang H, et al. HER-2 gene amplification by fluorescence in situ hybridization (FISH) compared with immunohistochemistry (IHC) in breast cancer: a study of 528 equivocal cases. Breast Cancer Res Treat. 2012;134(2):743–9.

144. Goud KI, et al. Evaluation of HER-2/neu status in breast cancer specimens using immunohistochemistry (IHC) & fluorescence in-situ hybridization (FISH) assay. Indian J Med Res. 2012;135:312–7.

145. Kemp JD, Royer MC. 2+ HER-2/neu IHC results: positively equivocal. J Cutan Pathol. 2010; 37(8): p. 915; author reply 916.

146. Hammond ME, et al. American Society of clinical oncology/college of American pathologists guideline recommendations for immunohistochemical testing of estrogen and progesterone receptors in breast cancer (unabridged version). Arch Pathol Lab Med. 2010;134(7):e48–72.

147. Hammond ME, et al. American Society of clinical oncology/college of American pathologists guideline recommendations for immunohistochemical testing of estrogen and progesterone receptors in breast cancer. J Clin Oncol. 2010;28(16):2784–95.

148. Penault-Llorca F, et al. Optimization of immunohistochemical detection of ERBB2 in human breast cancer: impact of fixation. J Pathol. 1994;173(1):65–75.

Chapter 10
Molecular Classification of Breast Cancer

Mohammed A. Aleskandarany, Ian O. Ellis and Emad A. Rakha

Introduction

Breast cancer represents a heterogeneous group of tumours with different histological appearances, molecular features, varied behaviour and response to therapy. Scrutiny of these parameters at the individual level should improve patient management and therefore improves both the quality of life and the overall survival of the patient. The management of breast cancer patients currently relies on robust well-validated traditional clinicopathological prognostic factors and a limited number of predictive biomarkers (namely hormone receptors and HER2). Clinicopathological variables were the earliest used classification systems with strong overall association with patients' outcome [1]. In addition to staging variables, histological grade, which represents morphological surrogate of tumour biological features has been validated by several independent studies as an independent prognostic stratifier in breast cancer [2]. Grade is incorporated into the well-validated Nottingham Prognostic Index (NPI) with equal weighting to that of lymph node stage to guide patients' management [3]. Histological type refers to the growth pattern of the breast cancer as per microscopic examination [4] has also recognised to have prognostic value and can provide complementary prognostic information with grade [5]. Other clinicopathological prognostic variables include lymphovascular invasion, patients' age, and menopausal status. Less validated variables include presence and extent of in situ component and tumour-associated inflammatory response.

M.A. Aleskandarany · I.O. Ellis · E.A. Rakha (⊠)
Department of Histopathology, Division of Cancer and Stem Cells, School of Medicine, The University of Nottingham and Nottingham University Hospitals NHS Trust, Nottingham City Hospital, Nottingham NG5 1PB, UK
e-mail: Emad.Rakha@nottingham.ac.uk

© Springer Science+Business Media New York 2015
A. Khan et al. (eds.), *Precision Molecular Pathology of Breast Cancer*,
Molecular Pathology Library 10, DOI 10.1007/978-1-4939-2886-6_10

There are several lines of evidence to suggest that the parameters currently available are insufficient to reflect fully the biological heterogeneity of tumours, and breast cancers of similar morphological appearances still vary in their behaviour and response to therapy. For instance, up to one-third of lymph node-negative breast cancer patients, classified as being within the good prognostic group, have been reported to develop recurrence later in their disease course [6]. Similarly, an equivalent proportion of node-positive patients, assigned into the poor prognosis group, remain free of distant metastases [7]. In addition, approximately 60 % of patients with breast cancer present as node negative, 80 % as oestrogen receptor positive and more than 40 % as grade 2 tumours. Further stratification of these cohorts is critically needed. Moreover, the widespread use of mammographic screening, improved understanding of the nature and biology of breast cancer and the increasing array of systemic therapy options (hormone, chemo and targeted therapy) [8] further emphasises our need to identify and stratify novel prognostic and predictive variables in breast cancer. This, in addition to the increasingly available systemic therapies and the move towards precision medicine have emphasised the need for identification of additional molecular prognostic classifiers that can reflect the degree of breast cancer biological and clinical heterogeneity.

Whenever possible, a molecular classifier test should be able to stratify patients into well-defined clinical outcome subgroups or into high positive and negative predictive response to a specific therapy. If assessment of a molecular marker does not lead to a decision in clinical practice, then its use in routine practice is discouraged [9]. Furthermore, recommendations for clinical introduction of molecular testing should be made only when the diagnostic methodologies are reliable, patients have access to the clinical services necessary to make informed decisions and interpret the results of testing, and it becomes clinically apparent how to utilise the results.

Biological variables in breast cancer can be assessed in routine practice using morphological surrogates such as tumour differentiation, proliferation status, and lymphovascular invasion or more accurately using molecular parameters such as assessment of gene/protein status individually or in consort (e.g. molecular profiling at the level of DNA, RNA or protein). Assessment of individual gene status in routine practice can be performed using different techniques such as immunohistochemistry (IHC; proteins), in situ hybridization (*HER*2) and enzyme-linked immunosorbent assay (tumour markers). Recent advances in human genome research, high-throughput molecular technologies and advances in bioinformatics have enabled the analysis of several hundreds and thousands of genes and gene products in one experiment and allowed the analysis of genes in the context of pathways and networks tackling the molecular complexity of breast cancer. Genome-wide profiling of chromosomal changes and rapid screening of genes for mutations/single nucleotide polymorphisms and methylation can be performed using techniques such as high-resolution single nucleotide polymorphism (SNP) arrays (SNP chips) [10], array comparative genomic hybridization (CGH) [11], multiplex polymerase chain reaction (PCR) and massively parallel sequencing (next-generation sequencing) [12]. Transcriptome and proteome profiling techniques include differential display [13], serial analysis of gene expression (SAGE) [14], gene expression microarrays (global gene expression profiling; GEP) [15] and massively parallel sequencing [16]. Massively parallel sequencing combines the high throughput of SAGE with the accuracy of EST sequencing. These molecular techniques hold promise for improving diagnosis, for the prediction of recurrence, and in aiding selection of therapies for individual patients.

Single Biomarker Classifiers

Of the individual molecular markers, the oestrogen receptor (ER), the progesterone receptor (PR) and the human epidermal growth factor receptor 2 genes (HER2) have proven predictive and prognostic value. ER, PR and HER2 status, which are essential part of the diagnostic workup of all breast cancer patients and they are routinely determined using a standardised technique and well-defined published guidelines [17–19]. It is currently recognised that the main consideration for treatment decision is endocrine responsiveness. Adjuvant endocrine therapy accounts for almost two-thirds of the overall benefit of adjuvant therapy in patients with ER-positive breast cancer. Use of anti-HER2 therapy is based on risk stratification and tumour HER2 status [20]. The current gold standard to asses ER status is IHC performed on formalin-fixed, paraffin-embedded cancer tissue. This diagnostic test is routinely used in the clinic, and major therapeutic decision-making dependent on the results; however, its reliability is not perfect. It has been reported that the existing IHC assays have only modest positive predictive value (30–60 %) for response to single-agent hormonal therapies. However, the negative predictive value of ER expression is high (i.e. ER-negativity which accounts for 20–30 % of breast cancer can identify the population of patients who will not benefit from endocrine therapy) [21–24]. Therefore, it is important to identify variables that allow identification of patients who can be safely spared adjuvant therapy or benefit from hormone therapy alone or combined with chemotherapy and/or targeted therapy. Approximately 40 % of ER-positive tumours are PR negative. Lack of PR expression in ER-positive tumours may be a surrogate marker of aberrant growth factor signalling that could contribute to tamoxifen resistance and that ER+/PR− tumours are generally less responsive than ER+/PR+ tumours [25, 26]. PR status can help to predict respond to hormone treatment, both in patients with metastatic disease [27] and in the adjuvant setting. Multiple studies have provided evidence for the prognostic and predictive importance of PR assessment in BC [26, 28–30].

Amplification of *HER2* gene occurs in 13–20 % of BC and more than half (approximately 55 %) of these cases are ER-negative [31, 32]. Numerous studies found that *HER2* gene amplification/protein overexpression is a predictor of poor prognosis and response for systemic chemotherapy [33–35]. Following the development of a humanised monoclonal antibody against HER2 and clinical trials demonstrating benefit of the use of anti-HER2 agents in patients with HER2 positive breast cancer [36], the reasons for establishing the HER2 status in routine clinical practice has changed, since it is a prerequisite for clinical use of anti-HER2 in patients with HER2-positive advanced disease as well as in the adjuvant setting for HER2-positive early stage disease.

Hormone receptor and HER2 are assessed in routine practice to provide information on response to endocrine therapy and anti-HER2 targeted therapy respectively. However, the expression of these biomarkers overlap and their prognostic and predictive value can be improved by using them in combination [37] or combined with the proliferation marker Ki67 [38]. Most IHC studies have also used a combination of ER, PR and HER2 as IHC surrogates to define the molecular classes initially identified by GEP. For instance, ER/PR positivity was used as a surrogate for luminal class and HER2 expression for HER2-positive tumours, while triple-negative (ER−, PR−, HER2−) phenotype is used to define the basal-like molecular class (BLBC) [39, 40]. In addition, some authors have classified HR-positive tumours that are also HER2-positive as the Luminal B subclass [39, 41]. Therefore, ER, PR and HER2 status provides an accessible biological molecular classifier of breast cancer with defined prognostic and predictive value and their value increases when they are used in combination where they can provide a valid practical surrogate of the GEP-defined molecular classes. Some other genes which are assessed individually in breast cancer such as Ki67 [42] have been proven of specific clinical utility. IHC expression of Ki67 is now widely used as an objective molecular measure of proliferation to overcome problems related to tumour fixation and mitotic figures identification [43, 44]. Although controversy regarding routine use of Ki67 in pathology practice, several studies have yielded promising results particularly its prognostic significance in node-negative [45, 46], ER-positive [47] and in histologic grade 2 tumours [48] and as a predictor of response to chemotherapy [49, 50].

Multigene Classifiers: Gene Expression Profiling and Molecular Taxonomy

Gene expression is a technical term to describe how a particular gene is active, or how many times it is expressed or transcribed, to produce the protein it encodes. This activity is measured by counting the number of mRNA molecules in a given cell type or tissue, though protein and not RNA is the functional product of genes. Although the first description of cDNA microarrays as a tool for profiling gene expressions was in 1987 [51], GEP technique was not widely used until advances in fluorescent labelling technologies, cDNA library construction and sequencing techniques have been achieved. The total gene expression pattern of a given sample is known as a gene expression profile and such expression data are often referred to as "signatures" or "portraits" as most tumours show certain expression profiles that are unique and related to a specific biological features [52, 53].

The introduction of the concept that breast cancer can be classified using GEP by Peru and colleagues in 2000 [54] has revolutionised breast cancer research and the number of studies classifying breast cancer using molecular classifiers have markedly exceeded our expectation. In fact GEP studies have not only contributed to our current understanding of breast cancer molecular complexity but also led to the identification of distinct molecular class of clinical relevance and the development of prognostic and predictive multigene signatures. Most GEP studies of breast cancer aimed at: (i) identifying specific molecular classes (class discovery; molecular taxonomy) that have biological and clinical relevance, which are unidentifiable by conventional means [54–56]. (ii) identifying specific molecular profile "gene signatures" that can predict tumour behaviour [57–60] and/or response to therapy [61–63] (class prediction). (iii) comparison of different "predefined" classes of breast cancer (class comparison) that aims to determine whether the expression profiles are different between these classes and, if so, to identify the differentially expressed genes [64–69].

Molecular taxonomy of breast cancer have been identified three main classes including (1) a luminal subgroup, which encompasses tumours that express ER and genes related to activation of the ER pathway; (2) a HER2 subgroup, which is characterised by overexpression of HER2 and by genes pertaining to HER2 amplicon; and (3) a subgroup of tumours that do not cluster with either luminal or HER2-positive tumours; the basal-like class, which is largely characterised by positive expression of basal cytokeratins and other genes that are characteristic of basal-like cells of the breast and by high proliferative activity [9–11, 19, 43]. Although HER2 positive and ER-positive luminal tumours were known before the advent of this GEP molecular taxonomy, BLBC class attracted attention as a novel class characterised not only by triple-negative phenotype (ER-negative, PR-negative and HER2-negative) but also by the a generally similar molecular profile (tumours clustered together at the molecular level) and the poor outcome [10, 11, 19]. Importantly, these classes showed distinct clinical outcome, with luminal subtype having the most favourable, HER2 overexpressing having the most detrimental and BLBC having poor prognosis, yet still relatively better than the HER2 overexpressing non-Herceptin treated cancers [55, 70]. The luminal class has further been classified into at least two subclasses; luminal A and luminal B with significant difference in molecular profile and clinical outcome. Luminal A tumours show high expression levels of ER-activated genes and low levels of proliferation related genes and have a good outcome whilst luminal B breast cancers show higher proliferation rates and/or HER2 expression with a significantly worse prognosis than luminal A tumours [71]. Other luminal subclasses have been described including luminal C [72] and luminal N [73] subclasses. Similarly, BLBC class has further been subclassified into subgroups such as claudin-low [74] and molecular apocrine subtype, which is characterised by androgen receptor (AR) expression and AR-related pathway with paradoxical expression of ER-related genes [75]. In addition, there are a few less defined molecular subtypes, such as normal breast-like class that displays a triple-negative phenotype but does not cluster with the basal-like centroid and is characterised by expression profiles similar to those found in normal breast tissue.

Early GEP studies suggest that the luminal class of breast cancer is characterised by ER positivity and other features characteristic of luminal mammary epithelial cells but is heterogeneous with respect to the expression of other genes and outcome. Subsequent studies [76] have demonstrated that that precise positioning of an individual within the spectrum of luminal breast cancer is based on expression of other genes. For instance luminal A tumours are characterised by high expression of luminal epithelial CKs and other luminal associated markers including ER and genes associated with ER function such as LIV1, hepatocyte nuclear factor 3 alpha (FOXA1), X-box binding protein 1 (XBP1) and GATA-binding protein 3 (GATA3) [77]. Whereas the luminal B group is characterised by low-to-moderate expression of the luminal A genes mentioned above, but is further distinguished by high expression of additional genes, mainly related to proliferation such as v-MYB, GGH, LAPTMB4, NSEP1 and CCNE1 [76]. Luminal tumour subclasses are also characterised by distinct type of genomic copy alteration and different level of amplification [78]. Although the class of breast cancer that is characterised by expression of markers characteristic of basal/myoepithelial cell was actually described many years ago [79, 80], they have attracted a lot of attention in recent years after their identification in GEP as a molecularly distinct subtype of breast cancer [54]. These tumours are known as BLBC represent 16 % up to 37 % of all breast cancer cases [68, 72, 81]. This class has received attention because of its nature as a poor prognostic group and as a good candidate for development of new targeted therapy. Most studies have shown that basal tumours are mainly included within a cluster in the ER-negative and HER2 negative tumours and are largely characterised by positive expression of basal cytokeratins (CK) and other genes characteristic of basal cells of the breast. Several basal class gene products identified are important structural elements of the basal cells of the breast [54, 82–84] and extracellular matrix (ECM) receptor proteins [85]. Other gene products included several proteins that activate signalling pathways, which are commonly deregulated in cancer [86] and gene products that have been implicated in cellular proliferation, suppression of apoptosis, cell migration, invasion and extracellular remodelling have been identified [87–89]. Basal class of breast cancer (BLBC) shows a high recurrence score and a poor 70-gene profile [90]. However, these results were not confined to BLBC and found also in the HER2 and Luminal-B subtypes. When BLBC were characterised using comparative genomic hybridisation (CGH) a greater genetic complexity with high frequency of DNA losses and gains was identified when compared to other breast cancer subtypes, suggesting a greater degree of genetic instability [91–93]. These tumours seem to harbour a dysfunctional BRCA1 pathway [94] and tumours arising in *BRCA*1 mutation carriers often display a basal-like phenotype [95, 96].

Although molecular taxonomy of breast cancer has attracted a lot of attention and speculation that this would result in dramatic improvements in breast cancer management, to date actual practical adoption appears limited. Certain critical issues have been raised such as validation, reproducibility and clinical utility. Most luminal tumours are ER-positive and can be identified in routine practice using IHC. ER expression and not luminal phenotype is recognised as a validated predictor to hormone therapy. The significance of luminal ER-negative tumours is not defined. Similarly, HER2-positive breast cancer patients are likely to be offered anti-HER2 therapy when indicated regardless of their molecular classification, while it is currently not justified to offer patients with cancers classified in the HER2-positive class if their tumours did not show evidence of HER2 gene amplification. Clinical relevance needs to be considered and factored into any emerging classification system to ensure that patients are treated appropriately. Furthermore, the so-called "normal breast-like" class is not well-defined [97] and the proportion of some classes defined by GEP varied substantially [98–100]. Moreover, it remains unknown how many molecular classes exist and more importantly how many classes can be reliably identified with the currently available data. From 4 [54] up to 10 [101] classes have been described. There remain major limitations in the ability to consistently assign a molecular class to new cases of breast cancer. The four main molecular classes frequently reported can be considered as an oversimplification of a novel molecular classification system and add little to our understanding of the biology and behaviour of breast cancer. The clinical difference between BLBC (GEP) and triple-negative (IHC) is disputed with triple-negativity provides more practical routinely applicable classification preferred by oncologists. Lumping of pure tubular carcinoma with micropapillary, invasive lobular or ductal NST carcinomas into a single "luminal" class or high-grade ductal NST, high-grade metaplastic and medullary carcinomas with low-grade adenosquamous and adenoid cystic carcinomas into "BLBC" class cannot be justified biologically or clinically.

It is also important to mention that other studies have reported different number and definition of molecular classes. For instance, in a study of 2000 breast cancers using an integrated approach of copy number and gene expression in a discovery and validation sets of 997 and 995 primary breast cancers, 10 novel molecular subgroups were reported [101]. These molecular classes were names as integrative clusters since they were defined based on both geneomic and transcriptomic profiles with consideration of the impact of somatic copy number variation on the transcriptome [101].

Microarray studies have primarily generated using invasive ductal carcinomas of no special type. However, subsequent studies have studied the gene expression pattern of some special types including medullary [102, 103], metaplastic [104], adenoid cystic carcinoma [105] and others [105]. Interestingly, tubular, mucinous and neuroendocrine carcinomas consistently displayed a luminal phenotype, whereas adenoid cystic, medullary and metaplastic carcinomas a basal-like phenotype [106]. For classification system that is applicable to all breast cancer patients, future studies of breast cancer classification should include samples of special types that comprise 25 % of breast cancer to provide standardised classification system and unravel the molecular basis of their specific morphologic patterns.

Multigene Signatures

In addition to the molecular classes, a number of multigene signatures have been identified through analysing GEP-derived data using different statistical/bioinformatics approaches. These gene signatures were developed based on the differential expression of a selected set of genes in a specific subgroup of tumours. Expression of these genes when analysed in combination can predict specific endpoint that is used to generate it. Multigene signatures include "prognostic gene signature" that can predict outcome. Other gene signatures were developed based on prediction of response to specific therapy and are used as predictive signatures. Prognostic signatures include the 70 gene signature or MammaPrint [81], the 76 gene signature [59], the genomic grade index (GGI) [107] and the Recurrence Scores (RS) of OncotypeDX^{TM} [108]. A common character shared by all these signatures is the use of combinations of genes, rather than using single genes, to predict a certain outcome which appears to reflect the overall genetic derangements underlying the complex tumour biology. Of critical importance is the very minimal to negligible degree of overlap between these signatures regarding their gene sets/lists [109]. This minimal overlap has mostly been attributed to the different/limited breast cancer tissue samples used in these studies, different gene chips utilised and varied approaches followed for data analysis [110]. Nonetheless, the widely accepted assumption is that although gene lists overlap minimally, distinct genes may track similar biological processes and the overall predictive power of different array-based models shows significant concordance [90, 111].

There is growing consensus that multigene prognostic tests provide useful complementary information to well-established traditional clinicopathological variables. Importantly, these tests primarily rely on quantification of ER and proliferation-associated genes and combine these into multivariate prediction models. Due to the higher proliferation rates in ER-negative cancers, the prognostic value of these tests in ER-negative cancers is limited. It is not surprising that clinically useful prognostic signatures for ER-negative cancers are still non-existing [112]. Therefore, these signatures have so far not replaced the currently used prognostic/predictive factors in the management of breast cancer. Nevertheless, the two currently clinically utilised assays, MammaPrint and OncotypeDX, are used in conjunction with the clinicopathologic factors [113, 114].

Immunohistochemical Molecular Classification

Due to the aforementioned technical, cost and reproducibility issues, some groups have pioneered the use of expression data of IHC biomarkers in the routinely utilised paraffin-embedded breast cancer tissue sections. Many studies, using surrogate immunohistochemical panels of markers, have recapitulated these prognostic classes with considerable success and reproducibility [115–118]. The feature common to GEP subtying and their IHC surrogates is the use of a group of genes in the former, or tissue markers in the latter to define classes which has proven to be prognostically more informative than using these genes/markers individually. The choice of these biomarker panels was essentially based on the realisation that the GEP-derived molecular subtypes are a reflection of the ER status, HER2 status and proliferation status in breast cancer [119].

Different authorities have utilised IHC expression data to classify breast cancer patients into distinct subtypes significantly different in prognosis. For instance, data for the expression levels for a selective panel of 25 BC-related biomarkers evaluated using IHC on tissue microarray (TMA) was analysed using supervised classification approaches and artificial neuronal network. Markers were those related to epithelial cell lineage, differentiation, hormone and growth factor receptors and gene products known to be altered in some forms of breast cancer. Six groups or BC classes were identified which were significantly different in clinico-pathological parameters and patient outcome in terms of overall and disease-free survival, independent of standard prognostic parameters; grade, tumour size and lymph node stage [117]. Of note, is the HER2 group was only 7 % of the studied patient population, which is below those reported in literature and in other studies.

Several groups have used IHC expression of ER, PR, HER2, basal cytokeratins (CKs) to devise a pragmatic molecular classification of breast cancer in routine practice. The resulting subtypes were classified as luminal, the HER2-overexpressing, and the triple negative/BLBC. The luminal subtype was subsequently subdivided into at least two subtypes, however, the criteria of defining luminal breast cancer subclasses are still based on different approaches utilising Ki67, PR expression and/or HER2 expression. It was initially proposed that those ER+ cancers overexpressing HER2 and being Ki67 high expressors ($\geq$14 %) as luminal B, while the ER+, HER2 negative, Ki67 low as luminal A [47]. Later on, the international expert panel gathered in the St Gallen International Breast Cancer Conference in 2013, have endorsed the use of PR positive expression ($\geq$20 %) to define luminal A breast cancer. They have recommended a Ki67 threshold of $\geq$20 % as an indicative of high Ki67 status in defining luminal B cancers [120].

The HER2 overexpressing/enriched breast cancers are those which showed evident unequivocal IHC expression of HER2 (3+), or those proven as *HER2* amplified as assessed by in situ hybridisation (ISH) techniques. Because *HER2* is an oncogene with the known impact of dismal outcome, based on the oncogene addiction theory [121], it has been proposed by many authorities, including our group, that HER2 overexpressing breast cancers should be allocated into the HER2 class/subtype irrespective of hormone receptor status [115]. The latter opinion, therefore, considers luminal B breast cancer to be those breast cancer characterised by high proliferative fraction as assessed by Ki67 expression at specific cut-off point. According to this definition, luminal B breast cancer has poorer outcome, and could benefit from adjuvant chemotherapy, which works better in tumour with high growth/proliferative fraction [122].

Probably, the most intensively debated issue within the topic IHC-defined breast cancer subtypes is BLBC. Although triple-negative breast cancer is defined by absence expression of ER, PR and HER2, there is no consensus definition, using IHC surrogate markers, for BLBC. Both TN and BLBC have poor clinical outcome and lack any modality of specific targeted therapy as those possessed by the HER2 overexpressing breast cancers. Different IHC markers have been used in defining the basal phenotype including: lack of ER, PR, HER2 expression (i.e. TN), and expressing one or more of the high-molecular-weight/basal CKs (CK5/6, CK14, or CK17) or being TN with expression of CK5/6 and/or EGFR and others [116, 123, 124]. However, comparative studies between the GEP-defined basal-like and IHC-defined BLBC are scarce [125]. This subtype is reported in the 15–20 % within most of the studied series. Therefore, this relatively low frequency hindered the development of consensus regarding BLBC. However, in their seminal meta-analysis of more than 10,000 breast cancer cases, Blows et al. reported the superior advantage of using five markers in definition of different molecular subtypes of breast cancer including the BLBC [118]. However, it is imperative that regardless of the panel of markers used in the characterisation of BLBC, most studies have reported poorer prognosis than the TN breast cancers [115, 116, 123].

The Nottingham Prognostic Index Plus (NPI+)

This algorithm devised by Abd El-Rehim et al. [56] was further refined through fuzzy rule induction algorithm to reduce the number of classifying markers/proteins to the minimum required to retain classification [126, 127]. Importantly, this approach used different multivariate clustering techniques, rather than a single clustering technique, with the main goal to derive a classification that is robust across different multivariate procedures. The initial step was dependent on the determination of the biological class of the tumour, through assessing the expression level of a ten biomarker panel; and the second step is the analysis of traditional clinicopathologic prognostic parameters. These ten biomarkers are ER, PR, HER2/c-erbB2, cytokeratin (CK) 5/6, CK7/8, p53, epidermal growth factor receptor (EGFR/HER1), c-erbB3/HER3, c-erbB4/HER4 and Mucin 1. These were selected from a large group of 25 markers of close relevance to breast cancer biology used in the original study [56] as the lowest number of markers that can preserve the same structure of the previous molecular classes [128]. This resulted in three main classes of luminal, basal and HER2, as previously established by Sorlie et al. [55] and with proportions consistent with breast cancer subtypes reported in other studies [116, 123]. Moreover, three further biologically and clinically relevant subclasses (luminal N, basal–p53 altered, and basal–p53 normal [73]) were identified. Using this panel of 10 IHC markers, we were able to subclassify unselected breast cancer series into seven distinct molecular classes that were biologically and clinically similar to those generated using 25 biomarkers [56]. These classes were used to develop a modified version of NPI by incorporating molecular and clinicopathological variables in a two-tier system [73]. Applying clinicopathological variables to each of the seven molecular classes using specific formulae generated novel prognostic index known as NPI-plus (NPI+), which improved patients' outcome stratification that is superior to the traditional NPI.

Molecular Classification Challenges

Molecular classification of breast cancer is still in evolution. With the increasing use of more sophisticated techniques such as next-generation sequencing and other high-throughput techniques, large amounts of data will continue to emerge, which could potentially lead to identification of more molecular types of breast cancer having prognostic/predictive utilities. However, transfer of these classifications and predictive algorithms from the bench to the bedside is a lengthy process requiring mounting clinical evidence and robust validation. Moreover, cost-effectiveness and quality control of such classifications/algorithms are additional challenges.

Currently, the lack of a "gold standard" definition of the luminal class combined with lack of evidence that luminal class diagnosis provides better biological refinement than ER positivity alone has resulted in continuation of treatment of these patients based on ER expression and HER2 status. In addition, although further prognostic markers are needed to refine classification of ER+ tumours, identification of predictive markers is equally important. As stated by Allred [129] new more powerful predictors of hormonal therapy response are needed, and they will most likely be based on multiple biomarkers. These are likely to be recognised by their relationship to a biological pathway or a therapeutic target, defined at either the transcriptional or biochemical level and have direct clinical therapeutic implications. Most of the previous GEP studies suffered from drawbacks in terms of the molecular approach employed, the size of cohorts, analytical method used and lack of detailed genetic, clinicopathological and immunophenotypical characterisation of the tumours [130, 131]. Although several studies have tried to develop molecular signatures that can identify a poor prognostic class within ER+ tumours [60, 108, 132–134], and define molecular pathways characteristic of luminal A tumours, debate remains over the validity of the predictors defined in most of these studies.

A common problem also noted with most of the prognostic gene signature stratifier is the limited insight into the oncogenic or biological pathways which drive tumours to progress, metastasise and develop resistance to therapy despite prognostic importance. So far studies have not been very successful in integrating data from both RNA and DNA partly as a result of the inherited difficulty in getting stable reproducible results from cancer genomes which are known to be unstable, and partly due to the low proportion of gene expression alteration which can be attributed to underlying variation in copy number in breast cancer [135]. Array-CGH is a powerful biological classifier in cancer [136] and using parallel analysis of data from both gene copy number (DNA) and gene expression using gene transcripts (RNA) and when possible proteins (i.e. IHC) may help to accurately stratify breast cancer into relevant molecular classes with improved clinical relevance in addition to identification of key molecules and potential therapeutic targets.

References

1. Elston CW, Ellis IO, Pinder SE. Pathological prognostic factors in breast cancer. Crit Rev Oncol Hematol. 1999;31(3):209–23.
2. Rakha EA, El-Sayed ME, Lee AH, Elston CW, Grainge MJ, Hodi Z, et al. Prognostic significance of Nottingham histologic grade in invasive breast carcinoma. J Clin Oncol. 2008;26(19):3153–8. PubMed PMID: 18490649. Epub 2008/05/21. eng.
3. Galea MH, Blamey RW, Elston CE, Ellis IO. The Nottingham Prognostic Index in primary breast-cancer. Breast Cancer Res Treat. 1992;22(3):207–19. PubMed PMID: ISI:A1992JQ41500005.
4. Sinn H-P, Kreipe H. A brief overview of the WHO classification of breast tumors, 4th edition, focusing on issues and updates from the 3rd edition. Breast Care. 2013;8(2):149–54. PubMed PMID: PMC3683948.
5. Rakha EA, El-Sayed ME, Menon S, Green AR, Lee AH, Ellis IO. Histologic grading is an independent prognostic factor in invasive lobular carcinoma of the breast. Breast Cancer Res Treat. 2008;111(1):121–7.
6. Cole BF, Gelber RD, Gelber S, Coates AS, Goldhirsch A. Polychemotherapy for early breast cancer: an overview of the randomised clinical trials with quality-adjusted survival analysis. The Lancet. 2001;358(9278):277–86.
7. Feng Y, Sun B, Li X, Zhang L, Niu Y, Xiao C, et al. Differentially expressed genes between primary cancer and paired lymph node metastases predict clinical outcome of node-positive breast cancer patients. Breast Cancer Res Treat. 2007;103(3):319–29.
8. Peto R, Boreham J, Clarke M, Davies C, Beral V. UK and USA breast cancer deaths down 25 % in year 2000 at ages 20–69 years. Lancet. 2000;355(9217):1822.
9. Hayes DF, Bast RC, Desch CE, Fritsche H Jr, Kemeny NE, Jessup JM, et al. Tumor marker utility grading system: a framework to evaluate clinical utility of tumor markers. J Natl Cancer Inst. 1996;88(20):1456–66.
10. Wang DG, Fan JB, Siao CJ, Berno A, Young P, Sapolsky R, et al. Large-scale identification, mapping, and genotyping of single-nucleotide polymorphisms in the human genome. Science. 1998;280(5366):1077–82.
11. Pinkel D, Segraves R, Sudar D, Clark S, Poole I, Kowbel D, et al. High resolution analysis of DNA copy number variation using comparative genomic hybridization to microarrays. Nat Genet. 1998;20(2):207–11.
12. Schweiger MR, Kerick M, Timmermann B, Albrecht MW, Borodina T, Parkhomchuk D, et al. Genome-wide massively parallel sequencing of formaldehyde fixed-paraffin embedded (FFPE) tumor tissues for copy-number- and mutation-analysis. PLoS ONE. 2009;4(5):e5548.
13. Liang P, Pardee AB. Differential display of eukaryotic messenger RNA by means of the polymerase chain reaction. Science. 1992;257(5072):967–71.
14. Velculescu VE, Zhang L, Vogelstein B, Kinzler KW. Serial analysis of gene expression. Science. 1995;270(5235):484–7.
15. Brown PO, Botstein D. Exploring the new world of the genome with DNA microarrays. Nat Genet. 1999;21(1 Suppl):33–7.
16. Torres TT, Metta M, Ottenwalder B, Schlotterer C. Gene expression profiling by massively parallel sequencing. Genome Res. 2008;18(1):172–7. PubMed PMID: 18032722. Pubmed Central PMCID: 2134766.
17. Rakha EA, Pinder SE, Bartlett JM, Ibrahim M, Starczynski J, Carder PJ, et al. Updated UK recommendations for HER2 assessment in breast cancer. J Clin Pathol. 2015;68(2):93–9. PubMed PMID: 25488926. Pubmed Central PMCID: 4316916.
18. Pathology reporting of breast disease. A Joint Document Incorporating the Third Edition of the NHS Breast Screening Programme's Guidelines for Pathology Reporting in Breast Cancer Screening and the Second Edition of The Royal College of Pathologists' Minimum Dataset for Breast Cancer Histopathology, Jan 2005. NHSBSP Pub. No 58 p.

19. Hammond ME, Hayes DF, Dowsett M, Allred DC, Hagerty KL, Badve S, et al. American Society of Clinical Oncology/College of American Pathologists guideline recommendations for immunohistochemical testing of estrogen and progesterone receptors in breast cancer. J Clin Oncol. 2010;28(16):2784–95.
20. Goldhirsch A, Glick JH, Gelber RD, Coates AS, Thurlimann B, Senn HJ. Meeting highlights: international expert consensus on the primary therapy of early breast cancer 2005. Ann Oncol. 2005;16(10):1569–83.
21. Effects of chemotherapy and hormonal therapy for early breast cancer on recurrence and 15-year survival: an overview of the randomised trials. Lancet. 2005;365(9472):1687–717. PubMed PMID: 15894097.
22. Effects of adjuvant tamoxifen and of cytotoxic therapy on mortality in early breast cancer. An overview of 61 randomized trials among 28,896 women. Early Breast Cancer Trialists' Collaborative Group. N Engl J Med. 1988;319(26):1681–92. PubMed PMID: 3205265.
23. Tamoxifen for early breast cancer: an overview of the randomised trials. Early Breast Cancer Trialists' Collaborative Group. Lancet. 1998;351(9114):1451–67. PubMed PMID: 9605801.
24. Fisher B, Dignam J, Bryant J, DeCillis A, Wickerham DL, Wolmark N, et al. Five versus more than five years of tamoxifen therapy for breast cancer patients with negative lymph nodes and estrogen receptor-positive tumors. J Natl Cancer Inst. 1996;88(21):1529–42.
25. Bardou VJ, Arpino G, Elledge RM, Osborne CK, Clark GM. Progesterone receptor status significantly improves outcome prediction over estrogen receptor status alone for adjuvant endocrine therapy in two large breast cancer databases. J Clin Oncol. 2003;21(10):1973–9.
26. Rakha EA, El-Sayed ME, Green AR, Paish EC, Powe DG, Gee J, et al. Biologic and clinical characteristics of breast cancer with single hormone receptor positive phenotype. J Clin Oncol. 2007;25(30):4772–8.
27. Ravdin PM, Green S, Dorr TM, McGuire WL, Fabian C, Pugh RP, et al. Prognostic significance of progesterone receptor levels in estrogen receptor-positive patients with metastatic breast cancer treated with tamoxifen: results of a prospective Southwest Oncology Group study. J Clin Oncol. 1992;10(8):1284–91.
28. Colomer R, Beltran M, Dorcas J, Cortes-Funes H, Hornedo J, Valentin V, et al. It is not time to stop progesterone receptor testing in breast cancer. J Clin Oncol. 2005;23(16):3868–9; author reply 9–70. PubMed PMID: 15923595.
29. Stendahl M, Ryden L, Nordenskjold B, Jonsson PE, Landberg G, Jirstrom K. High progesterone receptor expression correlates to the effect of adjuvant tamoxifen in premenopausal breast cancer patients. Clin Cancer Res. 2006;12(15):4614–8.
30. Regan MM, Viale G, Mastropasqua MG, Maiorano E, Golouh R, Carbone A, et al. Re-evaluating adjuvant breast cancer trials: assessing hormone receptor status by immunohistochemical versus extraction assays. J Natl Cancer Inst. 2006;98(21):1571–81.
31. Slamon DJ, Clark GM, Wong SG, Levin WJ, Ullrich A, McGuire WL. Human breast cancer: correlation of relapse and survival with amplification of the HER-2/neu oncogene. Science. 1987;235(4785):177–82.
32. Dandachi N, Dietze O, Hauser-Kronberger C. Chromogenic in situ hybridization: a novel approach to a practical and sensitive method for the detection of HER2 oncogene in archival human breast carcinoma. Lab Invest. 2002;82(8):1007–14.
33. Wolff AC, Hammond ME, Schwartz JN, Hagerty KL, Allred DC, Cote RJ, et al. American Society of Clinical Oncology/College of American Pathologists guideline recommendations for human epidermal growth factor receptor 2 testing in breast cancer. J Clin Oncol. 2007;25(1):118–45.
34. Bartlett J, Mallon E, Cooke T. The clinical evaluation of HER-2 status: which test to use? J Pathol. 2003;199(4):411–7.
35. Kaufmann M, von Minckwitz G, Bear HD, Buzdar A, McGale P, Bonnefoi H, et al. Recommendations from an international expert panel on the use of neoadjuvant

(primary) systemic treatment of operable breast cancer: new perspectives 2006. Ann Oncol. 2007;18(12):1927–34.

36. Ward S, Pilgrim H, Hind D. Trastuzumab for the treatment of primary breast cancer in HER2-positive women: a single technology appraisal. Health Technol Assess. 2009;13(Suppl 1):1–6.

37. Rakha EA, Reis-Filho JS, Ellis IO. Combinatorial biomarker expression in breast cancer. Breast Cancer Res Treat. 2010;120(2):293–308. PubMed PMID: 20107892. Epub 2010/01/29. eng.

38. Cuzick J, Dowsett M, Wale C, Salter J, Quinn E, Zabaglo L, et al. Prognostic value of a combined ER, PgR, Ki67, HER2 immunohistochemical (IHC4) score and comparison with the GHI recurrence score—results from TransATAC. Cancer Res. 2009;Suppl 24: Abstract 74.

39. Carey LA, Perou CM, Livasy CA, Dressler LG, Cowan D, Conway K, et al. Race, breast cancer subtypes, and survival in the Carolina Breast Cancer Study. J Am Med Assoc (JAMA). 2006;295(21):2492–502. PubMed PMID: ISI:000238057300024.

40. Kreike B, van Kouwenhove M, Horlings H, Weigelt B, Bartelink H, Van de Vijver MJ. Gene expression profiling and histopathological characterization of triple negative/basal-like breast carcinomas. Breast Cancer Res. 2007;9(5):R65.

41. Kurebayashi J, Moriya T, Ishida T, Hirakawa H, Kurosumi M, Akiyama F, et al. The prevalence of intrinsic subtypes and prognosis in breast cancer patients of different races. The Breast. 2007;16(2, Suppl 1):72–7.

42. Aleskandarany MA, Rakha EA, Macmillan RD, Powe DG, Ellis IO, Green AR. MIB1/Ki-67 labelling index can classify grade 2 breast cancer into two clinically distinct subgroups. Breast Cancer Res Treat. 2010;127(3):591–9.

43. Colozza M, Azambuja E, Cardoso F, Sotiriou C, Larsimont D, Piccart MJ. Proliferative markers as prognostic and predictive tools in early breast cancer: where are we now? 2005. p. 1723–39.

44. Viale G, Regan MM, Mastropasqua MG, Maffini F, Maiorano E, Colleoni M, et al. Predictive value of tumor Ki-67 expression in two randomized trials of adjuvant chemoendocrine therapy for node-negative breast cancer. J Natl Cancer Inst. 2008;100(3):207–12.

45. Baak JP, Gudlaugsson E, Skaland I, Guo LH, Klos J, Lende TH, et al. Proliferation is the strongest prognosticator in node-negative breast cancer: significance, error sources, alternatives and comparison with molecular prognostic markers. Breast Cancer Res Treat. 2009;115(2):241–54.

46. Yerushalmi R, Woods R, Ravdin PM, Hayes MM, Gelmon KA. Ki67 in breast cancer: prognostic and predictive potential. Lancet Oncol. 2010;11(2):174–83.

47. Cheang MC, Chia SK, Voduc D, Gao D, Leung S, Snider J, et al. Ki67 index, HER2 status, and prognosis of patients with luminal B breast cancer. J Natl Cancer Inst. 2009;101(10):736–50.

48. Aleskandarany MA, Rakha EA, Macmillan RD, Powe DG, Ellis IO, Green AR. MIB1/Ki-67 labelling index can classify grade 2 breast cancer into two clinically distinct subgroups. Breast Cancer Res Treat. 2010. PubMed PMID: 20623333. Epub 2010/07/14. Eng.

49. Aleskandarany MA, Green AR, Rakha EA, Mohammed RA, Elsheikh SE, Powe DG, et al. Growth fraction as a predictor of response to chemotherapy in node-negative breast cancer. Int J Cancer. 2010. PubMed PMID: 19711345.

50. Colleoni M, Orvieto E, Nole F, Orlando L, Minchella I, Viale G, et al. Prediction of response to primary chemotherapy for operable breast cancer. Eur J Cancer. 1999;35(4):574–9.

51. Augenlicht LH, Wahrman MZ, Halsey H, Anderson L, Taylor J, Lipkin M. Expression of cloned sequences in biopsies of human colonic tissue and in colonic carcinoma cells induced to differentiate in vitro. Cancer Res. 1987;47(22):6017–21. PubMed PMID: 3664505. Epub 1987/11/15. eng.

52. Bertucci F, Finetti P, Cervera N, Maraninchi D, Viens P, Birnbaum D. Gene expression profiling and clinical outcome in breast cancer. OMICS. 2006;10(4):429–43. PubMed PMID: 17233555. Epub 2007/01/20. eng.

53. Cowin PA, Anglesio M, Etemadmoghadam D, Bowtell DD. Profiling the cancer genome. Annu Rev Genomics Hum Genet. 2010;11:133–59. PubMed PMID: 20590430. Epub 2010/07/02. eng.

54. Perou CM, Sorlie T, Eisen MB, van de Rijn M, Jeffrey SS, Rees CA, et al. Molecular portraits of human breast tumours. Nature. 2000;406(6797):747–52. PubMed PMID: ISI:000088767700049.

55. Sorlie T, Perou CM, Tibshirani R, Aas T, Geisler S, Johnsen H. et al. Gene expression patterns of breast carcinomas distinguish tumor subclasses with clinical implications. Proc Natl Acad Sci USA. 2001;98(19):10869–74.

56. Abd El-Rehim DM, Ball G, Pinder SE, Rakha E, Paish C, Robertson JF, et al. High-throughput protein expression analysis using tissue microarray technology of a large well-characterised series identifies biologically distinct classes of breast cancer confirming recent cDNA expression analyses. Int J Cancer. 2005;116(3):340–50.

57. Foekens JA, Atkins D, Zhang Y, Sweep FC, Harbeck N, Paradiso A, et al. Multicenter validation of a gene expression-based prognostic signature in lymph node-negative primary breast cancer. J Clin Oncol. 2006;24(11):1665–71.

58. van 't Veer LJ, Dai H, van de Vijver MJ, He YD, Hart AA, Mao M, et al. Gene expression profiling predicts clinical outcome of breast cancer. Nature. 2002;415(6871):530–6.

59. Wang Y, Klijn JG, Zhang Y, Sieuwerts AM, Look MP, Yang F, et al. Gene-expression profiles to predict distant metastasis of lymph-node-negative primary breast cancer. Lancet. 2005;365(9460):671–9. PubMed PMID: 15721472.

60. Ma XJ, Wang Z, Ryan PD, Isakoff SJ, Barmettler A, Fuller A, et al. A two-gene expression ratio predicts clinical outcome in breast cancer patients treated with tamoxifen. Cancer Cell. 2004;5(6):607–16.

61. Zhang Y, Sieuwerts AM, McGreevy M, Casey G, Cufer T, Paradiso A, et al. The 76-gene signature defines high-risk patients that benefit from adjuvant tamoxifen therapy. Breast Cancer Res Treat. 2009;116(2):303–9.

62. Hess KR, Anderson K, Symmans WF, Valero V, Ibrahim N, Mejia JA, et al. Pharmacogenomic predictor of sensitivity to preoperative chemotherapy with paclitaxel and fluorouracil, doxorubicin, and cyclophosphamide in breast cancer. J Clin Oncol. 2006;24(26):4236–44.

63. Potti A, Dressman HK, Bild A, Riedel RF, Chan G, Sayer R, et al. Genomic signatures to guide the use of chemotherapeutics. Nat Med. 2006;12(11):1294–300.

64. Ma XJ, Salunga R, Tuggle JT, Gaudet J, Enright E, McQuary P, et al. Gene expression profiles of human breast cancer progression. Proc Natl Acad Sci USA. 2003;100(10):5974–9.

65. Schuetz CS, Bonin M, Clare SE, Nieselt K, Sotlar K, Walter M, et al. Progression-specific genes identified by expression profiling of matched ductal carcinomas in situ and invasive breast tumors, combining laser capture microdissection and oligonucleotide microarray analysis. Cancer Res. 2006;66(10):5278–86.

66. Korkola JE, DeVries S, Fridlyand J, Hwang ES, Estep AL, Chen YY, et al. Differentiation of lobular versus ductal breast carcinomas by expression microarray analysis. Cancer Res. 2003;63(21):7167–75.

67. Zhao H, Langerod A, Ji Y, Nowels KW, Nesland JM, Tibshirani R, et al. Different gene expression patterns in invasive lobular and ductal carcinomas of the breast. Mol Biol Cell. 2004;15(6):2523–36.

68. West M, Blanchette C, Dressman H, Huang E, Ishida S, Spang R, et al. Predicting the clinical status of human breast cancer by using gene expression profiles. Proc Natl Acad Sci USA. 2001;98(20):11462–7.

69. Huang E, Cheng SH, Dressman H, Pittman J, Tsou MH, Horng CF, et al. Gene expression predictors of breast cancer outcomes. Lancet. 2003;361(9369):1590–6.

70. Perou CM, Sorlie T, Eisen MB, van de Rijn M, Jeffrey SS, Rees CA, et al. Molecular portraits of human breast tumours. Nature. 2000;406(6797):747–52.

71. Habashy HO, Powe DG, Abdel-Fatah TM, Gee JM, Nicholson RI, Green AR, et al. A review of the biological and clinical characteristics of luminal-like oestrogen receptor-positive breast cancer. Histopathology. 2012;60(6):854–63. PubMed PMID: 21906125. Epub 2011/09/13. eng.

72. Sotiriou C, Neo SY, McShane LM, Korn EL, Long PM, Jazaeri A, et al. Breast cancer classification and prognosis based on gene expression profiles from a population-based study. Proc Natl Acad Sci USA. 2003;100(18):10393–8.

73. Rakha EA, Soria D, Green AR, Lemetre C, Powe DG, Nolan CC, et al. Nottingham Prognostic Index Plus (NPI+): a modern clinical decision making tool in breast cancer. Br J Cancer. 2014;110(7):1688–97. PubMed PMID: 24619074. Pubmed Central PMCID: 3974073.

74. Herschkowitz JI, Simin K, Weigman VJ, Mikaelian I, Usary J, Hu Z, et al. Identification of conserved gene expression features between murine mammary carcinoma models and human breast tumors. Genome Biol. 2007;8(5):R76. PubMed PMID: 17493263. Pubmed Central PMCID: 1929138.

75. Farmer P, Bonnefoi H, Becette V, Tubiana-Hulin M, Fumoleau P, Larsimont D, et al. Identification of molecular apocrine breast tumours by microarray analysis. Oncogene. 2005;24(29):4660–71.

76. Sorlie T, Tibshirani R, Parker J, Hastie T, Marron JS, Nobel A, et al. Repeated observation of breast tumor subtypes in independent gene expression data sets. Proc Natl Acad Sci USA. 2003;100(14):8418–23. PubMed PMID: ISI:000184222500069.

77. Sotiriou C, Neo SY, McShane LM, Korn EL, Long PM, Jazaeri A, et al. Breast cancer classification and prognosis based on gene expression profiles from a population-based study. Proc Natl Acad Sci USA. 2003;100(18):10393–8. PubMed PMID: ISI:000185119300048.

78. Anna Bergamaschi YHKPWTSTH-BPELRTA-LB-DJRP. Distinct patterns of DNA copy number alteration are associated with different clinicopathological features and gene-expression subtypes of breast cancer. Genes Chromosom Cancer. 2006;45(11):1033–40.

79. Dairkee SH, Ljung BM, Smith H, Hackett A. Immunolocalization of a human basal epithelium specific keratin in benign and malignant breast disease. Breast Cancer Res Treat. 1987;10(1):11–20.

80. Santini D, Ceccarelli C, Taffurelli M, Pileri S, Marrano D. Differentiation pathways in primary invasive breast carcinoma as suggested by intermediate filament and biopathological marker expression. J Pathol. 1996;179(4):386–91.

81. van de Vijver MJ, He YD, van't Veer LJ, Dai H, Hart AA, Voskuil DW, et al. A gene-expression signature as a predictor of survival in breast cancer. N Engl J Med. 2002;347(25):1999–2009.

82. Savage K, Lambros MB, Robertson D, Jones RL, Jones C, Mackay A, et al. Caveolin 1 is overexpressed and amplified in a subset of basal-like and metaplastic breast carcinomas: a morphologic, ultrastructural, immunohistochemical, and in situ hybridization analysis. Clin Cancer Res. 2007;13(1):90–101.

83. Yehiely F, Moyano JV, Evans JR, Nielsen TO, Cryns VL. Deconstructing the molecular portrait of basal-like breast cancer. Trends Mol Med. 2006;12(11):537–44.

84. Hu Z, Fan C, Oh DS, Marron JS, He X, Qaqish BF, et al. The molecular portraits of breast tumors are conserved across microarray platforms. BMC Genom. 2006;7:96.

85. Wilhelmsen K, Litjens SH, Sonnenberg A. Multiple functions of the integrin alpha6beta4 in epidermal homeostasis and tumorigenesis. Mol Cell Biol. 2006;26(8):2877–86.

86. Vogelstein B, Kinzler KW. Cancer genes and the pathways they control. Nat Med. 2004;10(8):789–99.

87. Koshikawa N, Giannelli G, Cirulli V, Miyazaki K, Quaranta V. Role of cell surface metalloprotease MT1-MMP in epithelial cell migration over laminin-5. J Cell Biol. 2000;148(3):615–24.

88. Hanahan D, Weinberg RA. The hallmarks of cancer. Cell. 2000;100(1):57–70.
89. Dumont N, Arteaga CL. Targeting the TGF beta signaling network in human neoplasia. Cancer Cell. 2003;3(6):531–6.
90. Fan C, Oh DS, Wessels L, Weigelt B, Nuyten DS, Nobel AB, et al. Concordance among gene-expression-based predictors for breast cancer. N Engl J Med. 2006;355(6):560–9.
91. Bergamaschi A, Kim YH, Wang P, Sorlie T, Hernandez-Boussard T, Lonning PE, et al. Distinct patterns of DNA copy number alteration are associated with different clinico-pathological features and gene-expression subtypes of breast cancer. Genes Chromosomes Cancer. 2006;45(11):1033–40.
92. Chin K, DeVries S, Fridlyand J, Spellman PT, Roydasgupta R, Kuo WL, et al. Genomic and transcriptional aberrations linked to breast cancer pathophysiologies. Cancer Cell. 2006;10(6):529–41.
93. Vincent-Salomon A, Gruel N, Lucchesi C, Mac Grogan G, Dendale R, Sigal-Zafrani B, et al. Identification of typical medullary breast carcinoma as a genomic sub-group of basal-like carcinomas, a heterogeneous new molecular entity. Breast Cancer Res. 2007;9(2):R24.
94. Rakha E, Reis-Filho JS. Basal-like breast carcinoma: from expression profiling to routine practice. Arch Pathol Lab Med. 2009;133(6):860–8. PubMed PMID: 19492878. Epub 2009/06/06. eng.
95. Turner NC, Reis-Filho JS. Basal-like breast cancer and the BRCA1 phenotype. Oncogene. 2006;25(43):5846–53.
96. Leidy J, Khan A, Kandil D. Basal-like breast cancer: update on clinicopathologic, immuno-histochemical, and molecular features. Arch Pathol Lab Med. 2014;138(1):37–43. PubMed PMID: 24377810. Epub 2014/01/01. eng.
97. Weigelt B, Baehner FL, Reis-Filho JS. The contribution of gene expression profiling to breast cancer classification, prognostication and prediction: a retrospective of the last decade. J Pathol. 2010;220(2):263–80.
98. Weigelt B, Mackay A, A'Hern R, Natrajan R, Tan DS, Dowsett M, et al. Breast cancer molecular profiling with single sample predictors: a retrospective analysis. Lancet Oncol. 2010;11(4):339–49.
99. Sorlie T, Tibshirani R, Parker J, Hastie T, Marron JS, Nobel A, et al. Repeated observation of breast tumor subtypes in independent gene expression data sets. Proc Natl Acad Sci U S A. 2003;100(14):8418–23.
100. Calza S, Hall P, Auer G, Bjohle J, Klaar S, Kronenwett U, et al. Intrinsic molecular signature of breast cancer in a population-based cohort of 412 patients. Breast Cancer Res. 2006;8(4):R34.
101. Curtis C, Shah SP, Chin SF, Turashvili G, Rueda OM, Dunning MJ, et al. The genomic and transcriptomic architecture of 2,000 breast tumours reveals novel subgroups. Nature. 2012;486(7403):346–52. PubMed PMID: 22522925. Pubmed Central PMCID: 3440846.
102. Bertucci F, Finetti P, Cervera N, Charafe-Jauffret E, Mamessier E, Adelaide J, et al. Gene expression profiling shows medullary breast cancer is a subgroup of basal breast cancers. Cancer Res. 2006;66(9):4636–44.
103. Vincent-Salomon A, Gruel N, Lucchesi C, MacGrogan G, Dendale R, Sigal-Zafrani B, et al. Identification of typical medullary breast carcinoma as a genomic sub-group of basal-like carcinomas, a heterogeneous new molecular entity. Breast Cancer Res. 2007;9(2):R24. PubMed PMID: 17417968. Pubmed Central PMCID: PMC1868916. Epub 2007/04/10. eng.
104. Weigelt B, Kreike B, Reis-Filho JS. Metaplastic breast carcinomas are basal-like breast cancers: a genomic profiling analysis. Breast Cancer Res Treat. 2009;117(2):273–80.
105. Weigelt B, Horlings HM, Kreike B, Hayes MM, Hauptmann M, Wessels LF, et al. Refinement of breast cancer classification by molecular characterization of histological special types. J Pathol. 2008;216(2):141–50.
106. Weigelt B, Geyer FC, Reis-Filho JS. Histological types of breast cancer: how special are they? Mol Oncol. 2010;4(3):192–208.

107. Sotiriou C, Wirapati P, Loi S, Harris A, Fox S, Smeds J, et al. Gene expression profiling in breast cancer: understanding the molecular basis of histologic grade to improve prognosis. J Natl Cancer Inst. 2006;98(4):262–72.

108. Paik S, Shak S, Tang G, Kim C, Baker J, Cronin M, et al. A multigene assay to predict recurrence of tamoxifen-treated, node-negative breast cancer. N Engl J Med. 2004;351(27):2817–26.

109. Wirapati P, Sotiriou C, Kunkel S, Farmer P, Pradervand S, Haibe-Kains B, et al. Meta-analysis of gene expression profiles in breast cancer: toward a unified understanding of breast cancer subtyping and prognosis signatures. Breast Cancer Res. 2008;10(4):R65.

110. Cheang MCU, van de Rijn M, Nielsen TO. Gene expression profiling of breast cancer. Annu Rev Pathol. 2008;3(1):67–97.

111. Prat A, Parker JS, Fan C, Cheang MC, Miller LD, Bergh J, et al. Concordance among gene expression-based predictors for ER-positive breast cancer treated with adjuvant tamoxifen. Ann Oncol. 2012;23(11):2866–73. PubMed PMID: 22532584. Pubmed Central PMCID: 3477878.

112. Gyorffy B, Hatzis C, Sanft T, Hofstatter E, Aktas B, Pusztai L. Multigene prognostic tests in breast cancer: past, present, future. Breast Cancer Res. 2015;17(1):11. PubMed PMID: doi:10.1186/s13058-015-0514-2.

113. Kim C, Paik S. Gene-expression-based prognostic assays for breast cancer. Nat Rev Clin Oncol. 2010;7(6):340–7. PubMed PMID: 20440284. Epub 2010/05/05. eng.

114. Azim HA, Jr., Michiels S, Zagouri F, Delaloge S, Filipits M, Namer M, et al. Utility of prognostic genomic tests in breast cancer practice: The IMPAKT 2012 Working Group Consensus Statement. Ann Oncol (official journal of the European Society for Medical Oncology/ESMO). 2013;24(3):647–54. PubMed PMID: 23337633. Epub 2013/01/23. eng.

115. Rakha EA, Elsheikh SE, Aleskandarany MA, Habashi HO, Green AR, Powe DG, et al. Triple-negative breast cancer: distinguishing between basal and nonbasal subtypes. Clin Cancer Res. 2009;15(7):2302–10.

116. Nielsen TO, Hsu FD, Jensen K, Cheang M, Karaca G, Hu Z, et al. Immunohistochemical and clinical characterization of the basal-like subtype of invasive breast carcinoma. Clin Cancer Res. 2004;10(16):5367–74.

117. Abd El-Rehim DM, Ball G, Pinder SE, Rakha E, Paish C, Robertson JFR, et al. High-throughput protein expression analysis using tissue microarray technology of a large well-characterised series identifies biologically distinct classes of breast cancer confirming recent cDNA expression analyses. Int J Cancer. 2005;116(3):340–50. PubMed PMID: ISI:000230466100002.

118. Blows FM, Driver KE, Schmidt MK, Broeks A, van Leeuwen FE, Wesseling J, et al. Subtyping of breast cancer by immunohistochemistry to investigate a relationship between subtype and short and long term survival: a collaborative analysis of data for 10,159 cases from 12 studies. PLoS Med. 2010;7(5):e1000279. PubMed PMID: 20520800. Pubmed Central PMCID: 2876119.

119. Rakha EA, El-Sayed ME, Reis-Filho JS, Ellis IO. Expression profiling technology: its contribution to our understanding of breast cancer. Histopathology. 2008;52(1):67–81.

120. Goldhirsch A, Winer EP, Coates AS, Gelber RD, Piccart-Gebhart M, Thurlimann B, et al. Personalizing the treatment of women with early breast cancer: highlights of the St Gallen International Expert Consensus on the Primary Therapy of Early Breast Cancer 2013. Ann Oncol (official journal of the European Society for Medical Oncology/ESMO). 2013;24(9):2206–23. PubMed PMID: 23917950. Pubmed Central PMCID: PMC3755334. Epub 2013/08/07. eng.

121. Weinstein IB, Joe A. Oncogene addiction. Cancer Res. 2008;68(9):3077–80.

122. Aleskandarany MA, Green AR, Benhasouna AA, Barros FF, Neal K, Reis-Filho JS, et al. Prognostic value of proliferation assay in the luminal, HER2-positive, and triple-negative biologic classes of breast cancer. Breast Cancer Res. 2012;14(1):R3. PubMed PMID: 22225836. Pubmed Central PMCID: PMC3496118. Epub 2012/01/10. eng.

123. Cheang MC, Voduc D, Bajdik C, Leung S, McKinney S, Chia SK, et al. Basal-like breast cancer defined by five biomarkers has superior prognostic value than triple-negative phenotype. Clin Cancer Res. 2008;14(5):1368–76.
124. Livasy CA, Karaca G, Nanda R, Tretiakova MS, Olopade OI, Moore DT, et al. Phenotypic evaluation of the basal-like subtype of invasive breast carcinoma. Mod Pathol. 2006;19(2):264–71.
125. Badve S, Dabbs DJ, Schnitt SJ, Baehner FL, Decker T, Eusebi V, et al. Basal-like and triple-negative breast cancers: a critical review with an emphasis on the implications for pathologists and oncologists. Mod Pathol. 2011;24(2):157–67.
126. Green AR, Powe DG, Rakha EA, Soria D, Lemetre C, Nolan CC, et al. Identification of key clinical phenotypes of breast cancer using a reduced panel of protein biomarkers. Br J Cancer. 2013;109(7):1886–94.
127. Soria D, Garibaldi Jm, Ambrogi F, Green AR, Powe D, Rakha E, Macmillan RD, et al. A methodology to identify consensus classes from clustering algorithms applied to immunohistochemical data from breast cancer patients. 2010 20100308 DCOM- 20100701(1879-0534 (Electronic)). eng.
128. Green AR, Powe DG, Rakha EA, Soria D, Lemetre C, Nolan CC, et al. Identification of key clinical phenotypes of breast cancer using a reduced panel of protein biomarkers. Br J Cancer. 2013;109(7):1886–94. PubMed PMID: 24008658. Pubmed Central PMCID: 3790179.
129. Allred DC. Commentary: hormone receptor testing in breast cancer: a distress signal from Canada. Oncologist. 2008;13(11):1134–6.
130. Simon R, Radmacher MD, Dobbin K, McShane LM. Pitfalls in the use of DNA microarray data for diagnostic and prognostic classification. J Natl Cancer Inst. 2003;95(1):14–8.
131. Forster T, Roy D, Ghazal P. Experiments using microarray technology: limitations and standard operating procedures. J Endocrinol. 2003;178(2):195–204.
132. Jansen MP, Foekens JA, van Staveren IL, Dirkzwager-Kiel MM, Ritstier K, Look MP, et al. Molecular classification of tamoxifen-resistant breast carcinomas by gene expression profiling. J Clin Oncol. 2005;23(4):732–40.
133. Loi S, Haibe-Kains B, Desmedt C, Wirapati P, Lallemand F, Tutt AM, et al. Predicting prognosis using molecular profiling in estrogen receptor-positive breast cancer treated with tamoxifen. BMC Genom. 2008;9:239.
134. Parker JS, Mullins M, Cheang MC, Leung S, Voduc D, Vickery T, et al. Supervised risk predictor of breast cancer based on intrinsic subtypes. J Clin Oncol. 2009;27(8):1160–7.
135. Pollack JR, Sorlie T, Perou CM, Rees CA, Jeffrey SS, Lonning PE, et al. Microarray analysis reveals a major direct role of DNA copy number alteration in the transcriptional program of human breast tumors. Proc Natl Acad Sci USA. 2002;99(20):12963–8.
136. Fritz B, Schubert F, Wrobel G, Schwaenen C, Wessendorf S, Nessling M, et al. Microarray-based copy number and expression profiling in dedifferentiated and pleomorphic liposarcoma. Cancer Res. 2002;62(11):2993–8.

Chapter 11
Triple-Negative Breast Cancer: Subtypes with Clinical Implications

Dina Kandil and Ashraf Khan

Background

Triple-negative breast cancers (TNBC) are a heterogeneous group of malignant breast tumors traditionally defined by their lack of expression of estrogen receptor (ER), progesterone receptor (PR), and over-expression of human epidermal growth factor receptor 2 (HER-2). TNBC accounts for about 10–15 % of all breast cancers. Population-based studies show that women with high body mass index and those who reported no recreational physical activity are at a higher risk for developing TNBC than women who are physically active and those with low body mass index [1, 2]. Interestingly, some factors that are known to decrease the risk of breast cancer in general, do increase the risk of TNBC. These include first childbirth at an early age and multiparity. Racial disparity is also well-documented with African-American women having the highest incidence rates for TNBC, followed by Hispanic women [3]. The negativity of these tumors for ER and PR as well as their lack of HER-2 over-expression, render them resistant to hormonal and trastuzumab (Herceptin) therapy, making treatment a challenging task. Although, by DNA microarray analysis, most TNBC will fall into the basal-like category of breast cancers, and therefore will theoretically have a poor prognosis compared to other subtypes, basal-like breast cancer is one of several "faces" of TNBC, albeit the "ugly face." In this chapter, we will discuss the different subtypes of TNBC, their morphological features, immunophenotype, molecular background and the clinical implications of these subtypes. The immunohistochemical and molecular characteristics are summarized in Table 11.1.

D. Kandil · A. Khan (✉)
Department of Pathology, University of Massachusetts Medical School,
UMassMemorial Medical Center, Three Biotech, One Innovation Drive,
Worcester, MA 01605, USA
e-mail: Ashraf.Khan@umassmemorial.org

© Springer Science+Business Media New York 2015
A. Khan et al. (eds.), *Precision Molecular Pathology of Breast Cancer*,
Molecular Pathology Library 10, DOI 10.1007/978-1-4939-2886-6_11

Table 11.1 Subtypes of TNBC with their characteristic immunohistochemical and molecular features

TNBC Subtype	Immunohistochemistry	Molecular characteristics
Adenoid cystic carcinoma	ER−/PR−/HER2− in >90 % C-KIT+, P63+, EGFR+HCM−, calponin—Ki67 low, TP53—low Topo IIα expression	t(6, 9)(q22–23;p23–24) MYB-NFIB fusion gene
		No EGFR gene amplification
		No KIT mutation
Metaplastic	ER−/PR−/HER2− in >90 %	Claudin-low associated
Carcinoma	Cytokeratin panel (CK903, AE1/AE3, CK903) variable P63+ (>90 %)	Low expression of GATA3-regulated genes and genes responsible for cell-cell adhesion
		Increase in markers linked to stem cell function
Carcinoma with apocrine	ER−/PR− usually HER2− (>50 %)	Gains in 1p, 1q and 2q
		Losses of 1p, 12q, 16q, 17q, and 22q19
Differentiation	GCDFP15+ (diffuse)	
	AR+, BCL2−	
Pleomorphic	ER−/PR− (all cases)	Aneuploidy and high S-phase
Carcinoma	HER2− (usually)	
	Pankeratin+, CAM 5.2+	
	EMA+ (weak and focal)	
	P53+ (71 %), Ki67 (high)	
	BCL2−	
Secretory carcinoma	ER−/PR−/HER2−. EMA+, S-100 protein+, E-cadherin+. CK5/6 and 14+	t(12, 15) ETV6-NTRK3 gene fusion. Alteration of the ETV6 gene in both the in situ and invasive components
Carcinoma with medullary features	ER−/PR−/HER2− in >90 %	EGFR gene amplification
	CK5/6, EGFR, TP53+ (variable)	TP53 gene mutation
	KI-67 high	BRCA1 gene mutations common
		Epstein-Barr virus infection?
Basal-like breast	ER−/PR−/HER2− (all cases)	TP53 mutation (83 %)
Carcinoma	CK5/6+, EGFR+ (45–70 %)	Alteration in BRCA-1 activity and loss of function
	CK14+, IMP3+, CKIT+ (45 %)	
	P53+. Others: VEGF+, maspin+	X-chromosome abnormalities
	osteopontin, Integrin β4	ID4 and cyclin E1 expression
	Caveolin1 and 2+	VEGF and Fascin expression

(+): Positive, (−): negative

Adenoid Cystic Carcinoma

Adenoid cystic carcinoma (ACC) of the breast is a rare and morphologically distinct form of breast cancer, comprising less than 1 % of all cases [4]. In contrast to other TNBC, the incidence of mammary ACC among Blacks is significantly lower than in Whites [5]. Histologically, these tumors are identical to their salivary gland counterparts. The tumor is composed of two cell types: cuboidal epithelial cells with rather abundant cytoplasm and pale nuclei lining tubular duct-like structures that contain neutral polysaccharides (PAS positive, diastase sensitive), and myoepithelial-like cells that elaborate acid mucopolysaccharides (alcian blue positive) and abundant basal lamina material. Mammary ACC can assume several architectural patterns including: solid, cribriform, tubular, and trabecular configurations. These patterns may not be distributed homogenously in a given tumor causing a potential diagnostic dilemma, especially on core needle biopsies. A predominant cribriform pattern may be confused with invasive or in situ cribriform carcinoma, and collagenous spherulosis (Fig. 11.1a). DCIS in association with ACC is seen in a minority of cases and may be difficult to distinguish from the surrounding nests of invasive carcinoma.

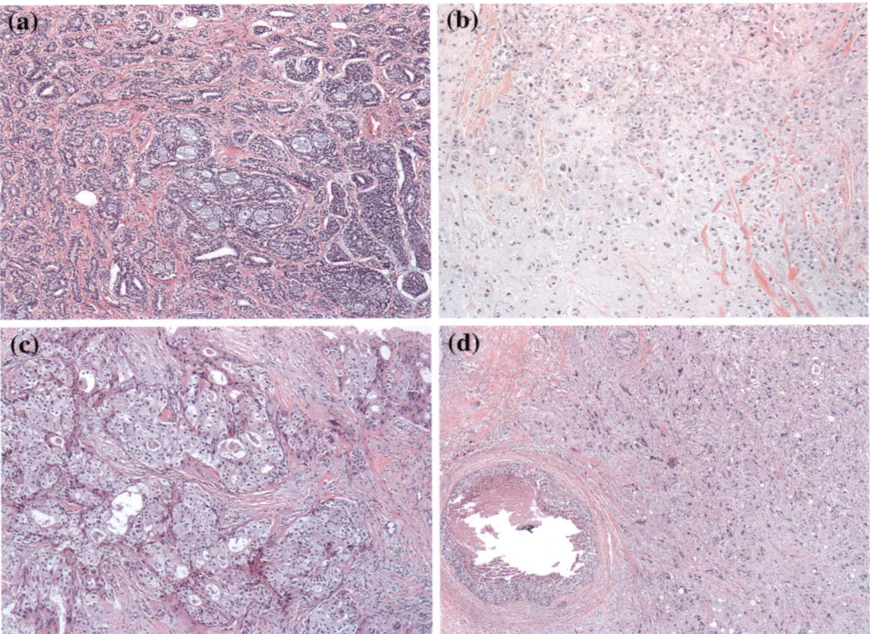

Fig. 11.1 **a** Adenoid cystic carcinoma, H&E 100×. **b** Metaplastic Carcinoma with mesenchymal differentiation, 100×. **c** Carcinoma with apocrine differentiation, 100×. **d** Pleomorphic carcinoma, 100×

Immunohistochemistry

Immunohistochemistry is helpful in cases of ACC, not only to confirm the diagnosis, but also to differentiate it from its mimickers. A panel including C-KIT (CD117), P63, heavy chain myosin, and calponin is very helpful [6]. ACC is usually positive for C-KIT and P63, and negative for both heavy chain myosin and calponin. Collagenous spherulosis and cribriform DCIS are positive for all myoepithelial cell markers but negative for C-KIT, while invasive cribriform carcinoma will not express any of those markers. Although, typically negative for ER, PR, and HER-2, up to 12 % of mammary ACC have been reported to be ER+/PR+ [5]. Other immunohistochemical studies dedicated solely to mammary ACC are identified in the literature, but are all limited by the small number of cases studied. These studies show a low proliferation index manifested by Ki-67, lack of P53 expression [7], and low Topoisomerase IIα expression, while demonstrating an over-expression of EGFR in 65 % of ACC cases [8].

Molecular Characteristics

Microarray-based gene expression studies have included ACC in the basal-like category due to their triple negative phenotype and expression of basal cell markers. However, studies focusing only on ACC show some molecular differences that distinguish ACC from the crowd of TNBC. ACC consistently displays t(6;9)(q22–23; pp 23–24) translocation, which generates a fusion transcript involving the MYB and NFIB genes [9]. This translocation is considered the key oncogenic mechanism in the pathogenesis of ACC. EGFR gene amplification which has been shown in some basal-like breast cancers, has not been demonstrated in ACC [8]. Similarly, C-KIT expression characteristic of ACC does not reflect an underlying KIT mutation.

Metaplastic Carcinoma

The term *metaplastic carcinoma* refers to a heterogeneous group of invasive breast carcinoma with microscopic features that diverge from glandular differentiation. These include either squamous or mesenchymal cell differentiation (e.g., spindle cell, chondroid, osseous, or myoid). Metaplastic carcinoma accounts for approximately 1 % of all invasive breast carcinomas. Clinically, patients present in a similar fashion to patients with invasive ductal carcinoma, NOS, in terms of their age at presentation and the manner in which the tumor is detected. The mammographic appearance of metaplastic carcinoma is not specific, except in tumors with osseous metaplasia, where bone-forming areas can be radiologically identified. Microscopically, metaplastic carcinoma varies in the type and extent of metaplastic change. In some tumors, the metaplastic foci may be present as isolated microscopic foci in an otherwise typical invasive ductal carcinoma. In other cases, particularly tumors with squamous and spindle cell metaplasia, the metaplastic component can present in a pure form without any recognizable glandular component. The latter may be difficult to differentiate from a malignant phyllodes tumor or a sarcoma on needle core biopsies. The most common heterologous elements in metaplastic carcinoma are osseous and chondroid differentiation (Fig. 11.1b). In these tumors, the bone and cartilage may appear histologically benign or frankly malignant, further raising the possibility of a sarcoma. The presence of DCIS in tumors with a predominant mesenchymal component, supports the diagnosis of metaplastic carcinoma.

Immunohistochemistry

The diagnosis of metaplastic carcinoma in challenging cases lies in the identification of the epithelial origin of the tumor cells. This may require the use of a panel of low-and high-molecular weight cytokeratins since many metaplastic carcinomas show only focal positivity for CK or may even be negative to some. CK903(34betaE12) and P63 have been reported as sensitive markers for metaplastic carcinomas [10]. As other members of the TNBC family, >90 % of metaplastic carcinomas are negative for ER, PR, and HER2.

Molecular Characteristics

Metaplastic carcinoma are thought to arise from altered epithelial and/or myoepithelial cells. This theory is supported by cytogenetic and molecular studies that demonstrate the same clonality in both the glandular and non-glandular components of the tumor, indicating a common stem cell origin [11, 12]. Collectively, metaplastic carcinomas fall into the category of basal-like breast cancer, however, recent studies suggested that a subset of these tumors displays transcriptomic features consistent with cells undergoing epithelial-to-mesenchymal transition. These are referred to as Claudin-low tumors. Metaplastic carcinomas and claudin-low tumors are shown by comparative genomic hybridization to have low expression of GATA3-regulated genes and of genes responsible for cell-cell adhesion with enrichment for markers linked to stem cell function [13].

Carcinomas with Apocrine Differentiation

Focal apocrine differentiation can be seen in many types of breast carcinoma including: lobular, ductal, tubular, micropapillary, and even medullary carcinoma. However, carcinomas with extensive apocrine differentiation represent approximately 4 % of breast cancer and are represented in this category [14]. Histologically, the majority of the tumor cells display features reminiscent of apocrine cells such as enlarged round nuclei with prominent nucleoli and abundant granular eosinophilic cytoplasm that is PAS-positive (Type A cells) (Fig. 11.1c). Some cells may have abundant foamy cytoplasm, which is referred to as Type B cells, while other tumors may have a combination of both.

Immunohistochemistry

A typical apocrine carcinoma shows diffuse positivity for GCDFP-15 [14], and BCL-2 negativity. Staining for ER, PR is usually negative. A portion of these tumors is also negative for HER2 protein over-expression (triple negative). Androgen receptor expression in ER-negative breast tumors was found to be associated with apocrine differentiation [15].

Molecular Characteristics

The immunophenotypic signature described above has inspired researchers to look for a similar *"apocrine molecular signature."* Microarray studies show increased androgen signaling and overlap with the HER2 group of tumors. However, this proposed molecular signature does not correlate well with apocrine morphology. Approximately, only half of carcinomas with apocrine differentiation show this molecular signature. Comparative genomic hybridization has identified several copy number alterations in carcinomas with apocrine differentiation including gains of 1p, 1q and 2q, as well as losses of 1p, 12q, 16q, 17q, and 22q [16]. However, these are also common alteration regions that are seen in breast carcinoma in general. This data suggests that although carcinomas with apocrine differentiation may have a characteristic morphology and immunophenotype, they do not represent a distinct molecular entity.

Pleomorphic Carcinoma

This unusual and rare tumor is considered a variant of high-grade invasive ductal carcinoma, NOS. Morphologically, it is characterized by proliferation of pleomorphic, bizarre cells with greater than sixfold variation in nuclear size. Multinucleated tumor giant cells are common and account for more than 50 % of the tumor cells. Areas of conventional adenocarcinoma may be present. However, pure pleomorphic carcinoma and cases associated with metaplastic carcinoma, especially of the spindle cell type, may be seen and can be misdiagnosed as sarcoma or metastatic tumors. The presence of adjacent foci of ductal carcinoma in situ supports a breast primary in challenging cases (Fig. 11.1d). Axillary lymph node metastases are present in almost half the cases.

Immunohistochemistry

In the original series by Silver and Tavassoli, all tumors showed strong, diffuse positivity for pan-cytokeratin and CAM 5.2, which is useful in differentiating these tumors from sarcomas. EMA was positive in areas of conventional ductal carcinoma, but was very weak and focal in the multinucleated tumor cells. All tumors were negative for ER and PR. HER-2 was also negative in the majority of cases, especially those with node-negative disease [17]. P53 expression was present in 71 %, but none expressed bcl-2. Ki-67 proliferation index was also increased with a mean of 33 %.

Molecular Characteristics

The data on pleomorphic carcinoma is very sparse due to the rarity of these tumors. Nevertheless, the majority of these tumors show aneuploid DNA content and high S-phase.

Secretory Carcinoma

Secretory carcinoma (SC) is an exceptionally rare, low-grade carcinoma accounting for <0.15 % of all breast cancers. They occur over a wide age range, but more commonly in children and young adults *"Juvenile carcinoma."* Clinically, they are well-circumscribed tumors, located close to the areola. Grossly, the tumor size ranges from 0.5 to 12 cm with an average of 3 cm. Microscopically, secretory carcinoma has pushing borders and is composed of polygonal cells with granular eosinophilic to foamy cytoplasm (Fig. 11.2a). A consistent finding is the presence of intracellular and extracellular, eosinophilic, secretory material that is positive for PAS and alcian blue (Fig. 11.2b, c). The tumor displays one or more of three growth patterns: solid, tubular, and microcyctic. The latter resembles thyroid follicles. Most tumors contain a mixture of all three patterns.

Immunohistochemistry

The tumor cells are negative for ER, PR, and HER-2, and frequently positive for epithelial membrane antigen (EMA), S-100 protein, and E-cadherin (Fig. 11.2d). Expression of basal cytokeratins (CK 5/6 and 14) was also identified in five out of

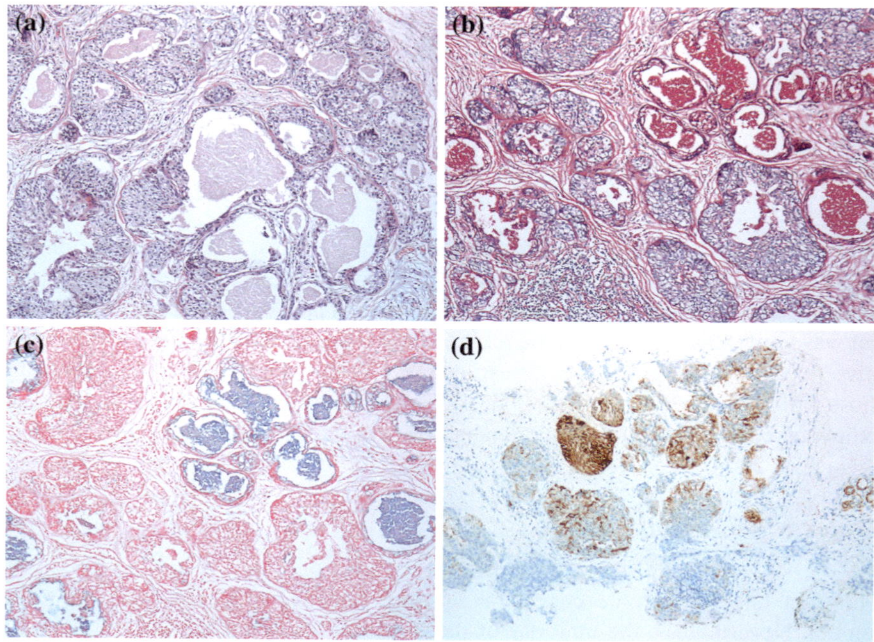

Fig. 11.2 Secretory carcinoma. **a** H&E, 100×. **b** Luminal secretions are strongly PAS-D positive. **c** Alcian blue positive. **d** S-100 protein is also strongly positive

six cases in one study, suggesting that secretory carcinoma belongs to the basal-like group of breast cancer [18].

Molecular Characteristics

In 2002, Tognon et al. [19] have shown that secretory carcinoma is characteristically associated with t(12, 15) that results in ETV6-NTRK3 gene fusion, the same translocation which was originally described in congenital fibrosarcoma and cellular mesoblastic nephroma. Additionally, FISH analysis shows alteration of the ETV6 gene in both the in situ and invasive components [18].

Carcinoma with Medullary Features

Classic medullary carcinoma (MC) is very rare, representing less than 1 % of all breast cancers. The diagnosis of classic MC requires stringent diagnostic criteria which include histological circumscription, lack of tubular formation with syncytial architecture in >75 % of the tumor, intense lymphoplasmacytic infiltration, and highly pleomorphic tumor cells with numerous mitoses. Tumors that lack some of these features are classified as "atypical medullary carcinoma" or "invasive ductal carcinoma with medullary features." However, these criteria are often difficult to apply resulting in a high interobserver variability. For the same reasons, the new <u>WHO Classification of Tumors of The Breast</u> has now grouped classic and atypical medullary as well as a subset of invasive carcinoma of no special type under "Carcinomas with medullary features". Foci of squamous metaplasia can also be seen in MC and should not be considered as a metaplastic carcinoma.

Immunohistochemistry

The majority (>90 %) of MC are negative for ER, PR, and HER-2, with variable expression of basal cytokeratin (CK5/6), EGFR, and P53. The intense lymphocytic infiltrate is predominantly CD3+T lymphocytes. Not surprisingly, MC shows a high proliferation index with Ki-67.

Molecular Characteristics

MC heirs a lot of its molecular features from its basal-like family of breast cancers, including EGFR gene amplification, TP53 gene mutation, and increased incidence in patients with BRCA1 gene mutations [20]. Some questioned the role of Epstein-Barr virus infection in MC given its morphologic similarities with lymphoepithelial carcinomas of other organs. Whereas, one study showed an association between Epstein-Barr virus and MC, another study failed to reproduce this link [21, 22].

Basal-like Breast Carcinoma

Basal-like breast carcinomas (BLBC) is a distinct group of breast carcinoma that has evolved as a separate molecular subtype from gene expression profiling studies [23, 24]. They usually present as rapidly growing breast masses, most probably as "interval breast cancers" (those diagnosed between annual mammograms) [25]. Radiologically, they are often ill-defined, oval, round, or lobulated masses. Extensive necrosis may give the impression of a partially solid and cystic mass on ultrasound. Except for circumscription and geographic necrosis, BLBC shares a lot of histologic features with medullary carcinoma. The tumor is usually grade III invasive ductal carcinoma with focal/absent in situ component, high nuclear grade, absence of tubular formation, and high-mitotic rate. There is usually a dense stromal lymphocytic infiltrate, a solid architecture with pushing borders and areas of

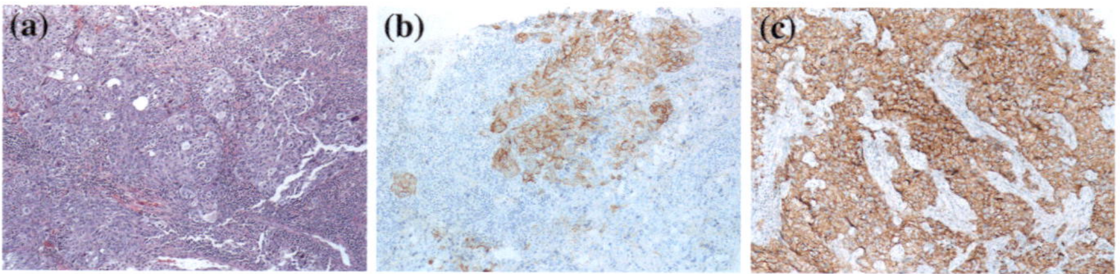

Fig. 11.3 Basal-like breast cancer. **a** H&E stain, 100×. **b** CK5/6 immunostain showing positive staining of the tumor cells. **c** IMP3 immunostain is diffusely positive

geographic necrosis (Fig. 11.3a). Like medullary carcinoma, BRCA-1 associated carcinomas are often BLBC.

Immunohistochemistry

Expression of basal cytokeratins, particularly CK5/6 and CK14 is considered the sine-qua-non of BLBC (Fig. 11.3b). CK17 is also present in approximately 50 % of cases, but may be focal and weak. The expression of EGFR in BLBC varies in several studies, ranging from 45 to 70 %. Since more than 80 % of BRCA-1 associated cancers cluster in the basal-like category, it is not surprising that basal CKs and EGFR expression are also observed in BRCA-1 associated breast cancers. However, attempts to use these markers together with hormone receptors to predict mutation status in these patients has not been successful due to the high overlap between both BRCA-1 and non BRCA-1 associated BLBC [26]. Various other immunohistochemical markers have been studied as a tool to recognize and further characterize this specific subset of tumors. Insulin-like growth factor-II mRNA-binding protein 3 (IMP3), which was first introduced as a marker of aggressive behavior in renal cell and urothelial carcinomas [27], has been demonstrated in 78 % of TNBC, and correlates with CK5/6 expression (Fig. 11.3c) [28]. C-KIT has been reported in approximately 45 % of BLBC. P53 over-expression is also more common in BLBC compared to all breast cancers. Vascular endothelial growth factor (VEGF), maspin, osteopontin, integrin β4, caveolin1 and 2 have all been reported to be preferentially expressed in BLBC [29–33]. However, the only IHC signature of BLBC that has been validated by expression profiling demonstrates that a panel composed of ER, HER2, CK 5/6, and EGFR can identify these tumors with 100 % specificity and 76 % sensitivity [34].

Molecular Characteristics

The literature has been enriched by many studies that focus on better understanding of the molecular background of BLBC, in attempt to translate this molecular phenotype into targeted therapy. TP53 mutation has been identified in up to 83 % BLBC cases. The mutation is thought to be an early event in tumorigenesis and is related to poor prognosis and resistance to chemotherapy [35, 36]. The link with BRCA-1 gene mutation is well established. More than 80 % of BRCA-1 associated cancers cluster in the basal-like category [37], and many sporadic BLBC were shown to have altered BRCA1 activity and loss of function. Approximately 10–20 % of BLBC show methylation of gene promoter, and some have decreased BRCA1 mRNA. X-chromosome abnormalities, including defects in inactivation, were also identified. Additionally, the dominant-negative transcriptional regulator ID4 has been shown to regulate *BRCA1* expression and to be preferentially expressed in BLBC [38–40]. Additionally, the loss of one *TP53* allele in mice with mammary-specific deletion of *BRCA1* dramatically accelerates mammary tumorigenesis, suggesting that TP53 mutations may act synergistically with BRCA1 defects in sporadic BLBC to drive tumor initiation.

The high-mitotic index and high rates of proliferation that characterize BLBC reflect the expression of several proliferation-related genes. EGFR is expressed in a large percentage of BLBC. A recent study on IMP-3 in BLBC showed it to be the effector of EGFR-mediated tumor migration and invasion suggesting a mechanism by which IMP-3 may be regulated in breast cancer. Cyclin E1 over-expression has also been shown in BLBC. ELISA studies reveal a three-fold increase in VEGF expression levels in TNBC compared to non-TNBC. Moreover, high VEGF-receptor2 expression was observed in a subset of TNBC and correlates with a shorter survival. The expression of Fascin, an invasion promoting gene, was observed in 54 % of BLBC, and in 83 % of BRCA1-associated carcinomas.

Prognosis

TNBC has gained a bad reputation as a tumor of poor prognosis largely because the terms TNBC and BLBC are often incorrectly used as synonyms. Studies have proven that this is not necessarily the case, and using the term TNBC to imply a badly behaving tumor will expose many patients to unnecessary treatments with ample side effects. Members of this diverse family of tumors behave differently and have variable prognoses.

Perhaps the most "innocent" member in this family is ACC. Despite its triple negative nature and paucity of treatment regimens, ACC is considered a low-grade carcinoma with an excellent prognosis. The data from the Surveillance, Epidemiology and End Results (SEER) program show that the 5-year, 10-year, and 15-year survival for patients with mammary ACC are 98, 95, and 91 %, respectively [5]. Many cases are treated with lumpectomy, but simple mastectomy is generally curative. Axillary dissection is unnecessary except for the very rare cases of nodal metastases. Local recurrence is rare, and is usually related to incomplete excision.

Prognostic data on patients with metaplastic carcinomas is somewhat limited due to the uncommon nature of the disease, and have been based largely on patients treated by mastectomy with axillary dissection. It is unclear if the type and amount of metaplasia has a significant effect on prognosis. However, specific subtypes such as low-grade adenosquamous carcinoma, have a good prognosis compared to other types of metaplastic carcinoma. On the contrary, recent data suggests that Claudin-low carcinomas may have a lower response rate to conventional chemotherapy and a worse clinical outcome than other metaplastic carcinomas [13].

With approximately 38 % mortality rate in the first 2 years, pleomorphic carcinoma has a very poor prognosis [17]. Conversely, secretory carcinoma has a favorable prognosis, especially in children and adolescents. In older patients, the tumor may take a more aggressive clinical course with late metastases [41]. Axillary lymph node and distant metastases are very rare and usually manifested in older patients.

Medullary carcinoma, when defined by strict morphologic criteria, also has a favorable prognosis. This may be related to the intense lymphocytic infiltration that represents the host immune response, the well circumscription that makes resection with wide clear margins a relatively easier task for surgeons, and the high mitotic rate that makes these tumors very sensitive to chemotherapy. Gene expression profiling studies have demonstrated that the expression levels of immune response genes are independent predictors of the outcome in patients with highly proliferative breast cancers. This suggests that the relatively good prognosis of tumors with medullary features may be attributed to the prominent lymphoplasmacytic stromal response. The 10-year survival for patients with pure MC is greater than 80 % in some reports. Axillary lymph node metastases are uncommon and, when present, are usually in fewer than four lymph nodes. However, patients with tumors larger than three cm or those with metastases to more than four lymph nodes do not have the same favorable prognosis. Additionally, patients with BRCA1 mutations who develop MC do not have the same prognosis as those without the mutation. The low level of reproducibility in diagnosing MC, and the concern for under calling an aggressive BLBC tumor as a MC, has led to a decrease in the number of reported MC cases and a marked shrinkage of this controversial subtype. Currently, it is a common practice to treat MC in a similarly aggressive fashion as BLBC.

BLBC represents the "ugly face" of TNBC. It is well-documented now that BLBC has the worst behavior amongst breast cancers. This poor prognosis may be attributable to the over expression of genes promoting proliferation, angiogenesis, and migration. Studies have shown a decreased disease-free survival and overall survival compared to other types of breast cancer. Patients with BLBC are at a higher risk for early relapse/recurrence. A large, central fibrotic scar, occasionally seen histologically, was suggested as a poor prognostic feature, associated with a higher risk of distant metastases [42]. Interestingly, BLBC has a different pattern of distant metastases. Brain metastases, which in itself carry a poor prognosis, are more common among patients with BLBC [43]. The expression of basal cytokeratins in breast cancer has been shown to be associated with a poor outcome [44]. Further, expression of these cytokeratins in node-negative breast carcinoma, is a poor prognostic factor, independent of tumor size and grade [44]. Multivariate analysis indicates that EGFR is also a significant, independent prognostic factor in breast cancer patients, whose expression is associated with shorter disease-free survival [45].

Of all the TNBC subtypes, treatment for BLBC remains the greatest challenge because of its clinically aggressive nature and limited therapeutic options. Traditionally, oncologists have used anthracycline and paclitaxel to treat these breast cancer patients. Even though neoadjuvant chemotherapy results in complete pathologic response in 15–25 % of BLBC [46], most patients continue to have residual disease and remain at a high risk for relapse and death within the first 5 years of diagnosis. Moreover, the nonspecific cytotoxicity of these agents may result in significant, dose-limiting side effects. Thus, the development of targeted therapies with improved therapeutic indices is of paramount importance. One approach was to explore platinum based chemotherapy agents (carboplatin, cisplatin, etc.). Platinum agents produce DNA cross-links, leading to DNA double-strand breaks, normally repaired by BRCA. Since many BLBC exhibits BRCA-1 gene defects, these cells become highly sensitive to the apoptosis induced by these agents. Cisplatin also promotes apoptosis in BLBC by disrupting a complex in the TP53 family that is present selectively in BLBC with mutant TP53. In a recent study, 22 % of patients with TNBC showed complete pathological remission with single-agent neoadjuvant cisplatin [47]. This rate is similar to that observed with non-platinum agents. Platinum agents appear to be the most promising therapy that may improve survival in BLBC.

BRCA1 pathway dysfunction is also the basis for treating BLBC with Poly (ADP) Ribose Polymerase Inhibitors (PARP-I). PARP is involved in base excision repair; an important pathway in the repair of single-strand breaks in DNA [48]. Single-strand breaks become double-strand breaks at replication forks, creating more DNA lesions to be repaired by homologous combination in the absence of functioning PARP. This occurs without increasing or affecting the process of homologous recombination [49]. Combined with the effects of BRCA-1 gene mutations on homologous recombination, increased numbers of DNA errors may lead to a cell cycle arrest and, potentially, permanent arrest and apoptosis in tumors. Cell lines with BRCA dysfunction have been proven to be extremely sensitive to PARP-I [50]. PARP-I are relatively nontoxic compared to general cytotoxic chemotherapy because they do not directly damage DNA, therefore, targeting cooperative pathways that may lead to the development of specific and less toxic therapy. Depending on whether the tumor is due to a BRCA germline mutation, or a sporadic mutation with BRCA-like effects, normal tissue outside the tumor maintains at least one copy of wild type BRCA, thus enabling the repair of normal cells affected by the PARP inhibition [50]. This approach uses the concept of *synthetic lethality* by targeting DNA repair pathways in a complementary manner, leading to a lethal combination [51].

Aberrant VEGF pathway activation shown in BLBC has led to the investigation of targeting anti-angiogenic therapeutic strategy to VEGF and its downstream receptors. Bevacizumab, the anti-VEGF antibody, was shown to increase disease-free survival when combined with paclitaxel in patients with TNBC by four months, compared to paclitaxel alone. However, the overall survival was unaffected [52]. Other small-molecule multikinase inhibitors have been developed as possible anti-angiogenic agents. These inhibit VEGFR and other receptor tyrosine kinases

[53]. Sunitinib (Sutent®) is a multi-targeted receptor tyrosine kinase inhibitor. Sunitinib inhibits cellular signaling by targeting multiple receptor tyrosine kinases (RTKs), including platelet-derived growth factor (PDGF-Rs) and VEGFRs, which play a role in both tumor angiogenesis and tumor cell proliferation. This simultaneous inhibition leads to reduced tumor vascularization, cancer cell death, and ultimately tumor shrinkage. Sunitinib was shown to induce an 11 % response rate when used as a single agent in patients with previously treated metastatic breast carcinoma. Fifteen percent of BLBC patients responded to treatment [54]. Other studies have demonstrated a response in one third of patients with metastatic or locally advanced BLBC to treatment with sunitinib added to paclitaxel. Other VEGFR multikinase inhibitors have not been as promising [55]. The currently demonstrated limited response to antiangiogenic agents is considered disappointing.

Since EGFR is upregulated in the majority of BLBC, it represents a potential therapeutic target. Lapatinib is a dual inhibitor of EGFR and HER2 tyrosine kinases [56]. In randomized trials, the use of lapatinib with placitaxel was shown to have a significant benefit in HER2-amplified tumors [57]. In contrast, patients with HER2-negative tumors and overexpression of EGFR did not benefit from the addition of lapatinib [56]. This suggests that although EGFR overexpression is present in the majority of BLBC, it may not be a helpful therapeutic target.

Multiple other downstream kinases are under consideration as targeted therapy for BLBC patients. Constitutive activity of these pathways downstream from EGFR may be an explanation for the lack of response to EGFR-targeted therapies. One such target currently being explored is the mitogen-activated protein kinase (MAPK)/extracellular signal-regulated kinase (ERK) kinase (MEK), a signaling pathway with a central role in promoting tumor initiation and progression [58]. Activation of this pathway has been shown to be associated with an increased risk of metastasis in breast cancer patients [59]. As a therapeutic target, early clinical studies have demonstrated a limited response [60, 61]. A more recent study has shown that BLBC appears to be particularly sensitive to MEK inhibitors. This study also elucidated the interaction and potential negative feedback loop between the MEK cascade and the phosphoindositide 3-kinase (PI3K)-PTEN-AKT signaling cascade, which counteracts the effects of MEK inhibition of cell cycle and apoptosis induction. These findings may, in part, explain why initial studies showed only a modest response to MEK inhibition and suggest concurrent treatment with both MEK and PI3K inhibitors is a promising therapeutic possibility [58].

Summary

TNBC is a heterogenous group of breast carcinoma with varying morphology, immunophenotype and molecular characteristics. Treatment and prognosis are highly variable amongst the group. Morphologic correlation with immunohistochemistry and molecular signature is the key to establish an accurate diagnosis, which will then dictate further management.

Key Points

- TNBC is a heterogeneous group of tumors accounting for about 10–15 % of all breast cancers.
- ACC is a low-grade carcinoma, morphologically identical to its salivary gland counterpart and has excellent prognosis.
- Claudin-low associated tumors are considered subsets of metaplastic carcinoma with low expression of GATA3-regulated genes and genes responsible for cell-cell adhesion.
- Carcinomas with apocrine differentiation have characteristic morphology and immunophenotype (GCDFP and AR positive), but do not represent a distinct molecular entity.
- Pleomorphic carcinomas are poorly differentiated tumors with highly pleomorphic, bizarre cells, and tumor giant cells mimicking sarcoma. These tumors have very poor prognosis.
- Secretory carcinoma has a favorable prognosis in children and young adults but can be aggressive in older patients.
- More than 80 % of BRCA-1 associated cancers cluster in the basal-like category.
- A panel of ER, HER2, CK 5/6, and EGFR can identify BLBC with 100 % specificity and 76 % sensitivity.
- MC are now commonly treated as BLBC due to the low level of reproducibility in its diagnosis and concern for under-treating an aggressive BLBC.

References

1. Trivers KF, Lund MJ, Porter PL, Liff JM, Flagg EW, Coates RJ, Eley JW. The epidemiology of triple-negative breast cancer, including race. Cancer Causes Control. 2009;20:1071–82.
2. Phipps AI, Chlebowski RT, Prentice R, McTiernan A, Stefanick ML, Wactawski-Wende J, Kuller LH, Adams-Campbell LL, Lane D, Vitolins M, Kabat GC, Rohan TE, Li CI. Body size, physical activity, and risk of triple-negative and estrogen receptor-positive breast cancer. Cancer Epidemiol Biomark Prev. 2011;20:454–63 (a publication of the American Association for Cancer Research, cosponsored by the American Society of Preventive Oncology).
3. Bauer KR, Brown M, Cress RD, Parise CA, Caggiano V. Descriptive analysis of estrogen receptor (er)-negative, progesterone receptor (pr)-negative, and her2-negative invasive breast cancer, the so-called triple-negative phenotype: A population-based study from the california cancer registry. Cancer. 2007;109:1721–8.
4. Sumpio BE, Jennings TA, Merino MJ, Sullivan PD. Adenoid cystic carcinoma of the breast. Data from the connecticut tumor registry and a review of the literature. Ann Surg. 1987;205:295–301.
5. Ghabach B, Anderson WF, Curtis RE, Huycke MM, Lavigne JA, Dores GM. Adenoid cystic carcinoma of the breast in the united states (1977 to 2006): A population-based cohort study. Breast Cancer Res. 2010;12:R54.
6. Rabban JT, Swain RS, Zaloudek CJ, Chase DR, Chen YY. Immunophenotypic overlap between adenoid cystic carcinoma and collagenous spherulosis of the breast: Potential diagnostic pitfalls using myoepithelial markers. Modern Pathol. 2006;19:1351–1357 (an official journal of the United States and Canadian Academy of Pathology, Inc).

7. Pastolero G, Hanna W, Zbieranowski I, Kahn HJ. Proliferative activity and p53 expression in adenoid cystic carcinoma of the breast. Modern Pathol. 1996;9:215–219 (an official journal of the United States and Canadian Academy of Pathology, Inc).

8. Vranic S, Frkovic-Grazio S, Lamovec J, Serdarevic F, Gurjeva O, Palazzo J, Bilalovic N, Lee LM, Gatalica Z. Adenoid cystic carcinomas of the breast have low topo IIα expression but frequently overexpress EGFR protein without EGFR gene amplification. Hum Pathol. 2010;41:1617–23.

9. Persson M, Andren Y, Mark J, Horlings HM, Persson F, Stenman G. Recurrent fusion of MYB and NFIB transcription factor genes in carcinomas of the breast and head and neck. Proc Natl Acad Sci USA. 2009;106:18740–4.

10. Dunne B, Lee AH, Pinder SE, Bell JA, Ellis IO. An immunohistochemical study of metaplastic spindle cell carcinoma, phyllodes tumor and fibromatosis of the breast. Hum Pathol. 2003;34:1009–15.

11. Teixeira MR, Qvist H, Bohler PJ, Pandis N, Heim S. Cytogenetic analysis shows that carcinosarcomas of the breast are of monoclonal origin. Genes Chromosom Cancer. 1998;22:145–51.

12. Wada H, Enomoto T, Tsujimoto M, Nomura T, Murata Y, Shroyer KR. Carcinosarcoma of the breast: Molecular-biological study for analysis of histogenesis. Hum Pathol. 1998;29:1324–8.

13. Hennessy BT, Gonzalez-Angulo AM, Stemke-Hale K, Gilcrease MZ, Krishnamurthy S, Lee JS, Fridlyand J, Sahin A, Agarwal R, Joy C, Liu W, Stivers D, Baggerly K, Carey M, Lluch A, Monteagudo C, He X, Weigman V, Fan C, Palazzo J, Hortobagyi GN, Nolden LK, Wang NJ, Valero V, Gray JW, Perou CM, Mills GB. Characterization of a naturally occurring breast cancer subset enriched in epithelial-to-mesenchymal transition and stem cell characteristics. Cancer Res. 2009;69:4116–24.

14. Eusebi V, Millis RR, Cattani MG, Bussolati G, Azzopardi JG. Apocrine carcinoma of the breast. A morphologic and immunocytochemical study. Am J Pathol. 1986;123:532–41.

15. Niemeier LA, Dabbs DJ, Beriwal S, Striebel JM, Bhargava R. Androgen receptor in breast cancer: Expression in estrogen receptor-positive tumors and in estrogen receptor-negative tumors with apocrine differentiation. Modern Pathol. 2010;23:205–212 (an official journal of the United States and Canadian Academy of Pathology, Inc).

16. Jones C, Damiani S, Wells D, Chaggar R, Lakhani SR, Eusebi V. Molecular cytogenetic comparison of apocrine hyperplasia and apocrine carcinoma of the breast. Am J Pathol. 2001;158:207–14.

17. Silver SA, Tavassoli FA. Pleomorphic carcinoma of the breast: Clinicopathological analysis of 26 cases of an unusual high-grade phenotype of ductal carcinoma. Histopathology. 2000;36:505–14.

18. Lae M, Freneaux P, Sastre-Garau X, Chouchane O, Sigal-Zafrani B, Vincent-Salomon A. Secretory breast carcinomas with ETV6-NTRK3 fusion gene belong to the basal-like carcinoma spectrum. Modern Pathol. 2009;22:291–298 (an official journal of the United States and Canadian Academy of Pathology, Inc).

19. Tognon C, Knezevich SR, Huntsman D, Roskelley CD, Melnyk N, Mathers JA, Becker L, Carneiro F, MacPherson N, Horsman D, Poremba C, Sorensen PH. Expression of the ETV6-NTRK3 gene fusion as a primary event in human secretory breast carcinoma. Cancer Cell. 2002;2:367–76.

20. Stratton M. RPathology of familial breast cancer: Differences between breast cancers in carriers of BRCA1 or BRCA2 mutations and sporadic cases. Breast cancer linkage consortium. Lancet. 1997;349:1505–1510.

21. Bonnet M, Guinebretiere JM, Kremmer E, Grunewald V, Benhamou E, Contesso G, Joab I. Detection of epstein-barr virus in invasive breast cancers. J Natl Cancer Inst. 1999;91:1376–81.

22. Lespagnard L, Cochaux P, Larsimont D, Degeyter M, Velu T, Heimann R. Absence of epstein-barr virus in medullary carcinoma of the breast as demonstrated by immunophenotyping, in situ hybridization and polymerase chain reaction. Am J Clin Pathol. 1995;103:449–52.

23. Perou CM, Sorlie T, Eisen MB, van de Rijn M, Jeffrey SS, Rees CA, Pollack JR, Ross DT, Johnsen H, Akslen LA, Fluge O, Pergamenschikov A, Williams C, Zhu SX, Lonning PE, Borresen-Dale AL, Brown PO, Botstein D. Molecular portraits of human breast tumours. Nature. 2000;406:747–52.
24. Sorlie T, Perou CM, Tibshirani R, Aas T, Geisler S, Johnsen H, Hastie T, Eisen MB, van de Rijn M, Jeffrey SS, Thorsen T, Quist H, Matese JC, Brown PO, Botstein D, Eystein Lonning P, Borresen-Dale AL. Gene expression patterns of breast carcinomas distinguish tumor subclasses with clinical implications. Proc Natl Acad Sci USA. 2001;98:10869–10874.
25. Kirsh VA, Chiarelli AM, Edwards SA, O'Malley FP, Shumak RS, Yaffe MJ, Boyd NF. Tumor characteristics associated with mammographic detection of breast cancer in the ontario breast screening program. J Natl Cancer Inst. 103:942–950.
26. Collins LC, Martyniak A, Kandel MJ, Stadler ZK, Masciari S. Miron A, Richardson AL, Schnitt SJ, Garber JE. Basal cytokeratin and epidermal growth factor receptor expression are not predictive of BRCA1 mutation status in women with triple-negative breast cancers. Am J Surg Pathol. 2009;33:1093–7.
27. Jiang Z, Chu PG, Woda BA, Rock KL, Liu Q, Hsieh CC, Li C, Chen W, Duan HO, McDougal S, Wu CL. Analysis of rna-binding protein IMP3 to predict metastasis and prognosis of renal-cell carcinoma: A retrospective study. Lancet Oncol. 2006;7:556–64.
28. Walter O, Prasad M, Lu S, Quinlan RM, Edmiston KL, Khan A. IMP3 is a novel biomarker for triple negative invasive mammary carcinoma associated with a more aggressive phenotype. Hum Pathol. 2009;40:1528–33.
29. Lu S, Simin K, Khan A, Mercurio AM. Analysis of integrin beta4 expression in human breast cancer: Association with basal-like tumors and prognostic significance. Clin Cancer Res. 2008;14:1050–8.
30. Ryden L, Jirstrom K, Haglund M, Stal O, Ferno M. Epidermal growth factor receptor and vascular endothelial growth factor receptor 2 are specific biomarkers in triple-negative breast cancer. Results from a controlled randomized trial with long-term follow-up. Breast Cancer Res Treat. 120:491–498.
31. Elsheikh SE, Green AR, Rakha EA, Samaka RM, Ammar AA, Powe D, Reis-Filho JS, Ellis IO. Caveolin 1 and caveolin 2 are associated with breast cancer basal-like and triple-negative immunophenotype. Br J Cancer. 2008;99:327–34.
32. Umekita YD, Ohi YD, Souda MD, Rai YD, Sagara YD, Sagara YD, Tamada SD, Tanimoto AD. Maspin expression is frequent and correlates with basal markers in triple-negative breast cancer. Diagn Pathol. 6:36.
33. Wang X, Chao L, Ma G, Chen L, Tian B, Zang Y, Sun J. Increased expression of osteopontin in patients with triple-negative breast cancer. Eur J Clin Invest. 2008;38:438–46.
34. Nielsen TO, Hsu FD, Jensen K, Cheang M, Karaca G, Hu Z, Hernandez-Boussard T, Livasy C, Cowan D, Dressler L, Akslen LA, Ragaz J, Gown AM, Gilks CB, van de Rijn M, Perou CM. Immunohistochemical and clinical characterization of the basal-like subtype of invasive breast carcinoma. Clin Cancer Res. 2004;10:5367–74.
35. Hollstein M, Sidransky D, Vogelstein B, Harris CC. P53 mutations in human cancers. Science. 1991;253:49–53.
36. Borresen-Dale AL. TP53 and breast cancer. Hum Mutat. 2003;21:292–300.
37. Waddell N, Arnold J, Cocciardi S, da Silva L, Marsh A, Riley J. Johnstone CN, Orloff M, Assie G, Eng C, Reid L, Keith P, Yan M, Fox S, Devilee P, Godwin AK, Hogervorst FB, Couch F, Grimmond S, Flanagan JM, Khanna K, Simpson PT, Lakhani SR, Chenevix-Trench G. Subtypes of familial breast tumours revealed by expression and copy number profiling. Breast Cancer Res Treat. 2010;123:661–77.
38. Schneider BP, Winer EP, Foulkes WD, Garber J, Perou CM, Richardson A, Sledge GW, Carey LA. Triple-negative breast cancer: Risk factors to potential targets. Clinical Cancer Res. 2008;14:8010–8 (an official journal of the American Association for Cancer Research).
39. Valentin MD, da Silva SD, Privat M, Alaoui-Jamali M, Bignon YJ. Molecular insights on basal-like breast cancer. Breast Cancer Res Treat. 2012;1:21–30.

40. Turner N, Tutt A, Ashworth A. Hallmarks of 'brcaness' in sporadic cancers. Nat Rev Cancer. 2004;4:814–9.
41. Krausz T, Jenkins D, Grontoft O, Pollock DJ, Azzopardi JG. Secretory carcinoma of the breast in adults: Emphasis on late recurrence and metastasis. Histopathology. 1989;14:25–36.
42. Van den Eynden GG, Smid M, Van Laere SJ, Colpaert CG, Van der Auwera I, Bich TX, van Dam P, den Bakker MA, Dirix LY, Van Marck EA, Vermeulen PB, Foekens JA. Gene expression profiles associated with the presence of a fibrotic focus and the growth pattern in lymph node-negative breast cancer. Clin Cancer Res. 2008;14:2944–52.
43. Hicks DG, Short SM, Prescott NL, Tarr SM, Coleman KA, Yoder BJ, Crowe JP, Choueiri TK, Dawson AE, Budd GT, Tubbs RR, Casey G, Weil RJ. Breast cancers with brain metastases are more likely to be estrogen receptor negative, express the basal cytokeratin CK 5/6, and overexpress HER2 or EGFR. Am J Surg Pathol. 2006;30:1097–104.
44. van de Rijn M, Perou CM, Tibshirani R, Haas P, Kallioniemi O, Kononen J, Torhorst J, Sauter G, Zuber M, Kochli OR, Mross F, Dieterich H, Seitz R, Ross D, Botstein D, Brown P. Expression of cytokeratins 17 and 5 identifies a group of breast carcinomas with poor clinical outcome. Am J Pathol. 2002;161:1991–6.
45. Liu D, He J, Yuan Z, Wang S, Peng R, Shi Y, Teng X, Qin T. EGFR expression correlates with decreased disease-free survival in triple-negative breast cancer: A retrospective analysis based on a tissue microarray. Med Oncol. 2012;29:401–405.
46. Rouzier R, Perou CM, Symmans WF, Ibrahim N, Cristofanilli M, Anderson K, Hess KR, Stec J, Ayers M, Wagner P, Morandi P, Fan C, Rabiul I, Ross JS, Hortobagyi GN, Pusztai L. Breast cancer molecular subtypes respond differently to preoperative chemotherapy. Clin Cancer Res. 2005;11:5678–85 (an official journal of the American Association for Cancer Research).
47. Silver DP, Richardson AL, Eklund AC, Wang ZC, Szallasi Z, Li Q, Juul N, Leong CO, Calogrias D, Buraimoh A, Fatima A, Gelman RS, Ryan PD, Tung NM, De Nicolo A, Ganesan S, Miron A, Colin C, Sgroi DC, Ellisen LW, Winer EP, Garber JE. Efficacy of neoadjuvant cisplatin in triple-negative breast cancer. J Clin Oncol. 2010;28:1145–53 (official journal of the American Society of Clinical Oncology).
48. Hoeijmakers JH. Genome maintenance mechanisms for preventing cancer. Nature. 2001;411:366–74.
49. Schultz N, Lopez E, Saleh-Gohari N, Helleday T. Poly(ADP-ribose) polymerase (PARP-1) has a controlling role in homologous recombination. Nucleic Acids Res. 2003;31:4959–64.
50. Farmer H, McCabe N, Lord CJ, Tutt AN, Johnson DA, Richardson TB, Santarosa M, Dillon KJ, Hickson I, Knights C, Martin NM, Jackson SP, Smith GC, Ashworth A. Targeting the DNA repair defect in BRCA mutant cells as a therapeutic strategy. Nature. 2005;434:917–21.
51. Ashworth A. A synthetic lethal therapeutic approach: Poly(ADP) ribose polymerase inhibitors for the treatment of cancers deficient in DNA double-strand break repair. J Clin Oncol. 2008;26:3785–90 (official journal of the American Society of Clinical Oncology).
52. Miller K, Wang M, Gralow J, Dickler M, Cobleigh M, Perez EA, Shenkier T, Cella D, Davidson NE. Paclitaxel plus bevacizumab versus paclitaxel alone for metastatic breast cancer. N Engl J Med. 2007;357:2666–76.
53. Ivy SP, Wick JY, Kaufman BM. An overview of small-molecule inhibitors of VEGFR signaling. Nat Rev Clin Oncol. 2009;6:569–79.
54. Burstein HJ, Elias AD, Rugo HS, Cobleigh MA, Wolff AC, Eisenberg PD, Lehman M, Adams BJ, Bello CL, DePrimo SE, Baum CM, Miller KD. Phase ii study of sunitinib malate, an oral multitargeted tyrosine kinase inhibitor, in patients with metastatic breast cancer previously treated with an anthracycline and a taxane. J Clin Oncol. 2008;26:1810–6 (official journal of the American Society of Clinical Oncology).
55. Moreno-Aspitia A, Morton RF, Hillman DW, Lingle WL, Rowland KM Jr, Wiesenfeld M, Flynn PJ, Fitch TR, Perez EA. Phase ii trial of sorafenib in patients with metastatic breast cancer previously exposed to anthracyclines or taxanes: North central cancer treatment group and mayo clinic trial n0336. J Clin Oncol. 2009;27(11):15 (official journal of the American Society of Clinical Oncology).

56. Finn RS, Press MF, Dering J, Arbushites M, Koehler M, Oliva C, Williams LS, Di Leo A. Estrogen receptor, progesterone receptor, human epidermal growth factor receptor 2 (her2), and epidermal growth factor receptor expression and benefit from lapatinib in a randomized trial of paclitaxel with lapatinib or placebo as first-line treatment in HER2-negative or unknown metastatic breast cancer. J Clin Oncol. 2009;27:3908–15 (official journal of the American Society of Clinical Oncology).
57. Geyer CE, Forster J, Lindquist D, Chan S, Romieu CG, Pienkowski T, Jagiello-Gruszfeld A, Crown J, Chan A, Kaufman B, Skarlos D, Campone M, Davidson N, Berger M, Oliva C, Rubin SD, Stein S, Cameron D. Lapatinib plus capecitabine for HER2-positive advanced breast cancer. N Engl J Med. 2006;355:2733–43.
58. Mirzoeva OK, Das D, Heiser LM, Bhattacharya S, Siwak D, Gendelman R, Bayani N, Wang NJ, Neve RM, Guan Y, Hu Z, Knight Z, Feiler HS, Gascard P, Parvin B, Spellman PT, Shokat KM, Wyrobek AJ, Bissell MJ, McCormick F, Kuo WL, Mills GB, Gray JW, Korn WM. Basal subtype and MAPK/ERK kinase (MEK)-phosphoinositide 3-kinase feedback signaling determine susceptibility of breast cancer cells to mek inhibition. Cancer Res. 2009;69:565–72.
59. Adeyinka A, Nui Y, Cherlet T, Snell L, Watson PH, Murphy LC. Activated mitogen-activated protein kinase expression during human breast tumorigenesis and breast cancer progression. Clin Cancer Res. 2002;8:1747–53 (an official journal of the American Association for Cancer Research).
60. Rinehart J, Adjei AA, Lorusso PM, Waterhouse D, Hecht JR, Natale RB, Hamid O, Varterasian M, Asbury P, Kaldjian EP, Gulyas S, Mitchell DY, Herrera R, Sebolt-Leopold JS, Meyer MB. Multicenter phase II study of the oral MEK inhibitor, CI-1040, in patients with advanced non-small-cell lung, breast, colon, and pancreatic cancer. J Clin Oncol. 2004;22:4456–62 (official journal of the American Society of Clinical Oncology).
61. Adjei AA, Cohen RB, Franklin W, Morris C, Wilson D, Molina JR, Hanson LJ, Gore L, Chow L, Leong S, Maloney L, Gordon G, Simmons H, Marlow A, Litwiler K, Brown S, Poch G, Kane K, Haney J, Eckhardt SG. Phase i pharmacokinetic and pharmacodynamic study of the oral, small-molecule mitogen-activated protein kinase kinase 1/2 inhibitor AZD6244 (ARRY-142886) in patients with advanced cancers. J Clin Oncol. 2008;26:2139–46 (official journal of the American Society of Clinical Oncology).

Chapter 12
Molecular-Based Diagnostic, Prognostic and Predictive Tests in Breast Cancer

Abir A. Muftah, Mohammed A. Aleskandarany,
Ian O. Ellis and Emad A. Rakha

Introduction

Generally speaking, a prognostic factor is any measurable parameter capable of providing information on patient clinical outcome, i.e. assessing the risk of disease recurrence at the time of primary diagnosis, independent of therapy. Prognostic factors are usually indicators of tumour growth, invasiveness and metastatic potential. A predictive factor is any measurable parameter capable of providing information on the likelihood of response to a particular therapeutic modality [1, 2]. A Prognostic/predictive factor could be either a single trait or signature of traits that can stratify patients into different population. Although prognostic and predictive factors could be separately classified, several factors in breast cancer provide both prognostic and predictive information [e.g. oestrogen receptor (ER) expression and human epidermal growth factor receptors 2 (HER2) overexpression]. Biological molecular prognostic and predictive variables are primary tumour molecular characteristics that reflect the underlying genetic abnormalities and their assessment, using different platforms, can be used to determine tumour behaviour and response to therapy.

ER, progesterone receptor (PR), HER2, tumour size, lymph node stage and histological grade are the existing practical prognostic and predictive parameters [3]. The last three prognostic parameters are combinatorially incorporated into the Nottingham Prognostic Index (NPI); [4], a well-recognised prognostic tool in

A.A. Muftah · M.A. Aleskandarany · I.O. Ellis · E.A. Rakha (⊠)
Department of Histopathology, Division of Cancer and Stem Cells, School of Medicine,
The University of Nottingham and Nottingham University Hospitals NHS Trust,
Nottingham City Hospital, Nottingham NG5 1PB, UK
e-mail: Emad.Rakha@nottingham.ac.uk

© Springer Science+Business Media New York 2015
A. Khan et al. (eds.), *Precision Molecular Pathology of Breast Cancer*,
Molecular Pathology Library 10, DOI 10.1007/978-1-4939-2886-6_12

"""

breast cancer because of its simplicity and clinical utility [5]. However, there are increasing concerns that these parameters are not sufficient to assess prognosis and response to therapy in view of the diversity and heterogeneity of breast cancer behaviour. In addition, although positivity of hormonal receptors and overexpression of HER2 in breast cancer provide prognostic information and act as predictive parameters for the response of hormonal therapy and anti-HER2 targeted agents, respectively [6–8], there remains a need for further refinement of management decision. In recent years, personalised systemic therapy has become an increasingly required in patient management, especially in early stage breast cancer. Accordingly, there is a need to develop or update the existing prognostic and predictive classifiers.

Gene-expression profiling studies have attracted attention by demonstrating the presence of different molecular classes with clinical relevance and that breast cancer morphologic heterogeneity can be linked to specific molecular profiles. Most of these molecular profiling studies have identified at least four distinctive molecular/biological subgroups: two luminal subtypes; namely luminal A and luminal B, the HER2-enriched and the basal-like types [9, 10].

Despite the prognostic relevance of molecular taxonomies and the well-documented prognostic power of certain gene signatures, there remain technical and cost-effectiveness issues regarding their incorporation into routine practice. Previous studies have demonstrated that the behaviour of well-established clinical parameters varies in the different molecular classes. Therefore, performance of current clinical prognostic indices may not provide the same information within the different molecular classes. Adjustment of the performance of the clinical parameters and prognostic indices to the most recent advancement in molecular classification of breast cancer is considered a way forward for personalised patient management. An additional problem with this approach is the cost and feasibility of microarray and chip gene expression technology for routine management of breast cancer. Alternatively, immunohistochemistry (IHC) is considered a practical, cost-effective and reliable technique for molecular classification and the gold standard in the routine assessment of the essential predictive molecular biomarkers; ER, PR and HER2 [11, 12].

Hormonal Receptors: Oestrogen Receptor (ER) and Progesterone Receptor (PR)

The expression of ER and PR acts as a prognostic and a predictive parameters and assessment of their expression is an established standard procedure in breast pathology. Oestrogen receptor is one of the steroid receptor families and localised predominantly in the nuclear compartment [13, 14]. These receptors stimulated by steroid hormones as oestrogen which both are taken part in several processes such as suppression of apoptosis, cellular proliferation, angiogenesis and invasion [15].

The oestrogen receptors, which are normally expressed in breast tissue, are two types ER-α [16] and ER-ß [17], ER-α, ER-α gene includes six functional domains and encodes a 67 KDa protein [11], is connected directly to the pathological processes which one of them is breast cancer [18].

Several studies assessed the prognostic value of ER negative status and its association with decrease in survival in node negative patients with breast cancer [19–22]. In addition, its expression in breast cancer has a high clinical importance as a predictive parameter and existence of oestrogen receptor confers favourable biology because the expression of ER by tumour cells was related to the benefit of hormonal therapy. Patient with ER-negative disease cannot benefit from endocrine therapy while the ER positive group does. For instance, the Early Breast Cancer Trialists' Collaborative Group represented that treatment of patients with tamoxifen; an anti-oestrogen therapy which can block cellular proliferation in breast cancer had an effect on the 5-years breast cancer mortality and recurrence [6]. Moreover, in a meta-analysis, tamoxifen and other selective oestrogen receptor modulators have shown an overall improvement by 38 % and 42 in the 10 years and 5 years follow-up, respectively [23]. Furthermore, several studies supported the relation between hormonal receptor status and response to chemotherapy as ER negative group (21–33 %) had a better response to necadjuvant chemotherapy than the hormonal receptors positive group (7–8 %) [24–26].

ER expressed in 60–80 % of breast cancer cases at the same time most of the oestrogen receptors cases express PRs as well [27, 28]. However, the discrepancy between PR and ER expression are sometimes present [28, 29]. PR is an ER-regulated gene; therefore the expression of this receptor is highly related to the existence of the ER. ER−/PR+ is an uncommon variety, constituting less than 1 % of all breast cancers [30]. Some benefits had been reported from tamoxifen therapy in this ER−/PR+ sub-group while no effect of PR receptor in oestrogen receptor positive cases [31].

Hormone receptor and HER2 also provide important diagnostic information in breast cancer. Hormone receptor positivity in primary or metastatic carcinoma is considered as strong diagnostic clue to breast origin. ER is expressed in both breast carcinomas and tumours of gynaecological origin. Although aberrant ER expression may be observed in other tissues such as lung carcinoma and colorectal carcinoma, the expression is usually weak and focal. For a diagnostic purpose, ER is often combined with other biomarkers based on initial assessment of the index tumour. Markers that can be used to determine origin of carcinoma with ER expression include CDX2 (colorectal), PAX8 (gynaecological tumours), TTF1 (lung and thyroid carcinoma), S100 and HMB45 (Melanoma). Interpretation of these markers is usually considered in combination together with morphology of the tumours and none of these markers alone can provide absolute specificity. Other diagnostic biomarkers for breast cancer include ER-related genes such as GATA3. As a diagnostic marker ER-alpha must be used; ER-beta is not specific to the breast and its expression can be seen in different organs. Other diagnostic breast biomarkers include GCDFP-15, mammaglobin and lactalbumin. Gross cystic disease fluid protein-15 (GCDFP-15) is a marker of apocrine differentiation that is considered to be specific to the breast, but it has low sensitivity and is also expressed in apocrine glands and submandibular salivary glands. Mammaglobin, a mammary-specific member of the uteroglobin family that is known to be overexpressed in human breast cancer; however, it is also expressed in some non-breast cancer sites such as endometroid carcinomas, endocervical adenocarcinoma in situ and sweat gland carcinomas.

Human Epidermal Growth Factor Receptor 2 (HER2)

HER2 is a member of the transmembrane receptors epidermal growth family (EGFR) of receptors; EGFR-/ErbB1, HER2/ErbB2, HER3/ErbB3 and HER4/ErbB4 [32]. Overexpression of HER2 occurs in 13–20 % of breast cancer cases, up to half of these cases are ER negative [33, 34]. Overexpression of HER2 is a well-established poor prognostic indicator of invasive breast cancer [27–29]. HER2 is the main predictive factor for anti-HER2 targeted therapy including Herceptin as well as other HER2 dual inhibitor tyrosine kinase such as Lapatinib which is dual inhibitor of HER2 and HER1 and HER dimerization inhibitor such as pertuzumab [35–37]. HER2 can also predict response to certain chemotherapeutic agents [38]. In addition to its prognostic value as a single marker with HER2 positive Herceptin naïve tumours show the worst outcome in breast cancer, HER2 when combined with hormone receptor with or without Ki67 can provide addition prognostic information similar to multiparameter prognostic gene signatures [39].

HER2 is also used to diagnose Paget's disease of the breast in which it is expressed in more than 90 % of Paget's cells; therefore, it can be used to differentiate Paget's disease from melanocytic lesion and Bowen's disease of the nipple. In addition *HER*2 amplification in breast tumours can be used to indicate malignancy as benign tumours do not show *HER*2 amplification. Some benign tumours show weak to moderate HER2 membrane staining.

Ki67 Expression

Cell proliferation is considered as one of the well-recognised prognostic factors in breast cancer [40]. Nuclear positivity of Ki67 protein is an indication of cellular proliferation and that the cells are in the proliferative pool/entered cell cycle but not necessarily in mitosis [41, 42]. Ki67 expression has long been reported as a prognostic marker in breast cancer [43–46]. Breast cancer positive for Ki67 is associated with worse prognosis than those tumours negative for Ki67. In retrospective analysis, we and others reported better response to adjuvant therapy in tumours with higher expression levels of Ki67 than those tumour having low levels of Ki67 [46, 47]. However, these results need validation on prospective basis. Importantly, Ki67 expression has been reported as an independent predictive factor for neoadjuvant chemotherapy in breast cancer patients [48, 49] as well as the neoadjuvant endocrine therapy in postmenopausal patients [50]. Patients with high post-treatment Ki67 expression levels were reported to have higher risk for disease relapse and death more than those with low or intermediate Ki67 expression [51]. In 2013, the St. Gallen International Breast Cancer Conference reinforced the addition of Ki67 into the definition of intrinsic subtype of breast cancer [52]. The most significant prognostic value of Ki67 in breast cancer is seen in ER+ luminal class and in grade 2 tumours. Ki67 has limited prognostic value in ER− and triple negative tumours. Consistent with its prognostic value, some centres have introduced Ki67 in the routine diagnostic practice.

Gene Expression Profiling

The introduction of modern technologies having the ability of simultaneous analysis of thousands of genes in a single assay combined with rigorous analytical approaches gave an opportunity for classifying breast cancer into distinct groups depend on gene expression profiles. This approach developed our understanding of breast cancer and opened new avenues for novel prognostic/predictive signatures in human breast cancer.

Breast Cancer Molecular Classes

Gene-expression profiling studies initially have led to invasive breast cancer classification into four distinctive molecular groups as discussed in Chap. 10. These molecularly classified subgroups have distinct clinical outcomes, with luminal A having the most favourable outcome, followed by luminal B, basal-like, and lastly the HER2-enriched [10, 53]. In addition to the prognostic value of this molecular classification, there is some evidences indicating that luminal A sub-group is particularly sensitive to endocrine therapy and it has a more positive natural history than HER2 and basal-like subgroups in spite of the sensitivity of HER2 subtype tumours to the chemotherapy [54]. Molecular classification of breast cancer was thought to provide predictive information superior to that provided by ER and HER2 alone. This concept was based on the fact that the classification of tumours within each class is based on several hundreds of genes reflecting the molecular portraits of the tumour. Global gene expression profiles are expected to provide more accurate information on the biological feature of the tumour and reflect the activity of important pathways and interaction of key driving molecules, and subsequently determine the behaviour of the tumour and response to specific therapy better than that provided by a single molecule. In addition, molecular classes were expected to provide information for resistance of some tumours to specific therapy such as HER2 positive tumours not responding to HER2 targeted therapy may be classified as luminal or basal tumours using gene expression profiling. Similar ER positive tumours that are assigned to basal or HER2 positive classes may explain resistance to endocrine therapy. However, the predictive value of molecular classes over ER and HER2 status remain limited and currently not used in clinical practice to predict response to targeted therapy. Molecular classification of breast does not have diagnostic value.

Prognostic Gene Signatures

Oncotype DX [21-Gene Genomic Health Recurrence Score (GHI-RS)]

A multistep approach was followed to develop a commercially available robust reverse transcriptase-polymerase chain reaction (RT-PCR) assay of 21 prospectively selected genes for invasive breast cancer. The initial step used a real-time RT-PCR to assess the gene expression from formalin-fixed paraffin-embedded (FFPE) tissue sections. The initial 250 genes were selected from genomic databases, along with review of literature and DNA array-based experiments (using fresh-frozen tissues). To test the correlation between recurrence of breast cancer and gene expressions of these 250 candidates, data from 447 patients from three independent clinical studies of breast cancer was analysed. Using the results of these studies, a panel of 21 genes (16 cancer-related genes and 5 other reference genes) was selected. Depending on the levels of expression of these genes, an algorithm was designed to calculate a recurrence score (RS) for each sample. The cancer-related genes include genes of the ER group (*ER, PR, SCUBE2* and *BCL2*), HER2 group (*HER2* and *GRB7*), cell proliferation group (*Ki67, CCNB1, Survivin, STK15* and *MYBL2*), invasion group (*MMP11* and *CTSL2*) and *GSTM1, BAG1* and *CD68*. The reference genes include *ACTB* (b-actin), *GAPDH, RPLPO, GUS* and *TFRC*. The expression of these 21 genes was presented as a recurrence score (RS); a continuous variable ranging between 0 and 100, where higher scores reflect a greater possibility of recurrence. The RS was divided into three categories: low risk (<18); intermediate risk ($\geq$18, but <31) and high risk ($\geq$31) [55]. The Oncotype DX breast cancer assay is designed to predict the 10-year risks of breast cancer recurrence in women with ER positive newly diagnosed node negative early stage (I–II) breast cancer, treated with tamoxifen. Oncotype DX is more than just a risk assessment tool: it can provide further information, including to what extent the woman would benefit from chemotherapy as well as tamoxifen therapy [56].

MammaPrint

MammaPrint is a diagnostic classifier developed by Van't Veer and colleagues, who identified a 70-gene signature significantly associated with prognosis in breast cancer patients using inkjet-synthesised oligonucleotide microarrays. The initial study was applied on 98 lymph node negative breast cancer patients younger than 55 years, with primary breast tumour size less than 5 cm [57]. The subsequent study of a cohort of 295 was validated for both lymph node negative and positive breast cancer cases [58]. MammaPrint can predict the probability of distant metastases within 5 years, and it can divide breast cancer patients into two groups with significantly different distant metastasis-free survival. In a good profile group, patients are more likely to remain free of distant metastases, while those classified as a poor profile group have a high risk of developing distant metastases [57, 59]. MammaPrint was the first FDA approved, gene expression-based prognostic test for stage I–II lymph node negative breast cancer [60].

Furthermore, an exploratory study resulted in the prediction that gene expression signatures (including the 70-gene signature) developed on frozen tissue showed a high level of concordance between fresh-frozen and FFPE matched pairs, [61] as validated by a subsequent study [62]. Recently in 2015, the MammaPrint as a breast cancer test using FFPE was FDA approved [63]. Importantly, the "Microarray in Node negative Disease may Avoid ChemoTherapy (MINDACT)" phase III randomised trial, prospectively tests the of MammaPrint assay, in parallel with Adjuvant! Online tool, on 6600 breast cancer patients form 9 countries [64]. The results of pilot study of MINDACT concludes that proportion of discordantly classified patients, the potential reduction in chemotherapy using the genomic signature, and compliance to treatment assignment are in accordance with the trial hypotheses are in accordance with the trial hypotheses [65].

Genomic Grade Index (GGI)

Sotiriou et al. used five datasets of gene expression with total number 661 breast cancer patients. They examined the association between the histologic grade and gene expression profiles of breast cancers for the reason of improving histologic grading by measuring the expression of 97 genes. Therefore, instead of the classic grades 1, 2 and 3, GGI divides histologic grade into low and high risk. The proposed gene expression grade index was able to reclassify the intermediate grade of ER positive cases into a high and low gene expression grade index [53]. Moreover, the GGI ability to predict response to neoadjuvant chemotherapy in ER positive and ER negative evaluated patients [66].

Breast Cancer Index (BCI)

It is a RT-PCR test of the ratio of two genes expression, *HOXB13* and *IL17BR*, joined with Molecular Grade Index (MGI) to test the risk of recurrence for ER+ and LN negative early invasive breast cancer patients. Initially, a genome-wide microarray analysis of frozen tumour specimens of 60 ER positive breast cancer patients treated with tamoxifen alone was performed [67]. Then, a two-gene expression ratio was identified which is highly predictive of clinical outcome. This expression ratio adapted to use analysis based on PCR of standard FFPE, which was established using an independent set of 20 FFPE tissues samples [68]. The BCI risk score ranges from 0 to 10 and divides patients into three categories, When the score is <5 (low risk group); between 5 and 6.3 (intermediate risk group); ≥6.4 (high risk group) [69]. Subsequent studies have demonstrated that both genes (*HOXB13* and *IL17BR*) have a prognostic as well as a predictive value [70–72].

PAM50 (Prediction Analysis of Microarray 50)

This a gene expression assay using 50 genes (PAM50), representing a reduced gene set assayed by quantitative real-time reverse transcription-PCR (qRT-PCR). It accurately identifies the four intrinsic biological/molecular subtypes of breast cancer and generates risk-of-relapse (ROR) scores. Moreover, its prognostic value in both untreated and tamoxifen-treated patient populations has been confirmed [73, 74]. A combined prognostic marker that includes the proliferation genes of PAM50 and tumour size identifies a subpopulation with an excellent outcome if treated with hormonal therapy alone and produces a score of estimating a probability of disease recurrence [75]. The PAM50 test was further adapted to be performed to develop a simplified workflow that could be easily and efficiently to measure gene expression in a local pathology lab (Prosigna™ Breast Cancer Gene Signature Assay, NanoString Technologies, Seattle) in frozen or FFPE tissues [76–78].

Next-Generation Sequencing (NGS)

Nucleic acid sequencing is a method for determining the exact order of nucleotides present in a given DNA or RNA molecule. Over the past decade, the use of nucleic acid sequencing has increased exponentially following attempt to complete human genome sequence and increasing demand for cheaper and faster sequencing methods. This demand has driven the development of next-generation sequencing (NGS) which perform massively parallel sequencing, during which millions of fragments of DNA from a single sample are sequenced in unison. NGS allows fast sequencing of the entire genome and it provides very sensitive quantifying applications including gene expression analysis more than traditional microarray-based methods. NGS can allow high-throughput sensitive analysis of the genome transcriptome and epigenome which is expected to provide important prognostic and predictive information. In addition it can provide information about the molecular nature of the tumour and detect previous unknown mutation that can useful in diagnosis and prediction of response to specific therapy. In breast, 45 regions of sequence alterations are demarcated by Curtis et al. to have a role in the development of the cancer [79]. The whole-genome sequencing data provide an overall view of individual tumour and understanding of the full catalogue of somatic genetic changes will be the way for personalised treatment of breast cancer patients [80].

Circulated Tumour Cells

Circulating tumour cells (CTC) are cells that originate from the primary tumour and circulate through blood stream and greatly contribute to the metastatic spread of cancer [81]. Currently, detection and molecular characterisation of CTCs in breast cancer patients is an active area of translational breast cancer research. Different detection systems have been developed for characterisation and enumeration of CTC with acceptable sensitivity and specificity. For instance, the protein-based CellSearch® system (FDA-USA cleared), the functional EPISPOT assay (for EPithelial ImmunoSPOT) [82], Ephesia-chip [83] and others [84, 85]. In addition, mRNA-based assays targeting specific mRNAs (e.g. CK19 mRNA), and the highly sensitive RT-qPCR assay (e.g. Adna-Test) [86], are the widely used alternatives to identify CTCs [87].

Different studies have reported CTC as a reliable prognostic factor in patients with early stage and metastatic breast cancer, irrespective of the CTC detection method and time point of blood sample withdrawal [88, 89]. Some studies also showed that CTC load in peripheral blood is associated with shorter survival in patients with early breast cancer [90, 91]. Moreover, CTC can be used as an effective independent prognostic factor before and after neoadjuvant chemotherapy [92]. CTC detection is able to monitor efficacy of adjuvant therapies [93], and assess therapeutic responses of advanced disease earlier than traditional imaging methods [94]. In addition to the analysis of peripheral blood CTC, some studies have assessed the prognostic value of breast cancer cells in bone marrow aspirates and demonstrated a correlation with outcome [95].

Tumour Markers

Some tumour markers are used in breast cancer diagnosis, prognosis and monitoring of the disease. Cancer antigen 15-3 (CA 15-3) and CA27.29, carcinoembryonic antigen (CEA) and cancer antigen 27.29 (CA 27.29) are found in a high proportion of patients with metastatic breast cancer. Elevated levels of these markers above certain limits can be used to indicate the presence of cancer hence diagnostic value. CA15-3 and CA27.29 are found on the surface of cancer cells and shed into the blood stream and can be used to monitor metastatic breast cancer. Urokinase plasminogen activator (uPA) and plasminogen activator inhibitor (PAI-1) play essential roles in tumour invasion and metastasis. High levels of uPA and PAI-1 are associated with poor prognosis in breast cancer [96].

Immunohistochemistry-Based Indices

Recently, instead of using a single marker approach, panels of biomarkers have been tested to predict the prognosis and to predict responses to specific therapies. Such an approach was adopted following the successful classification of breast cancer using global gene expression profiling, and the introduction of molecular classification based on the expression of several genes with clinical relevance. Multiple immunohistochemistry markers are used in combination to provide routine cost effective surrogates to gene expression profiling. Examples of IHC-based assays include Mammostrat, IHC4 and Nottingham Prognostic Index (NPI+).

Mammostrat

Ring et al. designed a multiple marker test using genes based on IHC assessment, and produced it to examine the likelihood of developing an IHC-based assay by using data from various gene expression studies. In this study, three retrospective breast cancer cohorts were used. The first cohort ($n = 466$) was a discovery cohort and other two ($n = 299$ and 344 patients, respectively) were independent validating cohorts. Using conventional FFPE samples, this primary study resulted in an IHC assay which calculates a relative risk of recurrence; currently commercially available as the Mammostrat assay [97]. Further validation of Mammostrat had been conducted by other investigators [98, 99]. Mammostrat uses five IHC markers: P53, SLC7A5 (solute carrier family 7 cationic amino acid transporter), NDRG1 (N-myc downstream-regulated gene 1), CEACAM5 (carcinoembryonic antigen cell adhesion molecule 5) and HTF9C (HpaII tiny fragments locus 9C), which stratify ER+ tamoxifen-treated breast cancer patients into three risk groups. Prognostic index ≤ 0 represents the low risk group; prognostic index >0 and ≤ 0.7 represents the moderate-risk group; and prognostic index >0.7 represents the high risk group [97, 98].

IHC4 Score

IHC4 is a prognostic score that assesses the levels of four widely measured proteins in breast cancer (ER, PR, HER2 and Ki67). Cuzick et al. developed IHC4 and compared it to the Oncotype DX to assess its utility on 1125 ER positive cases that had GHI-RS data and whether it can add a prognostic and predictive value to the classical prognostic parameters (tumour size, lymph node status and histological grade) in early stage breast cancer patients. The IHC4 score proved as an independent prognostic factor in addition to the existing classical variables. Importantly, the result provided by the IHC4 score were found to be identical to that presented by Oncotype DX. In addition, the IHC4 prognostic value was validated on an independent cohort of 786 patients with their outcome were equal as assessed by both Oncotype DX and IHC4 assay [100].

Nottingham Prognostic Index Plus (NPI+)

The NPI is an approved and widely accepted method for prognosis as well as survival prediction in operable cases of primary breast cancer [101]. It was one of the earliest indices to be developed. In 1982, it was applied throughout a retrospective study of 387 women with primary operable breast cancer using multivariate regression analysis; [102] and in 1991, the prognostic importance of NPI in breast cancer was initially expressed [103]. Then, after the long-term follow-up [4] and independent validation in different centres [104–106].

In their recently published study, Rakha et al. have devised an IHC marker-based prognostic index; NPI+ , by incorporating the IHC expression data of 10 markers along with the clinicopathological parameters, resulting in a structured NPI-like formulae for each class [107] (see Chap. 10). The NPI+ distinctive classes of breast cancer reveal a significant relationship with patient outcome. Additionally, they improve the prognostic value to the classic NPI [108, 109].

Online Prognostic Algorithms

Some prognostic algorithms have been developed and published online. These algorithms use molecular biomarkers mainly ER and HER2 and Ki67 combined with other well-established prognostic variables to predict breast cancer outcome in terms of probability of recurrences within specific period of time with or without consideration of hormone therapy. They main aim is to predict those who are likely to benefit from chemotherapy and those who should save such toxic drugs. They are not specifically predictive and they do not have any diagnostic value.

Adjuvant! Online

Adjuvant! Online is a free widely accepted prognostic and predictive online calculator for risk stratification of breast cancer patients (https://www.adjuvantonl ine.com). It allows the entry of a patient's age, comorbidity, menopausal status, tumour size and stage, number of positive lymph nodes and oestrogen receptor status in order to estimate mortality and disease recurrence at 10 years, as well as the potential benefit offered by adjuvant therapy [110]. The tool was established using a database that was recorded in the Surveillance, Epidemiology and End-results (SEER) registry. This model has been validated in USA, Canada, Asian and European studies [111–116].

Predict

It is a mathematical online model (http://www.predict.nhs.uk/predict.html), a prognostication tool to predict overall survival using cancer registration data identified by the Eastern Cancer Registration and Information Centre (ECRIC). The study population was 5694 breast cancer patients and was validated with another set of 5468 patients recorded in West Midlands Cancer Intelligence Unit (WMCIU) [117]. Wishart et al. incorporated the prognostic effect of HER2 status to produce the new version; PREDICT+, using the cohort cases from British Columbia which was used to validate the original PREDICT [111, 118]. It estimates the benefit of treatment from hormone treatment, chemotherapy and trastuzumab at 10-year time points. Improvement in the tool performance and clinical decision making for ER+ patients was achieved by adding Ki67 to PREDICT [119].

References

1. Gasparini G, Pozza F, Harris AL. Evaluating the potential usefulness of new prognostic and predictive indicators in node-negative breast cancer patients. J Natl Cancer Inst. 1993;85(15):1206–19.
2. Hayes DF, Trock B, Harris AL. Assessing the clinical impact of prognostic factors: when is "statistically significant" clinically useful? Breast Cancer Res Treat. 1998;52(1–3):305–19. PubMed PMID: 10066089. Epub 1999/03/05. eng.
3. Pathology reporting of breast disease. A Joint Document Incorporating the Third Edition of the NHS Breast Screening Programme's Guidelines for Pathology Reporting in Breast Cancer Screening and the Second Edition of The Royal College of Pathologists' Minimum Dataset for Breast Cancer Histopathology. NHSBSP Pub. No 58. 2005.
4. Galea MH, Blamey RW, Elston CE, Ellis IO. The Nottingham Prognostic Index in primary breast cancer. Breast Cancer Res Treat. 1992;22(3):207–19.
5. Elston CW, Ellis IO, Pinder SE. Pathological prognostic factors in breast cancer. Crit Rev Oncol Hematol. 1999;31(3):209–23.

6. Effects of chemotherapy and hormonal therapy for early breast cancer on recurrence and 15-year survival: an overview of the randomised trials. Lancet. 2005 May 14–20;365(9472):1687–717. PubMed PMID: 15894097.

7. Tamoxifen for early breast cancer: an overview of the randomised trials. Early Breast Cancer Trialists' Collaborative Group. Lancet. 1998 May 16;351(9114):1451–67. PubMed PMID: 9605801.

8. Mauri D, Pavlidis N, Polyzos NP, Ioannidis JP. Survival with aromatase inhibitors and inactivators versus standard hormonal therapy in advanced breast cancer: meta-analysis. J Natl Cancer Inst. 2006 Sep 20;98(18):1285–91. PubMed PMID: 16985247. Epub 2006/09/21. eng.

9. Perou CM, Sorlie T, Eisen MB, van de Rijn M, Jeffrey SS, Rees CA, et al. Molecular portraits of human breast tumours. Nature. 2000 Aug;406(6797):747–52. PubMed PMID: ISI:000088767700049.

10. Sorlie T, Perou CM, Tibshirani R, Aas T, Geisler S, Johnsen H, et al. Gene expression patterns of breast carcinomas distinguish tumor subclasses with clinical implications. Proc Natl Acad Sci USA. 2001 Sep 11;98(19):10869–74. PubMed PMID: 11553815. Pubmed Central PMCID: Pmc58566. Epub 2001/09/13. eng.

11. Badve S, Nakshatri H. Oestrogen-receptor-positive breast cancer: towards bridging histopathological and molecular classifications. J Clin Pathol. 2009;62(1):6–12.

12. Park D, Karesen R, Noren T, Sauer T. Ki-67 expression in primary breast carcinomas and their axillary lymph node metastases: clinical implications. Virchows Arch. 2007 Jul;451(1):11–8. PubMed PMID: 17554555. Epub 2007/06/08. eng.

13. King WJ, Greene GL. Monoclonal antibodies localize oestrogen receptor in the nuclei of target cells. Nature. 1984 Feb 23–29;307(5953):745–7. PubMed PMID: 6700704. Epub 1984/02/23. eng.

14. Welshons WV, Lieberman ME, Gorski J. Nuclear localization of unoccupied oestrogen receptors. Nature. 1984 Feb 23–29;307(5953):747–9. PubMed PMID: 6700705. Epub 1984/02/23. eng.

15. Snoj NDP, Bedard P, Sotiriou C. Molecular biology of breast cancer. In: Coleman WB, Tsongalis GJ, editors. Essential concepts in molecular pathology. San Diego: Elsevier Press; 2012.

16. Green S, Walter P, Kumar V, Krust A, Bornert JM, Argos P, et al. Human oestrogen receptor cDNA: sequence, expression and homology to v-erb-A. Nature. 1986 Mar 13–19;320(6058):134–9. PubMed PMID: 3754034. Epub 1986/03/13. eng.

17. Mosselman S, Polman J, Dijkema R. ER beta: identification and characterization of a novel human estrogen receptor. FEBS Lett. 1996;392:49–53. (Netherlands).

18. Li X, Huang J, Yi P, Bambara RA, Hilf R, Muyan M. Single-chain estrogen receptors (ERs) reveal that the ERalpha/beta heterodimer emulates functions of the ERalpha dimer in genomic estrogen signaling pathways. Mol Cell Biol. 2004 Sep;24(17):7681–94. PubMed PMID: 15314175. Pubmed Central PMCID: Pmc506997. Epub 2004/08/18. eng.

19. Crowe JP, Hubay CA, Pearson OH, Marshall JS, Rosenblatt J, Mansour EG, et al. Estrogen receptor status as a prognostic indicator for stage I breast cancer patients. Breast Cancer Res Treat. 1982;2(2):171–6. PubMed PMID: 7171837. Epub 1982/01/01. eng.

20. Fisher B, Redmond C, Fisher ER, Caplan R. Relative worth of estrogen or progesterone receptor and pathologic characteristics of differentiation as indicators of prognosis in node negative breast cancer patients: findings from National Surgical Adjuvant Breast and Bowel Project Protocol B-06. J Clin Oncol. 1988 Jul;6(7):1076–87. PubMed PMID: 2856862. Epub 1988/07/01. eng.

21. Pichon MF, Broet P, Magdelenat H, Delarue JC, Spyratos F, Basuyau JP, et al. Prognostic value of steroid receptors after long-term follow-up of 2257 operable breast cancers. Br J Cancer. 1996;73(12):1545–51.

22. Railo M, Lundin J, Haglund C, von Smitten K, von Boguslawsky K, Nordling S. Ki-67, p53, Er-receptors, ploidy and S-phase as prognostic factors in T1 node negative breast cancer. Acta Oncol. 1997;36(4):369–74. PubMed PMID: 9247096. Epub 1997/01/01. eng.

23. Cuzick J, Sestak I, Bonanni B, Costantino JP, Cummings S, DeCensi A, et al. Selective oestrogen receptor modulators in prevention of breast cancer: an updated meta-analysis of individual participant data. Lancet. 2013 May 25;381(9880):1827–34. PubMed PMID: 23639488. Pubmed Central PMCID: PMC3671272. Epub 2013/05/04. eng.
24. von Minckwitz G, Untch M, Nuesch E, Loibl S, Kaufmann M, Kummel S, et al. Impact of treatment characteristics on response of different breast cancer phenotypes: pooled analysis of the German neo-adjuvant chemotherapy trials. Breast Cancer Res Treat. 2011;125(1):145–56.
25. Ring AE, Smith IE, Ashley S, Fulford LG, Lakhani SR. Oestrogen receptor status, pathological complete response and prognosis in patients receiving neoadjuvant chemotherapy for early breast cancer. Br J Cancer. 2004 Dec 13;91(12):2012–7. PubMed PMID: 15558072. Pubmed Central PMCID: Pmc2409783. Epub 2004/11/24. eng.
26. Colleoni M, Viale G, Zahrieh D, Pruneri G, Gentilini O, Veronesi P, et al. Chemotherapy is more effective in patients with breast cancer not expressing steroid hormone receptors: a study of preoperative treatment. Clin Cancer Res. 2004 Oct 1;10(19):6622–8. PubMed PMID: 15475452. Epub 2004/10/12. eng.
27. Dobrescu A, Chang M, Kirtani V, Turi GK, Hennawy R, Hindenburg AA. Study of estrogen receptor and progesterone receptor expression in breast ductal carcinoma in situ by immunohistochemical staining in ER/PgR-negative invasive breast cancer. ISRN Oncol. 2011;2011:673790. PubMed PMID: 22091428. Pubmed Central PMCID: 3200125.
28. Cui X, Schiff R, Arpino G, Osborne CK, Lee AV. Biology of progesterone receptor loss in breast cancer and its implications for endocrine therapy. J Clin Oncol. 2005 Oct 20;23(30):7721–35. PubMed PMID: 16234531. Epub 2005/10/20. eng.
29. Rakha EA, El-Sayed ME, Green AR, Paish EC, Powe DG, Gee J, et al. Biologic and clinical characteristics of breast cancer with single hormone receptor positive phenotype. J Clin Oncol. 2007;25(30):4772–8.
30. Hefti MM, Hu R, Knoblauch NW, Collins LC, Haibe-Kains B, Tamimi RM, et al. Estrogen receptor negative/progesterone receptor positive breast cancer is not a reproducible subtype. Breast Cancer Res. 2013 Aug 23;15(4):R68. PubMed PMID: 23971947. Epub 2013/08/27. eng.
31. Dowsett M, Houghton J, Iden C, Salter J, Farndon J, A'Hern R, et al. Benefit from adjuvant tamoxifen therapy in primary breast cancer patients according oestrogen receptor, progesterone receptor, EGF receptor and HER2 status. Ann Oncol. 2006;17(5):818–26.
32. Prenzel N, Fischer OM, Streit S, Hart S, Ullrich A. The epidermal growth factor receptor family as a central element for cellular signal transduction and diversification. Endocr Relat Cancer. 2001 Mar;8(1):11–31. PubMed PMID: 11350724. Epub 2001/05/15. eng.
33. Slamon DJ, Clark GM, Wong SG, Levin WJ, Ullrich A, McGuire WL. Human breast cancer: correlation of relapse and survival with amplification of the HER-2/neu oncogene. Science. 1987;235(4785):177–82.
34. Slamon DJ, Godolphin W, Jones LA, Holt JA, Wong SG, Keith DE, et al. Studies of the HER-2/neu proto-oncogene in human breast and ovarian cancer. Science. 1989;244(4905):707–12.
35. Cortes J, Fumoleau P, Bianchi GV, Petrella TM, Gelmon K, Pivot X, et al. Pertuzumab monotherapy after trastuzumab-based treatment and subsequent reintroduction of trastuzumab: activity and tolerability in patients with advanced human epidermal growth factor receptor 2-positive breast cancer. J Clin Oncol. 2012;30(14):1594–600.
36. Baselga J, Bradbury I, Eidtmann H, Di Cosimo S, de Azambuja E, Aura C, et al. Lapatinib with trastuzumab for HER2-positive early breast cancer (NeoALTTO): a randomised, open-label, multicentre, phase 3 trial. Lancet. 2012;379(9816):633–40.
37. Blackwell KL, Burstein HJ, Storniolo AM, Rugo HS, Sledge G, Aktan G, et al. Overall survival benefit with lapatinib in combination with trastuzumab for patients with human epidermal growth factor receptor 2-positive metastatic breast cancer: final results from the EGF104900 Study. J Clin Oncol. 2012;30(21):2585–92.

38. Tolaney SM, Barry WT, Dang CT, Yardley DA, Moy B, Marcom PK, et al. Adjuvant pacli-taxel and trastuzumab for node-negative, HER2-positive breast cancer. N Engl J Med. 2015 Jan 8;372(2):134–41. PubMed PMID: 25564897. Pubmed Central PMCID: 4313867.
39. Dowsett M, Sestak I, Lopez-Knowles E, Sidhu K, Dunbier AK, Cowens JW, et al. Comparison of PAM50 risk of recurrence score with oncotype DX and IHC4 for predicting risk of distant recurrence after endocrine therapy. J Clin Oncol. 2013;31(22):2783–90.
40. Clahsen PC, van de Velde CJ, Duval C, Pallud C, Mandard AM, Delobelle-Deroide A, et al. The utility of mitotic index, oestrogen receptor and Ki-67 measurements in the crea-tion of novel prognostic indices for node-negative breast cancer. Eur J Surg Oncol. 1999 Aug;25(4):356–63. PubMed PMID: 10419704. Epub 1999/07/27. eng.
41. Lehr HA, Hansen DA, Kussick S, Li M, Hwang H, Krummenauer F, et al. Assessment of proliferative activity in breast cancer: MIB-1 immunohistochemistry versus mitotic figure count. Hum Pathol. 1999 Nov;30(11):1314–20. PubMed PMID: 10571511. Epub 1999/11/26. eng.
42. Thor AD, Liu S, Moore DH, 2nd, Edgerton SM. Comparison of mitotic index, in vitro bro-modeoxyuridine labeling, and MIB-1 assays to quantitate proliferation in breast cancer. J Clin Oncol. 1999 Feb;17(2):470–7. PubMed PMID: 10080587. Epub 1999/03/18. eng.
43. Trihia H, Murray S, Price K, Gelber RD, Golouh R, Goldhirsch A, et al. Ki-67 expression in breast carcinoma: its association with grading systems, clinical parameters, and other prog-nostic factors–a surrogate marker? Cancer. 2003;97(5):1321–31.
44. Domagala W, Markiewski M, Harezga B, Dukowicz A, Osborn M. Prognostic significance of tumor cell proliferation rate as determined by the MIB-1 antibody in breast carcinoma: its relationship with vimentin and p53 protein. Clin Cancer Res. 1996 Jan;2(1):147–54. PubMed PMID: 9816101. Epub 1996/01/01. eng.
45. de Azambuja E, Cardoso F, de Castro G, Jr., Colozza M, Mano MS, Durbecq V, et al. Ki-67 as prognostic marker in early breast cancer: a meta-analysis of published studies involv-ing 12,155 patients. Br J Cancer. 2007 May 21;96(10):1504–13. PubMed PMID: 17453008. Pubmed Central PMCID: Pmc2359936. Epub 2007/04/25. eng.
46. Viale G, Giobbie-Hurder A, Regan MM, Coates AS, Mastropasqua MG, Dell'Orto P, et al. Prognostic and predictive value of centrally reviewed Ki-67 labeling index in post-menopausal women with endocrine-responsive breast cancer: results from Breast International Group Trial 1-98 comparing adjuvant tamoxifen with letrozole. J Clin Oncol. 2008;26(34):5569–75.
47. Aleskandarany MA, Green AR, Rakha EA, Mohammed RA, Elsheikh SE, Powe DG, et al. Growth fraction as a predictor of response to chemotherapy in node negative breast cancer. Int J Cancer. 2009 Aug 26. PubMed PMID: 19711345.
48. Brown JR, DiGiovanna MP, Killelea B, Lannin DR, Rimm DL. Quantitative assessment Ki-67 score for prediction of response to neoadjuvant chemotherapy in breast cancer. Lab Invest. 2014 Jan;94(1):98–106. PubMed PMID: 24189270. Epub 2013/11/06. eng.
49. Ingolf J-B, Russalina M, Simona M, Julia R, Gilda S, Bohle RM, et al. Can Ki-67 play a role in prediction of breast cancer patients' response to Neoadjuvant chemotherapy? BioMed Res Int. 2014 03/25 01/13/received 02/11/accepted;2014:628217. PubMed PMID: PMC3982412.
50. Takei H, Kurosumi M, Yoshida T, Hayashi Y, Higuchi T, Uchida S, et al. Neoadjuvant endo-crine therapy of breast cancer: which patients would benefit and what are the advantages? Breast Cancer (Tokyo, Japan). 2011 Apr;18(2):85–91. PubMed PMID: 21104350. Epub 2010/11/26. eng.
51. von Minckwitz G, Schmitt WD, Loibl S, Muller BM, Blohmer JU, Sinn BV, et al. Ki67 measured after neoadjuvant chemotherapy for primary breast cancer. Clin Cancer Res. 2013 Aug 15;19(16):4521–31. PubMed PMID: 23812670. Epub 2013/07/03. eng.
52. Goldhirsch A, Wood WC, Coates AS, Gelber RD, Thurlimann B, Senn HJ, et al. Strategies for subtypes-dealing with the diversity of breast cancer: highlights of the St. Gallen inter-national expert consensus on the primary therapy of early breast cancer 2011. Ann Oncol. 2011;22:1736–47. (England).

53. Sotiriou C, Wirapati P, Loi S, Harris A, Fox S, Smeds J, et al. Gene expression profiling in breast cancer: understanding the molecular basis of histologic grade to improve prognosis. J Natl Cancer Inst. 2006;98(4):262–72.

54. Rouzier R, Perou CM, Symmans WF, Ibrahim N, Cristofanilli M, Anderson K, et al. Breast cancer molecular subtypes respond differently to preoperative chemotherapy. Clin Cancer Res. 2005;11(16):5678–85.

55. Paik S, Shak S, Tang G, Kim C, Baker J, Cronin M, et al. A multigene assay to predict recurrence of tamoxifen-treated, node-negative breast cancer. N Engl J Med. 2004;351(27):2817–26.

56. Paik S, Tang G, Shak S, Kim C, Baker J, Kim W, et al. Gene expression and benefit of chemotherapy in women with node-negative, estrogen receptor-positive breast cancer. J Clin Oncol. 2006;24(23):3726–34.

57. van 't Veer LJ, Dai H, van de Vijver MJ, He YD, Hart AA, Mao M, et al. Gene expression profiling predicts clinical outcome of breast cancer. Nature. 2002;415:530–6. (England).

58. van de Vijver MJ, He YD, van't Veer LJ, Dai H, Hart AA, Voskuil DW, et al. A gene-expression signature as a predictor of survival in breast cancer. N Engl J Med. 2002;347:1999–2009. (United States: 2002 Massachusetts Medical Society).

59. van de Vijver MJ, He YD, van't Veer LJ, Dai H, Hart AA, Voskuil DW, et al. A gene-expression signature as a predictor of survival in breast cancer. N Engl J Med. 2002 Dec 19;347(25):1999–2009. PubMed PMID: 12490681.

60. Li X, Quigg RJ, Zhou J, Gu W, Nagesh Rao P, Reed EF. Clinical utility of microarrays: current status, existing challenges and future outlook. Curr Genomics. 2008 07/25/received 08/11/revised 08/14/accepted;9(7):466–74. PubMed PMID: PMC2691672.

61. Mittempergher L, de Ronde JJ, Nieuwland M, Kerkhoven RM, Simon I, Rutgers EJ, et al. Gene expression profiles from formalin fixed paraffin embedded breast cancer tissue are largely comparable to fresh frozen matched tissue. PLoS One. 2011;6(2):e17163. PubMed PMID: 21347257. Pubmed Central PMCID: PMC3037966. Epub 2011/02/25. eng.

62. Sapino A, Roepman P, Linn SC, Snel MH, Delahaye LJ, van den Akker J, et al. MammaPrint molecular diagnostics on formalin-fixed, paraffin-embedded tissue. J Mol Diagn. 2014 Mar;16(2):190–7. PubMed PMID: 24378251. Epub 2014/01/01. eng.

63. http://www.agendia.com/agendia-receives-new-fda-clearance-for-mammaprint-ffpe-breast-cancer-test/ 2015 [cited 2015 09/04].

64. Bogaerts J, Cardoso F, Fau-Buyse M, Buyse M, Fau-Braga S, Braga S, Fau-Loi S, Loi S, Fau-Harrison JA, Harrison Ja, Fau-Bines J, et al. Gene signature evaluation as a prognostic tool: challenges in the design of the MINDACT trial. 2006 20061004 DCOM-20061024(1743-4262 (Electronic)). eng.

65. Rutgers E, Piccart-Gebhart MJ, Bogaerts J, Delaloge S, Veer LV, Rubio IT, et al. The EORTC 10041/BIG 03-04 MINDACT trial is feasible: results of the pilot phase. Eur J Cancer. 2011 Dec;47(18):2742–9. PubMed PMID: 22051734. Epub 2011/11/05. eng.

66. Filho OM, Ignatiadis M, Sotiriou C. Genomic Grade Index: An important tool for assessing breast cancer tumor grade and prognosis. Crit Rev Oncol/Hematol. 2011 1//;77(1):20–9.

67. Ma XJ, Salunga R, Dahiya S, Wang W, Carney E, Durbecq V, et al. A five-gene molecular grade index and HOXB13:IL17BR are complementary prognostic factors in early stage breast cancer. Clin Cancer Res. 2008;14(9):2601–8.

68. Ma XJ, Wang Z, Ryan PD, Isakoff SJ, Barmettler A, Fuller A, et al. A two-gene expression ratio predicts clinical outcome in breast cancer patients treated with tamoxifen. Cancer Cell. 2004;5:607–16. (United States).

69. Jerevall PL, Ma XJ, Li H, Salunga R, Kesty NC, Erlander MG, et al. Prognostic utility of HOXB13:IL17BR and molecular grade index in early-stage breast cancer patients from the Stockholm trial. Br J Cancer. 2011;104:1762–9. (England).

70. Ma XJ, Hilsenbeck SG, Wang W, Ding L, Sgroi DC, Bender RA, et al. The HOXB13:IL17BR expression index is a prognostic factor in early-stage breast cancer. J Clin Oncol. 2006;24:4611–9. (United States).

71. Goetz MP, Suman VJ, Ingle JN, Nibbe AM, Visscher DW, Reynolds CA, et al. A two-gene expression ratio of homeobox 13 and interleukin-17B receptor for prediction of recurrence and survival in women receiving adjuvant tamoxifen. Clin Cancer Res. 2006;12:2080–7. (United States).
72. Jerevall PL, Brommesson S, Strand C, Gruvberger-Saal S, Malmstrom P, Nordenskjold B, et al. Exploring the two-gene ratio in breast cancer-independent roles for HOXB13 and IL17BR in prediction of clinical outcome. Breast Cancer Res Treat. 2008 Jan;107(2):225–34. PubMed PMID: 17453342. Epub 2007/04/25. eng.
73. Nielsen TO, Parker JS, Leung S, Voduc D, Ebbert M, Vickery T, et al. A comparison of PAM50 intrinsic subtyping with immunohistochemistry and clinical prognostic factors in tamoxifen-treated estrogen receptor-positive breast cancer. Clin Cancer Res. 2010 Nov 1;16(21):5222–32. PubMed PMID: 20837693. Pubmed Central PMCID: 2970720.
74. Parker JS, Mullins M, Cheang MC, Leung S, Voduc D, Vickery T, et al. Supervised risk predictor of breast cancer based on intrinsic subtypes. J Clin Oncol. 2009;27(8):1160–7.
75. Nielsen TO, Parker JS, Leung S, Voduc D, Ebbert M, Vickery T, et al. A comparison of PAM50 intrinsic subtyping with immunohistochemistry and clinical prognostic factors in tamoxifen-treated estrogen receptor-positive breast cancer. Clin Cancer Res. 2010 Aacr.; 2010;16:5222–32. (United States).
76. Geiss GK, Bumgarner RE, Birditt B, Dahl T, Dowidar N, Dunaway DL, et al. Direct multiplexed measurement of gene expression with color-coded probe pairs. Nature Biotechnol. 2008 Mar;26(3):317–25. PubMed PMID: 18278033. Epub 2008/02/19. eng.
77. Reis PP, Waldron L, Goswami RS, Xu W, Xuan Y, Perez-Ordonez B, et al. mRNA transcript quantification in archival samples using multiplexed, color-coded probes. BMC Biotechnol. 2011;11:46. PubMed PMID: 21549012. Pubmed Central PMCID: PMC3103428. Epub 2011/05/10. eng.
78. Nielsen T, Wallden B, Schaper C, Ferree S, Liu S, Gao D, et al. Analytical validation of the PAM50-based Prosigna breast cancer prognostic gene signature assay and nCounter analysis system using formalin-fixed paraffin-embedded breast tumor specimens. BMC Cancer. 2014;14(1):177. PubMed PMID: doi:10.1186/1471-2407-14-177.
79. Curtis C, et al. The genomic andtranscriptomic architecture of 2000 breast tumours reveals novel subgroups. Nature. 2012;346–52. (England).
80. Bieche I, Lidereau R. Genome-based and transcriptome-based molecular classification of breast cancer. Curr Opin Oncol. 2011 Jan;23(1):93–9. PubMed PMID: 21076301. Epub 2010/11/16. eng.
81. Aceto N, Bardia A, Miyamoto DT, Donaldson MC, Wittner BS, Spencer JA, et al. Circulating tumor cell clusters are oligoclonal precursors of breast cancer metastasis. Cell. 2014 Aug 28;158(5):1110–22. PubMed PMID: 25171411. Pubmed Central PMCID: PMC4149753. Epub 2014/08/30. eng.
82. Alix-Panabieres C. EPISPOT assay: detection of viable DTCs/CTCs in solid tumor patients. Recent results in cancer research Fortschritte der Krebsforschung Progres dans les recherches sur le cancer. 2012;195:69–76. PubMed PMID: 22527495. Epub 2012/04/25. eng.
83. Saliba AE, Saias L, Psychari E, Minc N, Simon D, Bidard FC, et al. Microfluidic sorting and multimodal typing of cancer cells in self-assembled magnetic arrays. Proc Natl Acad Sci USA. 2010 Aug 17;107(33):14524–9. PubMed PMID: 20679245. Pubmed Central PMCID: PMC2930475. Epub 2010/08/04. eng.
84. Pecot CV, Bischoff FZ, Mayer JA, Wong KL, Pham T, Bottsford-Miller J, et al. A novel platform for detection of CK+ and CK− CTCs. Cancer discovery. 2011 Dec;1(7):580–6. PubMed PMID: 22180853. Pubmed Central PMCID: PMC3237635. Epub 2011/12/20. eng.
85. Issadore D, Chung J, Shao H, Liong M, Ghazani AA, Castro CM, et al. Ultrasensitive clinical enumeration of rare cells ex vivo using a micro-hall detector. Science translational medicine. 2012 Jul 4;4(141):141ra92. PubMed PMID: 22764208. Pubmed Central PMCID: PMC3603277. Epub 2012/07/06. eng.

86. Andreopoulou E, Yang LY, Rangel KM, Reuben JM, Hsu L, Krishnamurthy S, et al. Comparison of assay methods for detection of circulating tumor cells in metastatic breast cancer: AdnaGen AdnaTest BreastCancer Select/Detect versus Veridex CellSearch system. Int J Cancer. 2012 Apr 1;130(7):1590–7. PubMed PMID: 21469140. Epub 2011/04/07. eng.

87. Pantel K, Alix-Panabières C. Detection methods of circulating tumor cells. J Thoracic Dis. 2012 07/20/received 08/23/accepted;4(5):446–7. PubMed PMID: PMC3461061.

88. Zhang L, Riethdorf S, Wu G, Wang T, Yang K, Peng G, et al. Meta-analysis of the prognostic value of circulating tumor cells in breast cancer. Clin Cancer Res. 2012 Oct 15;18(20):5701–10. PubMed PMID: 22908097. Epub 2012/08/22. eng.

89. Giuliano M, Giordano A, Jackson S, De Giorgi U, Mego M, Cohen EN, et al. Circulating tumor cells as early predictors of metastatic spread in breast cancer patients with limited metastatic dissemination. Breast Cancer Res. 2014;16(5):440. PubMed PMID: 25223629. Pubmed Central PMCID: PMC4303121. Epub 2014/09/17. eng.

90. Stathopoulou A, Vlachonikolis I, Mavroudis D, Perraki M, Kouroussis C, Apostolaki S, et al. Molecular detection of cytokeratin-19-positive cells in the peripheral blood of patients with operable breast cancer: evaluation of their prognostic significance. J Clin Oncol. 2002;20(16):3404–12.

91. Zach O, Kasparu H, Wagner H, Krieger O, Lutz D. Prognostic value of tumour cell detection in peripheral blood of breast cancer patients. Acta Med Austriaca Suppl. 2002;59:32–4.

92. Rack B, Schindlbeck C, Jückstock J, Andergassen U, Hepp P, Zwingers T, et al. Circulating tumor cells predict survival in early average-to-high risk breast cancer patients. J Nat Cancer Inst. 2014 May 1;106(5).

93. Bardia A, Haber DA. Solidifying liquid biopsies: can circulating tumor cell monitoring guide treatment selection in breast cancer? J Clin Oncol. 2014 November 1;32(31):3470–1.

94. Budd GT, Cristofanilli M, Ellis MJ, Stopeck A, Borden E, Miller MC, et al. Circulating tumor cells versus imaging—predicting overall survival in metastatic breast cancer. Clin Cancer Res. 2006 November 1;12(21):6403–9.

95. Funke I, Schraut W. Meta-analyses of studies on bone marrow micrometastases: an independent prognostic impact remains to be substantiated. J Clin Oncol. 1998;16(2):557–66.

96. Look MP, van Putten WL, Duffy MJ, Harbeck N, Christensen IJ, Thomssen C, et al. Pooled analysis of prognostic impact of urokinase-type plasminogen activator and its inhibitor PAI-1 in 8377 breast cancer patients. J Natl Cancer Inst. 2002;94(2):116–28.

97. Ring BZ, Seitz RS, Beck R, Shasteen WJ, Tarr SM, Cheang MC, et al. Novel prognostic immunohistochemical biomarker panel for estrogen receptor-positive breast cancer. J Clin Oncol. 2006;24(19):3039–47.

98. Ross DT, Kim CY, Tang G, Bohn OL, Beck RA, Ring BZ, et al. Chemosensitivity and stratification by a five monoclonal antibody immunohistochemistry test in the NSABP B14 and B20 trials. Clin Cancer Res. 2008;14:6602–9. (United States).

99. Bartlett JM, Thomas J, Ross DT, Seitz RS, Ring BZ, Beck RA, et al. Mammostrat as a tool to stratify breast cancer patients at risk of recurrence during endocrine therapy. Breast Cancer Res. 2010;12:R47. (England).

100. Cuzick J, Dowsett M, Pineda S, Wale C, Salter J, Quinn E, et al. Prognostic value of a combined estrogen receptor, progesterone receptor, Ki-67, and human epidermal growth factor receptor 2 immunohistochemical score and comparison with the Genomic Health recurrence score in early breast cancer. J Clin Oncol. 2011;29(32):4273–8.

101. Blamey RW, Pinder SE, Ball GR, Ellis IO, Elston CW, Mitchell MJ, et al. Reading the prognosis of the individual with breast cancer. Eur J Cancer. 2007;43(10):1545–7.

102. Haybittle JL, Blamey RW, Elston CW, Johnson J, Doyle PJ, Campbell FC, et al. A prognostic index in primary breast cancer. Br J Cancer. 1982;45(3):361–6.

103. Elston CW, Ellis IO. Pathological prognostic factors in breast cancer. I. The value of histological grade in breast cancer: experience from a large study with long-term follow-up. Histopathology. 1991;19(5):403–10.

104. Balslev I, Axelsson CK, Zedeler K, Rasmussen BB, Carstensen B, Mouridsen HT. The Nottingham Prognostic Index applied to 9,149 patients from the studies of the Danish Breast Cancer Cooperative Group (DBCG). Breast Cancer Res Treat. 1994;32(3):281–90.
105. D'Eredita G, Giardina C, Martellotta M, Natale T, Ferrarese F. Prognostic factors in breast cancer: the predictive value of the Nottingham Prognostic Index in patients with a long-term follow-up that were treated in a single institution. Eur J Cancer. 2001;37(5):591–6.
106. Brown J, Jones M, Benson EA. Comment on the Nottingham Prognostic Index. Breast Cancer Res Treat. 1993;25(3):283. PubMed PMID: 8267734. Epub 1993/01/01. eng.
107. Rakha EA, Soria D, Green AR, Lemetre C, Powe DG, Nolan CC, et al. Nottingham Prognostic Index Plus (NPI+): a modern clinical decision making tool in breast cancer. 2014 20140402 DCOM- 20140530(1532-1827 (Electronic)). eng.
108. Green AR, Powe DG, Rakha EA, Soria D, Lemetre C, Nolan CC, et al. Identification of key clinical phenotypes of breast cancer using a reduced panel of protein biomarkers. Br J Cancer. 2013 Oct 1;109(7):1886–94. PubMed PMID: 24008658. Pubmed Central PMCID: 3790179.
109. Rakha EA, Soria D, Green AR, Lemetre C, Powe DG, Nolan CC, et al. Nottingham Prognostic Index Plus (NPI+): a modern clinical decision making tool in breast cancer. Br J Cancer. 2014 Mar 11. PubMed PMID: 24619074. Epub 2014/03/13. Eng.
110. Ravdin PM, Siminoff LA, Davis GJ, Mercer MB, Hewlett J, Gerson N, et al. Computer program to assist in making decisions about adjuvant therapy for women with early breast cancer. J Clin Oncol. 2001;19(4):980–91.
111. Olivotto IA, Bajdik CD, Ravdin PM, Speers CH, Coldman AJ, Norris BD, et al. Population-based validation of the prognostic model ADJUVANT! for early breast cancer. J Clin Oncol. 2005;23(12):2716–25.
112. Mook S, Schmidt MK, Rutgers EJ, van de Velde AO, Visser O, Rutgers SM, et al. Calibration and discriminatory accuracy of prognosis calculation for breast cancer with the online Adjuvant! program: a hospital-based retrospective cohort study. Lancet Oncol. 2009;10(11):1070–6.
113. Hajage D, de Rycke Y, Bollet M, Savignoni A, Caly M, Pierga JY, et al. External validation of Adjuvant! Online breast cancer prognosis tool. Prioritising recommendations for improvement. PLoS One. 2011;6:e27446. (United States).
114. Bhoo-Pathy N, Yip CH, Hartman M, Saxena N, Taib NA, Ho GF, et al. Adjuvant! Online is overoptimistic in predicting survival of Asian breast cancer patients. Eur J Cancer. 2012;48:982–9. (England: 2012 Elsevier Ltd).
115. Campbell HE, Taylor MA, Harris AL, Gray AM. An investigation into the performance of the Adjuvant! Online prognostic programme in early breast cancer for a cohort of patients in the United Kingdom. Br J Cancer. 2009;101:1074–84. (England).
116. Engelhardt EG, Garvelink MM, de Haes JH, van der Hoeven JJ, Smets EM, Pieterse AH, et al. Predicting and communicating the risk of recurrence and death in women with early-stage breast cancer: a systematic review of risk prediction models. J Clin Oncol. 2014;32:238–50. (United States).
117. Wishart GC, Azzato EM, Greenberg DC, Rashbass J, Kearins O, Lawrence G, et al. PREDICT: a new UK prognostic model that predicts survival following surgery for invasive breast cancer. Breast Cancer Res. 2010;12:R1. (England).
118. Wishart GC, Bajdik CD, Dicks E, Provenzano E, Schmidt MK, Sherman M, et al. PREDICT Plus: development and validation of a prognostic model for early breast cancer that includes HER2. Br J Cancer. 2012;107:800–7. (England).
119. Wishart GC, Rakha E, Green A, Ellis I, Ali HR, Provenzano E, et al. Inclusion of KI67 significantly improves performance of the PREDICT prognostication and prediction model for early breast cancer. BMC Cancer. 2014;14:908. (England).

Chapter 13
Role of MicroRNAs in Breast Cancer

Jennifer L. Clark, Dina Kandil, Ediz F. Cosar and Ashraf Khan

Introduction

MicroRNAs (miRNAs) are short noncoding RNAs involved in post-transcriptional gene silencing. Deregulation of miRNA expression has been implicated in the initiation and progression of many human cancers, including breast. Expression profiling in many breast cancer subtypes and characterization of deranged miRNA expression has lead to the development of multiple miRNA expression signatures with implications for diagnosis, treatment, and prognostication. These small RNAs will be important targets in the development of novel molecular classification systems for the individualized treatment of breast cancer.

Biology of MicroRNA

miRNAs are noncoding single-stranded RNAs approximately 22 nucleotides (nt) in length, ranging from 20 to 25 nt [1, 2]. Altogether, genes encoding miRNAs comprise 1 % of the human genome, predicted to encode more than 1000 miRNAs [3, 4]. These genes are highly conserved and generally located in noncoding intergenic regions or within introns in a protein coding region [5]. The target of a miRNA is an mRNA transcript, leading to the degradation of the transcript and inhibition of protein translation [1, 3]. Though miRNAs bind their targets through

J.L. Clark · D. Kandil · E.F. Cosar · A. Khan (✉)
Department of Pathology, University of Massachusetts Medical School, UMassMemorial
Medical Center, Three Biotech, One Innovation Drive, Worcester, MA 01605, USA
e-mail: Ashraf.Khan@umassmemorial.org

© Springer Science+Business Media New York 2015
A. Khan et al. (eds.), *Precision Molecular Pathology of Breast Cancer*,
Molecular Pathology Library 10, DOI 10.1007/978-1-4939-2886-6_13

sequence complementarity, a single miRNA is capable of targeting a multitude of genes, and a single gene may be repressed by multiple miRNAs [6].

Though a mature miRNA measures only ~22 nt in length, miRNA precursors are longer and undergo a maturation process involving trimming and cleavage of the primary transcript [3]. The initial transcription of a miRNA gene results in a long primary miRNA (pri-miRNA) measuring several kilobases in length and containing a stem-loop secondary structure or hairpin [7]. The hairpin portion is isolated through trimming of the 5′ and 3′ ends by the nuclear ribonuclease Drosha, resulting in a precursor miRNA (pre-miRNA) approximately 60–100 nt in total length [8]. The pre-miRNA is exported out of the nucleus for further processing by the nuclear transport receptor exportin-5 [9–11]. Once in the cytoplasm, the hairpin loop structure of the pre-miRNA is cleaved off by the cytoplasmic ribonuclease DICER, resulting in a 22 nt miRNA duplex [7]. See Fig. 13.1 for a schematic demonstrating miRNA processing.

The miRNA duplex is then incorporated into the RNA-induced silencing complex (RISC) where the two strands are separated and the nonselected passenger strand degraded, resulting in a mature miRNA guide strand which is loaded into the complex [7]. This requires the core component argonaute protein and possibly an additional unidentified helicase [7, 12]. The guide strand in association with the RISC complex binds to the complementary sequence on the target mRNA transcript. This interaction acts to either repress translation or promote cleavage and

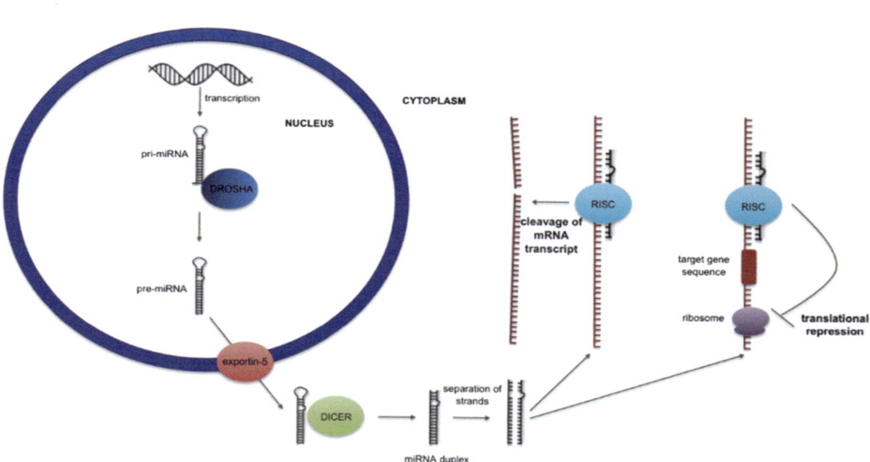

Fig. 13.1 MicroRNA processing and the RISC complex. The gene encoding the microRNA is transcribed to produce a pri-miRNA which is cleaved by DROSHA to produce a pre-miRNA. The pre-miRNA is exported from the nucleus to the cytoplasm via exportin-5. In the cytoplasm, the pre-miRNA is cleaved again by DICER to produce a miRNA duplex. The leading strand then separates from the duplex and associates with the RISC complex at the target gene sequence on mRNA transcripts. The target gene is silenced through cleavage of the mRNA transcript and/or suppression of translation

degradation of the mRNA transcript, effectively resulting in suppression of the targeted gene [7]. See Fig. 13.1 for schematic demonstrating miRNA-mediated gene silencing through incorporation into the RISC complex.

The cellular outcomes of gene silencing by miRNAs vary widely depending on the function of the target gene and physiological context. Initial studies of miRNA investigated the role of these molecules in worm development. A number of miRNAs have been identified in *C. elegans* which target specific transcription factors expressed only in early stages of development whose downregulation hastens transition to the next step in the developmental program (i.e., lin-4, let-7) [7]. In other physiological processes, the role of miRNAs is often more complex. For example, a miRNA might target a gene encoding a suppressor of a particular signaling pathway. Silencing of this gene by a miRNA will decrease production of the suppressor and lead ultimately to upregulation of the signaling pathway. For example, miR-210 represses COX10, relieving its suppression of the production of reactive oxygen species in the developing placenta [13]. Other miRNAs play vital roles in complex negative feedback loops, holding signals in dynamic balance depending on cellular and environmental context. The role of miR-146 in regulation of NF-κB signaling is a notable example [14, 15]. See Fig. 13.2 for a schematic outlining possible outcomes of deranged miRNA expression.

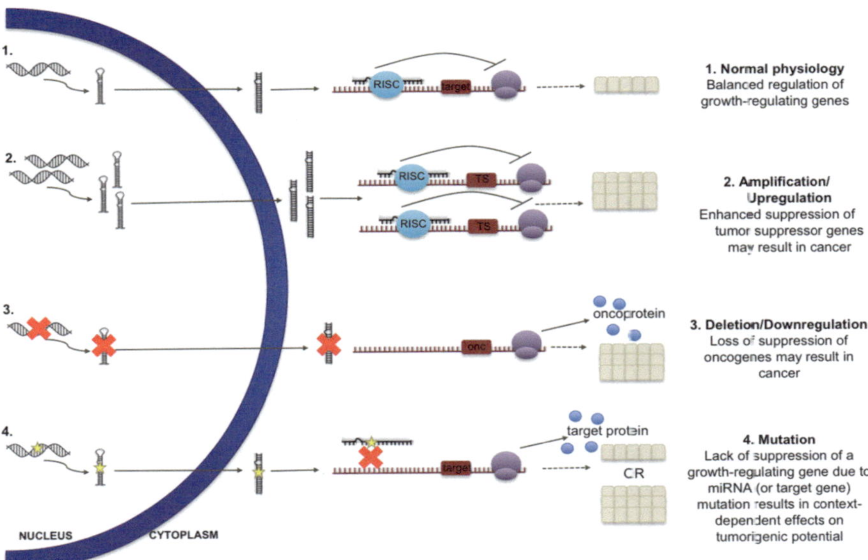

Fig. 13.2 MicroRNA defects contributing to carcinogenesis. In normal physiology, miRNA regulate growth in a balanced fashion. Amplification or upregulation of miRNAs which target tumor suppressor genes and deletion or downregulation of miRNAs which target oncogenes may result in cancer. Mutation of miRNAs or their target sequences may result in context-dependent effects on tumorigenesis

Roles of miRNAs and Associated Proteins in Cancer Biology

As with genes encoding protein products, those encoding miRNAs are also subject to amplification, deletion, mutation, and other derangements which may contribute to human disease (see Fig. 13.2). Indeed, miRNAs and associated proteins have been implicated in both hematologic and solid tumor malignancies. Consistent with increased "genetic activity" in cancer, miRNAs are globally downregulated in the malignant cell [16]. However, particular miRNAs, as well as components of the miRNA processing machinery, have been shown to play varied roles in tumor initiation and disease progression.

A variety of miRNAs have been shown to be upregulated in cancer. Similar in concept to "oncogenes," such miRNAs are termed "oncomiRs" [14]. These oncomiRs generally exert their oncogenic effect by suppressing genes encoding antiproliferative, proapoptotic, or other antitumor factors. One of the first examples of an oncomiR and the first example of oncomiR addiction was miR-21, a miRNA found to be overexpressed in human tumors [17–20]. Several groups have shown in mouse models that forced overexpression of miR-21 or expression in the presence of an oncogene such as Kras results in malignancy [17, 21]. Furthermore, deleting miR-21 or restoring normal levels of miR-21 expression results in reduced cancer incidence or regression of primary tumors, respectively [17, 22]. In order to exert its oncogenic effects, miR-21 is thought to repress PTEN and other targets to suppress proapoptotic pathways [14, 23]. Another notable example is the miR-17–92 cluster, a group of miRNAs expressed polycistronically, which is amplified in a number of human malignancies [24–27]. Its targets include the proapoptotic gene BCL-2-like protein 11 (BIM) and tumor suppressor PTEN [28].

Many miRNAs have tumor suppressive properties, suppressing genes with oncogenic potential. Similar to tumor suppressor proteins, loss of a tumor suppressive miRNA through deletion or mutation increases susceptibility to malignancy. Such miRNAs are often downregulated or absent in malignant cells. The first miR-NAs implicated in such a role were miR-15 and miR-16a, both members of the miR-15–16 cluster [29]. The cluster is located within a fragile site which is frequently deleted in B-cell chronic lymphocytic leukemia [29]. The cluster normally exerts tumor suppressive effects through suppression of cyclin D1, and restoration of miR-15–16 indeed results in decreased cellular proliferation [30–32].

In many cases, miRNAs have context-dependent roles in cancer. As mentioned previously, miR-146 plays a complex role in signaling through NF-κB which may have oncogenic or tumor suppressive effects depending on the interplay of other signaling pathways [14]. Similarly, miR-29 has been shown to have tumor suppressive effects in aggressive CLL by targeting the oncogenes such as TCL1, but recent evidence suggests that miR-29 might also act as an oncomiR by targeting the tumor suppressor peroxidasin [33–35]. More generally, the functions of various miRNAs may be altered through mutation of the miRNA itself or mutations in the sequence of potential target genes, with various effects on tumorigenicity.

Proteins involved in miRNA processing and function have also been implicated in tumorigenesis. A number of perturbations in the miRNA processing machinery have been identified which contribute to human cancers. DICER has been most studied in this context as the central molecule in miRNA processing due to the observed global downregulation of miRNA in cancer [16]. Indeed, DICER is often hemizygously deleted or downregulated in human tumors [36–45]. Interestingly, homozygous deletion does not increase tumorigenicity though miRNA expression is absent, suggesting that DICER itself is a haploinsufficient tumor suppressor [36, 46].

Association of miRNAs with Breast Cancer

In the normal physiology of breast, the expression of various miRNAs directs different stages of mammary gland development, as well as the transition from the mature breast to lactation and involution [47, 48]. Deregulation of physiologic miRNA expression and aberrant suppression or upregulation of various miRNAs may contribute to tumorigenesis, disease progression, and response to therapy. Those miRNAs which have been most widely studied are mentioned here. A more complete, though not exhaustive, list can be found in Tables 13.1 and 13.2.

OncomiRs

As previously discussed, though miRNAs are generally considered to have suppressive properties, multiple miRNAs have been implicated as oncomiRs in breast cancer, most of which function through the suppression of tumor suppressors. One such oncomiR is miR-155, a miRNA which targets the tumor suppressor SOCS1 directly, thereby indirectly activating JAK-STAT signaling [49]. Similarly, miR-181 directly targets the tumor suppressor ATM and has been shown to support malignant transformation and tumorigenesis in both cell culture and mouse models, respectively [50]. Other potential oncomiRs have been identified as biomarkers. miR-21 was initially identified as a biomarker in breast cancer and subsequently shown to target a number of tumor suppressors to promote breast tumorigenesis and metastasis [51–53]. See Table 13.1 for a partial list of miRNAs identified as oncomiRs in breast cancer.

Tumor Suppressive miRNAs

In line with the suppressive functions of miRNAs, a larger number have been identified as potential tumor suppressors in breast cancer. One of the first miRNAs ever identified and one of the first to be designated a *bona fide* tumor suppressor in

Table 13.1 Example MicroRNAs with significance in breast cancer

MicroRNA	Significance	Example gene targets	References
let-7	Generally downregulated, upregulated in lymph node negative disease, expression associated with luminal subtypes	ERα, IL-6	[109–112]
miR-10b	Downregulated	HOXD1, Tiam1	[65, 110, 113]
miR-16	Upregulation sensitizes HER2+/ER+ cancer to tamoxifen, downregulation associated with tamoxifen resistance	MYB, WIP1	[114–116]
miR-17–92	Frequently deleted, upregulated in ER-lymph node negative cancer	HIF1, STAT3, AIB1, BRCA1, ERα	[117–123]
miR-21	Upregulated	PTEN, PDCD4, TIMP3, RHOB, BCL2	[110, 124–128]
miR-26	Upregulated in ER+ disease	EZH2, MTDH, MCL-1	[110, 129, 130]
miR-27	Upregulated in disease progression	FOXO1, ZBTB10, CYP1B1	[131–133]
miR-29	Upregulated in both ER+ and PR+ disease, reduced expression associated with basal-like subtype	SPARC, TTP, DNMT3b	[110, 134–136]
miR-30	Upregulated in both ER+ and PR+ disease	UBC9, ITGB3, FOXD1, AVEN	[110, 137–139]
miR-125	Downregulated	ERBB2, ERBB3, BAK1, MUC1	[61, 95, 110, 140]
miR-126	Downregulated in cancer and metastatic disease	VEGF-A, PIK3R2, IRS1	[66, 141, 142]
miR-145	Downregulated	MUC1, ERα	[110, 143, 144]
miR-146	Context-dependent effects as outlined in text	IRAK1, TRAF6, BRCA1, BRCA2	[145–147]
miR-155	Upregulated, associated with chemoresistance	FOXO3, SOCS1, RHOA	[49, 93, 110, 148]
miR-185	Downregulated in ER+ disease	SIX1	[110, 149]
miR-200	Downregulated in epithelial–mesenchymal transition	ZEB1, ZEB2	[57, 59]
miR-205	Downregulated in cancer and epithelial-mesenchymal transition, expression associated with ductal morphology	ZEB1, VEGF-A, ERBB3	[59, 111, 150, 151]
miR-206	Generally upregulated, downregulated in ER+	ERα, GATA3, SRC3	[110, 152–154]
miR-210	Upregulated in cancer and triple negative disease, associated with invasiveness	MNT, RAD52	[110, 155–158]

(continued)

Table 13.1   (continued)

MicroRNA	Significance	Example gene targets	References
miR-221	Generally downregulated, upregulation in invasive disease, associated with tamoxifen resistance	ERα, p27KIP1, TRPS1	[91, 92, 159, 160]
miR-326	Downregulated in late stage disease, associated with chemoresistance	MRP-1	[161]
miR-335	Downregulated in metastatic disease	SOX4, TNC	[66, 162]
miR-373	Upregulated in metastatic lesions	CD44, TXNIP, RABEP1	[163, 164]
miR-375	Upregulated in progressive lobular carcinoma, downregulated in tamoxifen resistance	MTDH, RASD1	[165–167]
miR-520	Upregulated in metastatic lesions	CD44, TGFBR2	[163, 168]

Table 13.2   Example circulating MicroRNAs associated with breast cancer

MicroRNA	Significance	References
let-7	Serum biomarker for breast cancer	[169]
miR-10	Increased serum concentration associated with metastatic disease, specific for bone metastasis	[85, 170, 171]
miR-19	Serum biomarker for inflammatory breast cancer, higher levels associated with improved outcome in HER2+ metastatic disease	[172]
miR-21	Serum biomarker for breast cancer, serum levels correlated to distant metastasis and lymph node positivity	[77, 81]
miR-30	Serum biomarker for breast cancer (decreased levels)	[86]
miR-34	Increased serum concentration associated with metastatic disease	[170]
miR-92	Serum biomarker for breast cancer (decreased levels), decreased serum levels associated with lymph node positivity	[81]
miR-122	Increased serum concentration associated with metastatic recurrence	[173]
miR-125	Increased serum levels associated with chemoresistance	[83]
miR-155	Higher serum levels in PR+ breast cancer	[174]
miR-181	Serum biomarker for breast cancer (decreased levels)	[175]
miR-182	Serum biomarker for breast cancer, higher serum levels in PR− breast cancer	[88]
miR-195	Serum biomarker for breast cancer, differentiates breast from other malignancies	[169, 176]
miR-210	Serum biomarker for breast cancer, increased serum levels associated with lymph node positivity and resistance to traztuzumab	[82]
miR-214	Serum biomarker for breast cancer, increased serum levels associated with lymph node positivity	[177]
miR-373	Increased serum concentration associated with lymph node positivity	[85]

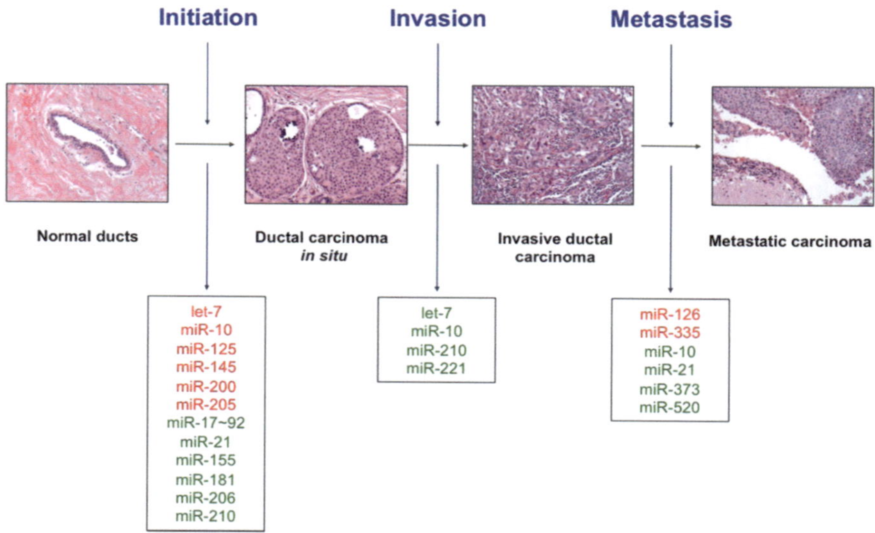

Fig. 13.3 MicroRNAs in tumor progression. Various miRNAs contribute to breast tumor initiation, progression to invasive disease, and metastasis to distant sites. Those miRNAs which are downregulated at each step are marked in *red*, and those miRNAs which are upregulated at each step are marked in *green*

breast cancer was let-7 [54]. Let-7 targets the oncogene RAS and is a regulator of the mammary stem cell population [54, 55]. Upregulation of this miRNA forces stem cells to exit the self-renewing population thought to harbor cancer-initiating cells [55]. Another regulator of the stem cell population is miR-200 which functions in a similar manner [56]. miR-200 also suppresses tumorigenesis by promoting mesenchymal–epithelial transition (MET) and targeting the AKT prosurvival pathway [57–60]. Another identified tumor suppressor is miR-125 which was shown to directly target HER2 in this aggressive subtype of breast carcinoma [61]. See Table 13.1 for a partial list of miRNAs identified as tumor suppressors in breast cancer. See Fig. 13.3 for a list of miRNAs involved in breast carcinogenesis and disease progression.

Context-Dependent miRNAs

In addition, to the context-dependent miRNAs discussed previously, many miRNAs have been shown to have varied and conflicting roles in breast cancer. A notable example is the miR-17–92 cluster, originally identified as a tumor suppressor in breast cancer by targeting cyclin D1 and IL-8 to inhibit the aggressive features of cancer, including proliferation, motility, and invasion [62, 63]. However, more recent studies have found an oncogenic role for this cluster, suggesting that it may have tumor suppressive or oncogenic effects depending on cellular context [64]. It is likely that many miRNAs will ultimately be determined to have multiple and conflicting roles in breast cancer in a context-dependent manner.

miRNAs Involved in Disease Progression

Many miRNAs with no identified role in breast tumorigenesis have been implicated specifically in disease progression and metastasis. Best studied is miR-10b which, though absent or downregulated in primary tumors, is upregulated in metastatic lesions as it is induced by the epithelial–mesenchymal transition (EMT) transcription factor Twist. Homeobox D10 (HOXD10) is targeted by miR-10b, indirectly inducing RAS homolog C (RHOC) to promote invasion and motility [65]. Other miRNAs such as miR-335 and miR-126 have been identified which are suppressed in metastatic lesions and likely inhibit disease progression by targeting genes involved in invasion and motility [66]. In experimental models, reconstituting expression of these miRNAs can suppress carcinoma cell migration and inhibit metastasis in mice [66]. A partial list of miRNAs involved in disease progression can be found in Table 13.1.

miRNAs Associated with Histologic Phenotypes

Though there is currently little evidence associating particular miRNAs with the various morphologies of breast carcinoma, many miRNAs have been associated more broadly with histopathologic phenotypes. For example, a number of miR-NAs have been associated with hormone receptor status, an immensely important clinicopathologic feature in predicting prognosis and guiding treatment. For example, miR-191 is upregulated in estrogen receptor (ER) positive cancer compared to ER negative breast cancer [67, 68]. Other miRNAs have been associated with HER2 status, molecular or intrinsic subtypes (to be discussed further in the next section), and broad morphologic categories (i.e., ductal vs. lobular). Many of these are mentioned in Table 13.1.

miRNA Signatures Associated with Breast Cancer

Advancements in microarray technology have made molecular profiling of large numbers of specimens possible. While the molecular profile of a tumor may hint at particular miRNAs which might play a role in tumor initiation and progression, the greatest strength of miRNA profiling technology is the ability to efficiently analyze a large number of tumors to identify miRNA signatures associated with important clinicopathologic variables. A large number of studies have identified miRNA signatures which may predict the clinical behavior of breast tumors. Those best validated will be discussed here.

The Cancer Genome Atlas Network (TCGA) published their landmark study in 2012 outlining the molecular profile of more than 500 breast tumors and approximately 20 normal breast samples [69]. In addition to whole genome sequencing, the study included gene expression analysis and reported on both mRNA and miRNA expression. Clustering analysis revealed 7 subtypes of tumors within the tested tumor subset correlating to mRNA profiling subsets (particularly those correlating to the basal-like intrinsic subtype as predicted by PAM50), hormone receptor status, and HER2 status [69].

Other groups have used this same patient cohort to identify miRNA signatures with clinical significance. These identified signatures are then applied to data from other existing cohorts to assess applicability more broadly. To date, miRNA and integrated miRNA/mRNA signatures have been validated in multiple cohorts to predict both distant relapse-free and overall survival, invasiveness or risk of transition from ductal carcinoma in situ (DCIS) to invasive carcinoma, aggressiveness in inflammatory breast carcinoma, likelihood of metastasis based on tumor-initiating properties, and possibly others [70–73]. The greatest promise seems to lie with the integrated 9 miRNA/11 mRNA signature developed by Volinia and Croce which demonstrated a higher prognostic value in early stage tumors than the popular Oncotype DX and MammaPrint assays [70].

Clinical Relevance of miRNA Expression Data

Though miRNA expression analysis and miRNA profiling of tumors is used widely in cancer research, these methodologies are not currently used in the standard treatment of breast cancer. Many academic groups and commercial companies are exploring the clinical usefulness of miRNA expression data in the diagnosis and management of breast cancer and other malignancies. Though evaluation of single miRNAs with known diagnostic or prognostic significance may prove clinically useful, miRNA signatures will likely be more widely used in the future.

Diagnosis

Though analysis of particular miRNAs or miRNA signatures in breast tumor samples will be useful in patient management once validated, detection and accurate diagnosis of breast cancer remains an invasive process involving biopsy and/or lumpectomy. Much recent work in diagnostics has focused on noninvasive means of detection in order to detect breast cancers early and avoid unnecessary invasive procedures. The miRNAs expressed in normal and malignant tissues are frequently detectable in the body fluids of patients. As miRNAs are remarkably stable in the serum and detection methodologies advancing, it is possible that a simple blood test could detect cancer-associated miRNAs with high sensitivity and specificity [74–76]. In particular, miR-21 has been used in several studies to differentiate patients with and without breast cancer, suggesting this may be a promising candidate serum biomarker [77–81]. A variety of other miRNAs have been identified in the serum whose expression levels correlate to various clinicopathologic features [82–88].

Prognosis

Great advances in molecular pathology have revolutionized breast cancer medicine, identifying particular biomarkers with prognostic significance such as ER/PR and HER2. However, the management dilemma remains that prediction of relapse-free and overall survival is not perfect, and many patients with low risk cancer based on ER and PR positivity, for example, will experience local or distant relapse at various timepoints after the initial diagnosis. New diagnostic molecular assays such as Oncotype DX and Mammaprint attempt to bridge that gap with some success. miRNA and integrated miRNA/mRNA analysis to identify certain prognostic signatures as discussed previously show great promise as alternative or additional tests to determine which patients are most likely to relapse and require more aggressive treatment. Such tests may become commercially available in the near future.

Treatment Response

Resistance to standard chemotherapy is currently one of the major areas of focus in breast cancer research. Though certain markers are known to associate with sensitivity to particular therapies, such as HER2 for Herceptin or ER for tamoxifen, we do not currently have markers of resistance in widespread clinical use. A number of large studies have identified genetic signatures associated with treatment response, including a study that identified miRNA signatures associated with sensitivity to several commonly used chemotherapeutics [89]. A variety of other studies have used miRNA profiling to identify particular miRNAs which are up- and downregulated in drug-sensitive versus drug-resistant cell lines [90–95]. Many of these are mentioned in Table 1. In the study of treatment resistance, miRNAs have become attractive targets, as more therapeutic options exist for overcoming resistance associated with these genetic elements [96]. Current studies have not used this information in clinical decision-making, and further characterization of identified miRNAs and miRNA signatures will be required to apply this data in patient studies.

miRNA Therapeutics

As investigation continues to develop new therapeutics for resistant and difficult-to-treat cancer (i.e., triple negative), miRNAs have recently become attractive targets for therapy. These molecules are minimally antigenic compared to protein and carbohydrate biological drugs and small enough to penetrate a cell as a nanoparticle, liposome, or exosome without the need for potentially dangerous viral vectors [47]. However, tumor-specific drug delivery is a major concern, as systemic exposure to a miRNA or antagomiR (antisense oligonucleotide specific to a particular miRNA) could have unforeseen consequences in other organ systems. Tumor-specific antibody- and ligand-mediated systems will likely help to solve this major challenge [47].

Though miRNA therapeutics have not yet been studied in human patients, a number of potential therapies have been successfully tested in animal models. AntagomiR-10b has been used by Weinberg's group to inhibit motility and invasiveness of a mouse mammary tumor cell line in a mouse model without adverse effect [97]. AntagomiR-21 has also been used to inhibit angiogenesis and induce apoptosis in a murine breast cancer model [98]. Other groups have used antagomiRs to treat neuroblastoma and cardiac hypertrophy, among others [99–101]. Though only one study has explored miRNA replacement therapy in breast cancer cells in vitro for radio-sensitization, miRNA replacement therapy has been tested with some success in cancers of the liver, colon, and lung using adenoviral, nanoparticle, or lipid-based delivery systems [102–106]. Unfortunately, tumor-specific delivery was not possible in these studies. However, successful treatment without major adverse effects is promising for the development of safe, effective new miRNA-based therapeutics in the near future.

Laboratory Methods

Knowledge of the techniques through which miRNA are purified and analyzed is vital for the accurate interpretation of miRNA data gathered from clinical specimens.

Detection and Quantitation

The analysis of miRNA expression requires isolation of RNA from clinical specimens, including plasma samples, fine needle aspirates, and formalin-fixed tissues. There is a remarkable stability of small RNAs in the blood, particularly in the exosomal fraction, and miRNA can be isolated from the plasma with relative ease [107]. Most commonly, RNA is isolated using commercial kits and reagents, though the underlying methodology is the same. In brief, organic components are isolated through fluid phase separation by centrifugation. Chloroform and phenol in an aqueous buffer are added to the sample prior to centrifugation. A denaturing reagent, often guanidinium isothiocyanate, is also added to denature ribonucleoproteins which may complex with RNA, as well as RNAases. Following centrifugation, nucleic acids (DNA and RNA) will be found in the aqueous phase, lipids in the chloroform interphase, and other organic molecules in the phenol organic phase. The aqueous phase is then mixed with ethanol or isopropanol to precipitate nucleic acids. This mixture can then be applied to a silica-based column (i.e., RNeasy) to isolate total RNA (see Fig. 13.4) [74].

Though isolation of RNA from plasma is relatively rapid and simple, miRNA analysis of a tumor often requires fine needle aspirates of the lesion or formalin-fixed paraffin-embedded (FFPE) tissue blocks, as fresh tissue is not frequently available in the clinical setting. Fortunately, the small size of miRNAs is relatively protective against the damaging effects of formalin. Tissue is isolated from paraffin tissue curls treated with xylene by centrifugation. The resulting tissue pellet is treated with the broad specificity enzyme proteinase K to degrade contaminating

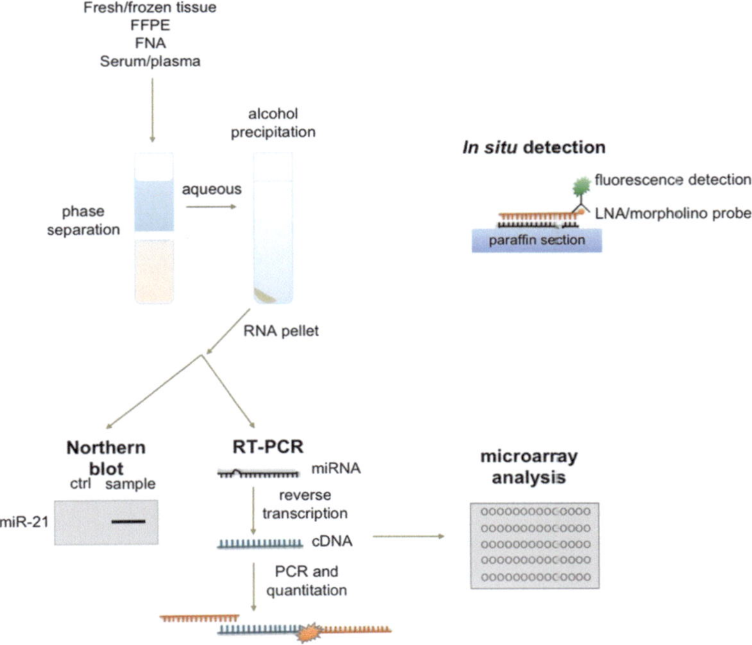

Fig. 13.4 Laboratory methods for microRNA detection in clinical samples. Total RNA may be isolated from tissues and body fluids through phase separation and precipitation in alcohol. Individual miRNAs may be detected using Northern blot or RT-PCR. Microarray analysis can be used to profile a large of miRNAs from a single sample. In paraffin-embedded tissues, individual miRNAs may be detected using fluorescent in situ hybridization and visualized through fluorescent microscopy

proteins in the preparation. Nucleic acids are then precipitated in ethanol and total RNA isolated as previously discussed, usually using a commercially available silica-based column (see Fig. 13.4) [74].

As these techniques separate total RNA from the tissue specimen, miRNAs of interest must then be specifically detected. This is normally accomplished in one of two ways: (1) Northern blot or (2) real-time reverse transcriptase polymerase chain reaction (RT-PCR). In Northern blotting, total RNA extracts are separated by charge and size in an agarose or polyacrylamide gel, transferred to a nylon membrane, hybridized to sequence-specific probes, and detected radiographically or by chemiluminescence. While blotting is semiquantitative and best for determining qualitatively whether a miRNA is expressed, RT-PCR is truly quantitative. First, extracted RNA is reverse transcribed by the enzyme reverse transcriptase in a thermal cycler to produced complementary DNA (cDNA). Next, traditional PCR is used to amplify the target miRNA sequence using specific primers. A variety of fluorescent dyes and sequence-specific oligonucleotide probes are commercially available for detection of amplified miRNA sequences which utilize straight fluorescence or Förster resonance energy transfer (FRET), respectively. Direct detection of miRNAs in situ is also possible using locked nucleic acid (LNA) or Morpholino oligonucleotide probes (see Fig. 13.4) [74, 108].

Microarray Analysis

Though the ability to detect specific miRNAs has allowed great advances in our understanding of these molecules in human disease, microarray analysis has allowed the simultaneous investigation of hundreds of miRNAs. Briefly, extracted RNA from a clinical sample is applied to a chip containing hundreds of specific oligonucleotide probes to which miRNAs in the sample will hybridize, allowing detection and quantitation of many miRNAs at once in a single sample. By utilizing probes for housekeeping genes in the microarray, the resulting data can be normalized, allowing comparison of multiple clinical samples. For example, it is possible to determine which miRNAs are up- or downregulated in tumor samples compared to normal tissue or identify miRNA signatures associated with a particular tumor subtype, hinting at potential biomarkers and pharmacological targets (see Fig. 13.4) [74].

Key Points

- MicroRNAs are small, noncoding RNAs measuring ~22 nucleotides in length which are processed by the ribonucleases Drosha and DICER from longer transcripts containing a hairpin structure
- Mature microRNAs silence genes containing complementary sequences through the RISC silencing complex

- A single microRNA may silence multiple genes, and a single gene may be silenced by multiple microRNAs
- OncomiRs are microRNAs with oncogenic properties, often through silencing of a tumor suppressor gene
- Tumor suppressive microRNAs generally exert suppressive effects by silencing an oncogene
- MicroRNAs have a number of context-dependent roles in tumor initiation, disease progression, prognosis, and response to therapy
- MicroRNAs are readily detectable in the blood and other body fluids, FNA material, and FFPE blocks
- Microarray technology has made possible the detection of hundreds of microRNAs at once in large numbers of tumors, allowing for the development of microRNA signatures associated with various clinical parameters
- Though not currently in clinical use, detection of particular microRNAs and microRNA profiling of blood and tumor samples may soon contribute to clinical decision-making as an adjunct to traditional pathologic evaluation
- AntagomiRs (antisense oligonucleotides) and miRNA replacement therapy have been used successfully in animal models and are potential candidates for new therapeutics in breast cancer

References

1. Ambros V. microRNAs: tiny regulators with great potential. Cell. 2001;107(7):823–6.
2. Ambros V, et al. A uniform system for microRNA annotation. RNA. 2003;9(3):277–9.
3. Kim VN. MicroRNA biogenesis: coordinated cropping and dicing. Nat Rev Mol Cell Biol. 2005;6(5):376–85.
4. Kozomara A, Griffiths-Jones S. miRBase: annotating high confidence microRNAs using deep sequencing data. Nucleic Acids Res. 2014;42(1):D68–73.
5. Lau NC, et al. An abundant class of tiny RNAs with probable regulatory roles in *Caenorhabditis elegans*. Science. 2001;294(5543):858–62.
6. Lewis BP, et al. Prediction of mammalian microRNA targets. Cell. 2003;115(7):787–98.
7. Bartel DP. MicroRNAs: genomics, biogenesis, mechanism, and function. Cell. 2004;116(2):281–97.
8. Lee Y, et al. The nuclear RNase III Drosha initiates microRNA processing. Nature. 2003;425(6956):415–9.
9. Lund E, et al. Nuclear export of microRNA precursors. Science. 2004;303(5654):95–8.
10. Yi R, et al. Exportin-5 mediates the nuclear export of pre-microRNAs and short hairpin RNAs. Genes Dev. 2003;17(24):3011–6.
11. Bohnsack MT, Czaplinski K, Gorlich D. Exportin 5 is a RanGTP-dependent dsRNA-binding protein that mediates nuclear export of pre-miRNAs. RNA. 2004;10(2):185–91.
12. Tang G. siRNA and miRNA: an insight into RISCs. Trends Biochem Sci. 2005;30(2):106–14.
13. Doridot L, et al. Trophoblasts, invasion, and microRNA. Front Genet. 2013;4:248.
14. Kasinski AL, Slack FJ. Epigenetics and genetics. MicroRNAs en route to the clinic: progress in validating and targeting microRNAs for cancer therapy. Nat Rev Cancer. 2011;11(12):849–64.
15. Taganov KD, et al. NF-kappaB-dependent induction of microRNA miR-146, an inhibitor targeted to signaling proteins of innate immune responses. Proc Natl Acad Sci USA. 2006;103(33):12481–6.

16. Sassen S, Miska EA, Caldas C. MicroRNA: implications for cancer. Virchows Arch. 2008;452(1):1–10.
17. Medina PP, Nolde M, Slack FJ. OncomiR addiction in an in vivo model of microRNA-21-induced pre-B-cell lymphoma. Nature. 2010;467(7311):86–90.
18. Chan JA, Krichevsky AM, Kosik KS. MicroRNA-21 is an antiapoptotic factor in human glioblastoma cells. Cancer Res. 2005;65(14):6029–33.
19. Landgraf P, et al. A mammalian microRNA expression atlas based on small RNA library sequencing. Cell. 2007;129(7):1401–14.
20. Volinia S, et al. A microRNA expression signature of human solid tumors defines cancer gene targets. Proc Natl Acad Sci USA. 2006;103(7):2257–61.
21. Hatley ME, et al. Modulation of K-Ras-dependent lung tumorigenesis by MicroRNA-21. Cancer Cell. 2010;18(3):282–93.
22. Ma X, et al. Loss of the miR-21 allele elevates the expression of its target genes and reduces tumorigenesis. Proc Natl Acad Sci USA. 2011;108(25):10144–9.
23. Meng F, et al. MicroRNA-21 regulates expression of the PTEN tumor suppressor gene in human hepatocellular cancer. Gastroenterology. 2007;133(2):647–58.
24. He L, et al. A microRNA polycistron as a potential human oncogene. Nature. 2005;435(7043):828–33.
25. Hayashita Y, et al. A polycistronic microRNA cluster, miR-17-92, is overexpressed in human lung cancers and enhances cell proliferation. Cancer Res. 2005;65(21):9628–32.
26. Rinaldi A, et al. Concomitant MYC and microRNA cluster miR-17-92 (C13orf25) amplification in human mantle cell lymphoma. Leuk Lymphoma. 2007;48(2):410–2.
27. Reichek JL, et al. Genomic and clinical analysis of amplification of the 13q31 chromosomal region in alveolar rhabdomyosarcoma: a report from the Children's Oncology Group. Clin Cancer Res. 2011;17(6):1463–73.
28. Xiao C, et al. Lymphoproliferative disease and autoimmunity in mice with increased miR-17-92 expression in lymphocytes. Nat Immunol. 2008;9(4):405–14.
29. Calin GA, et al. Frequent deletions and down-regulation of micro-RNA genes miR15 and miR16 at 13q14 in chronic lymphocytic leukemia. Proc Natl Acad Sci USA. 2002;99(24):15524–9.
30. Deshpande A, et al. 3′UTR mediated regulation of the cyclin D1 proto-oncogene. Cell Cycle. 2009;8(21):3584–92.
31. Salerno E, et al. Correcting miR-15a/16 genetic defect in New Zealand Black mouse model of CLL enhances drug sensitivity. Mol Cancer Ther. 2009;8(9):2684–92.
32. Klein U, et al. The DLEU2/miR-15a/16-1 cluster controls B cell proliferation and its deletion leads to chronic lymphocytic leukemia. Cancer Cell. 2010;17(1):28–40.
33. Pekarsky Y, et al. Tcl1 expression in chronic lymphocytic leukemia is regulated by miR-29 and miR-181. Cancer Res. 2006;66(24):11590–3.
34. Pekarsky Y, Croce CM. Is miR-29 an oncogene or tumor suppressor in CLL? Oncotarget. 2010;1(3):224–7.
35. Santanam U, et al. Chronic lymphocytic leukemia modeled in mouse by targeted miR-29 expression. Proc Natl Acad Sci USA. 2010;107(27):12210–5.
36. Kumar MS, et al. Dicer1 functions as a haploinsufficient tumor suppressor. Genes Dev. 2009;23(23):2700–4.
37. Tokumaru S, et al. let-7 regulates Dicer expression and constitutes a negative feedback loop. Carcinogenesis. 2008;29(11):2073–7.
38. Pampalakis G, et al. Down-regulation of dicer expression in ovarian cancer tissues. Clin Biochem. 2010;43(3):324–7.
39. Wu JF, et al. Down-regulation of Dicer in hepatocellular carcinoma. Med Oncol. 2011;28(3):804–9.
40. Dedes KJ, et al. Down-regulation of the miRNA master regulators Drosha and Dicer is associated with specific subgroups of breast cancer. Eur J Cancer. 2011;47(1):138–50.
41. Torres A, et al. Major regulators of microRNAs biogenesis Dicer and Drosha are down-regulated in endometrial cancer. Tumour Biol. 2011;32(4):769–76.

42. Faggad A, et al. Down-regulation of the microRNA processing enzyme Dicer is a prognostic factor in human colorectal cancer. Histopathology. 2012;61(4):552–61.
43. Zhu DX, et al. Downregulated Dicer expression predicts poor prognosis in chronic lymphocytic leukemia. Cancer Sci. 2012;103(5):875–81.
44. Wu D, et al. Downregulation of Dicer, a component of the microRNA machinery, in bladder cancer. Mol Med Rep. 2012;5(3):695–9.
45. Kitagawa N, et al. Downregulation of the microRNA biogenesis components and its association with poor prognosis in hepatocellular carcinoma. Cancer Sci. 2013;104(5):543–51.
46. Lambertz I, et al. Monoallelic but not biallelic loss of Dicer1 promotes tumorigenesis in vivo. Cell Death Differ. 2010;17(4):633–41.
47. Liu H. MicroRNAs in breast cancer initiation and progression. Cell Mol Life Sci. 2012;69(21):3587–99.
48. Piao HL, Ma L. Non-coding RNAs as regulators of mammary development and breast cancer. J Mammary Gland Biol Neoplasia. 2012;17(1):33–42.
49. Jiang S, et al. MicroRNA-155 functions as an OncomiR in breast cancer by targeting the suppressor of cytokine signaling 1 gene. Cancer Res. 2010;70(8):3119–27.
50. Wang Y, et al. Transforming growth factor-beta regulates the sphere-initiating stem cell-like feature in breast cancer through miRNA-181 and ATM. Oncogene. 2011;30(12):1470–80.
51. Yan LX, et al. MicroRNA miR-21 overexpression in human breast cancer is associated with advanced clinical stage, lymph node metastasis and patient poor prognosis. RNA. 2008;14(11):2348–60.
52. Qian B, et al. High miR-21 expression in breast cancer associated with poor disease-free survival in early stage disease and high TGF-beta1. Breast Cancer Res Treat. 2009;117(1):131–40.
53. Buscaglia LE, Li Y. Apoptosis and the target genes of microRNA-21. Chin J Cancer. 2011;30(6):371–80.
54. Johnson SM, et al. RAS is regulated by the let-7 microRNA family. Cell. 2005;120(5):635–47.
55. Ibarra I, et al. A role for microRNAs in maintenance of mouse mammary epithelial progenitor cells. Genes Dev. 2007;21(24):3238–43.
56. Shimono Y, et al. Downregulation of miRNA-200c links breast cancer stem cells with normal stem cells. Cell. 2009;138(3):592–603.
57. Park SM, et al. The miR-200 family determines the epithelial phenotype of cancer cells by targeting the E-cadherin repressors ZEB1 and ZEB2. Genes Dev. 2008;22(7):894–907.
58. Korpal M, et al. The miR-200 family inhibits epithelial-mesenchymal transition and cancer cell migration by direct targeting of E-cadherin transcriptional repressors ZEB1 and ZEB2. J Biol Chem. 2008;283(22):14910–4.
59. Gregory PA, et al. The miR-200 family and miR-205 regulate epithelial to mesenchymal transition by targeting ZEB1 and SIP1. Nat Cell Biol. 2008;10(5):593–601.
60. Hyun S, et al. Conserved MicroRNA miR-8/miR-200 and its target USH/FOG2 control growth by regulating PI3K. Cell. 2009;139(6):1096–108.
61. Scott GK, et al. Coordinate suppression of ERBB2 and ERBB3 by enforced expression of micro-RNA miR-125a or miR-125b. J Biol Chem. 2007;282(2):1479–86.
62. Yu Z, et al. A cyclin D1/microRNA 17/20 regulatory feedback loop in control of breast cancer cell proliferation. J Cell Biol. 2008;182(3):509–17.
63. Yu Z, et al. microRNA 17/20 inhibits cellular invasion and tumor metastasis in breast cancer by heterotypic signaling. Proc Natl Acad Sci USA. 2010;107(18):8231–6.
64. Li H, et al. miR-17-5p promotes human breast cancer cell migration and invasion through suppression of HBP1. Breast Cancer Res Treat. 2011;126(3):565–75.
65. Ma L, Teruya-Feldstein J, Weinberg RA. Tumour invasion and metastasis initiated by micro-RNA-10b in breast cancer. Nature. 2007;449(7163):682–8.
66. Tavazoie SF, et al. Endogenous human microRNAs that suppress breast cancer metastasis. Nature. 2008;451(7175):147–52.

67. Di Leva G, et al. Estrogen mediated-activation of miR-191/425 cluster modulates tumorigenicity of breast cancer cells depending on estrogen receptor status. PLoS Genet. 2013;9(3):e1003311.
68. Nagpal N, et al. MicroRNA-191, an estrogen-responsive microRNA, functions as an oncogenic regulator in human breast cancer. Carcinogenesis. 2013;34(8):1889–99.
69. Network TCGA. Comprehensive molecular portraits of human breast tumours. Nature. 2012;490(7418):61–70.
70. Volinia S, Croce CM. Prognostic microRNA/mRNA signature from the integrated analysis of patients with invasive breast cancer. Proc Natl Acad Sci USA. 2013;110(18):7413–7.
71. Volinia S, et al. Breast cancer signatures for invasiveness and prognosis defined by deep sequencing of microRNA. Proc Natl Acad Sci USA. 2012;109(8):3024–9.
72. Lerebours F, et al. miRNA expression profiling of inflammatory breast cancer identifies a 5-miRNA signature predictive of breast tumor aggressiveness. Int J Cancer. 2013;133(7):1614–23.
73. Wang L, et al. A microRNA expression signature characterizing the properties of tumor-initiating cells for breast cancer. Oncol Lett. 2012;3(1):119–24.
74. Sethi S, et al. Clinical implication of MicroRNAs in molecular pathology. Clin Lab Med. 2013;33(4):773–86.
75. Gallo A, et al. The majority of microRNAs detectable in serum and saliva is concentrated in exosomes. PLoS ONE. 2012;7(3):e30679.
76. Cuk K, et al. Plasma microRNA panel for minimally invasive detection of breast cancer. PLoS ONE. 2013;8(10):e76729.
77. Asaga S, et al. Direct serum assay for microRNA-21 concentrations in early and advanced breast cancer. Clin Chem. 2011;57(1):84–91.
78. Wang B, Zhang Q. The expression and clinical significance of circulating microRNA-21 in serum of five solid tumors. J Cancer Res Clin Oncol. 2012;138(10):1659–66.
79. Gao J, et al. Clinical significance of serum miR-21 in breast cancer compared with CA153 and CEA. Chin J Cancer Res. 2013;25(6):743–8.
80. Kumar S, et al. Overexpression of circulating miRNA-21 and miRNA-146a in plasma samples of breast cancer patients. Indian J Biochem Biophys. 2013;50(3):210–4.
81. Si H, et al. Circulating microRNA-92a and microRNA-21 as novel minimally invasive biomarkers for primary breast cancer. J Cancer Res Clin Oncol. 2013;139(2):223–9.
82. Jung EJ, et al. Plasma microRNA 210 levels correlate with sensitivity to trastuzumab and tumor presence in breast cancer patients. Cancer. 2012;118(10):2603–14.
83. Wang H, et al. Circulating MiR-125b as a marker predicting chemoresistance in breast cancer. PLoS ONE. 2012;7(4):e34210.
84. Sun Y, et al. Serum microRNA-155 as a potential biomarker to track disease in breast cancer. PLoS ONE. 2012;7(10):e47003.
85. Chen W, et al. The level of circulating miRNA-10b and miRNA-373 in detecting lymph node metastasis of breast cancer: potential biomarkers. Tumour Biol. 2013;34(1):455–62.
86. Zeng RC, et al. Down-regulation of miRNA-30a in human plasma is a novel marker for breast cancer. Med Oncol. 2013;30(1):477.
87. Eichelser C, et al. Deregulated serum concentrations of circulating cell-free microRNAs miR-17, miR-34a, miR-155, and miR-373 in human breast cancer development and progression. Clin Chem. 2013;59(10):1489–96.
88. Wang PY, et al. Higher expression of circulating miR-182 as a novel biomarker for breast cancer. Oncol Lett. 2013;6(6):1681–6.
89. Salter KH, et al. An integrated approach to the prediction of chemotherapeutic response in patients with breast cancer. PLoS ONE. 2008;3(4):e1908.
90. Kovalchuk O, et al. Involvement of microRNA-451 in resistance of the MCF-7 breast cancer cells to chemotherapeutic drug doxorubicin. Mol Cancer Ther. 2008;7(7):2152–9.
91. Miller TE, et al. MicroRNA-221/222 confers tamoxifen resistance in breast cancer by targeting p27Kip1. J Biol Chem. 2008;283(44):29897–903.

92. Zhao JJ, et al. MicroRNA-221/222 negatively regulates estrogen receptor alpha and is associated with tamoxifen resistance in breast cancer. J Biol Chem. 2008;283(45):31079–86.

93. Kong W, et al. MicroRNA-155 regulates cell survival, growth, and chemosensitivity by targeting FOXO3a in breast cancer. J Biol Chem. 2010;285(23):17869–79.

94. Pogribny IP, et al. Alterations of microRNAs and their targets are associated with acquired resistance of MCF-7 breast cancer cells to cisplatin. Int J Cancer. 2010;127(8):1785–94.

95. Zhou M, et al. MicroRNA-125b confers the resistance of breast cancer cells to paclitaxel through suppression of pro-apoptotic Bcl-2 antagonist killer 1 (Bak1) expression. J Biol Chem. 2010;285(28):21496–507.

96. Weidhaas JB, et al. MicroRNAs as potential agents to alter resistance to cytotoxic anticancer therapy. Cancer Res. 2007;67(23):11111–6.

97. Ma L, et al. Therapeutic silencing of miR-10b inhibits metastasis in a mouse mammary tumor model. Nat Biotechnol. 2010;28(4):341–7.

98. Zhao D, et al. In vivo monitoring of angiogenesis inhibition via down-regulation of mir-21 in a VEGFR2-luc murine breast cancer model using bioluminescent imaging. PLoS ONE. 2013;8(8):e71472.

99. Fontana L, et al. Antagomir-17-5p abolishes the growth of therapy-resistant neuroblastoma through p21 and BIM. PLoS ONE. 2008;3(5):e2236.

100. Ge YF, et al. AntagomiR-27a targets FOXO3a in glioblastoma and suppresses U87 cell growth in vitro and in vivo. Asian Pac J Cancer Prev. 2013;14(2):963–8.

101. Care A, et al. MicroRNA-133 controls cardiac hypertrophy. Nat Med. 2007;13(5):613–8.

102. Liang Z, et al. MicroRNA-302 replacement therapy sensitizes breast cancer cells to ionizing radiation. Pharm Res. 2013;30(4):1008–16.

103. Kota J, et al. Therapeutic microRNA delivery suppresses tumorigenesis in a murine liver cancer model. Cell. 2009;137(6):1005–17.

104. Ibrahim AF, et al. MicroRNA replacement therapy for miR-145 and miR-33a is efficacious in a model of colon carcinoma. Cancer Res. 2011;71(15):5214–24.

105. Trang P, et al. Regression of murine lung tumors by the let-7 microRNA. Oncogene. 2010;29(11):1580–7.

106. Wiggins JF, et al. Development of a lung cancer therapeutic based on the tumor suppressor microRNA-34. Cancer Res. 2010;70(14):5923–30.

107. Mraz M, et al. MicroRNA isolation and stability in stored RNA samples. Biochem Biophys Res Commun. 2009;390(1):1–4.

108. Lagendijk AK, Moulton JD, Bakkers J. Revealing details: whole mount microRNA in situ hybridization protocol for zebrafish embryos and adult tissues. Biol Open. 2012;1(6):566–9.

109. Iliopoulos D, Hirsch HA, Struhl K. An epigenetic switch involving NF-kappaB, Lin28, Let-7 MicroRNA, and IL6 links inflammation to cell transformation. Cell. 2009;139(4):693–706.

110. Iorio MV, et al. MicroRNA gene expression deregulation in human breast cancer. Cancer Res. 2005;65(16):7065–70.

111. Quesne JL, et al. Biological and prognostic associations of miR-205 and let-7b in breast cancer revealed by in situ hybridization analysis of micro-RNA expression in arrays of archival tumour tissue. J Pathol. 2012;227(3):306–14.

112. Zhao Y, et al. Let-7 family miRNAs regulate estrogen receptor alpha signaling in estrogen receptor positive breast cancer. Breast Cancer Res Treat. 2011;127(1):69–80.

113. Moriarty CH, Pursell B, Mercurio AM. miR-10b targets Tiam1: implications for Rac activation and carcinoma migration. J Biol Chem. 2010;285(27):20541–6.

114. Cittelly DM, et al. Oncogenic HER2Δ16 suppresses miR-15a/16 and deregulates BCL-2 to promote endocrine resistance of breast tumors. Carcinogenesis. 2010;31(12):2049–57.

115. Chung EY, et al. c-Myb oncoprotein is an essential target of the dleu2 tumor suppressor microRNA cluster. Cancer Biol Ther. 2008;7(11):1758–64.

116. Zhang X, et al. Oncogenic Wip1 phosphatase is inhibited by miR-16 in the DNA damage signaling pathway. Cancer Res. 2010;70(18):7176–86.

117. Zhang L, et al. microRNAs exhibit high frequency genomic alterations in human cancer. Proc Natl Acad Sci USA. 2006;103(24):9136–41.
118. Janssen EA, et al. Biologic profiling of lymph node negative breast cancers by means of microRNA expression. Mod Pathol. 2010;23(12):1567–76.
119. Taguchi A, et al. Identification of hypoxia-inducible factor-1 alpha as a novel target for miR-17-92 microRNA cluster. Cancer Res. 2008;68(14):5540–5.
120. Brock M, et al. Interleukin-6 modulates the expression of the bone morphogenic protein receptor type II through a novel STAT3-microRNA cluster 17/92 pathway. Circ Res. 2009;104(10):1184–91.
121. Hossain A, Kuo MT, Saunders GF. Mir-17-5p regulates breast cancer cell proliferation by inhibiting translation of AIB1 mRNA. Mol Cell Biol. 2006;26(21):8191–201.
122. Shen J, Ambrosone CB, Zhao H. Novel genetic variants in microRNA genes and familial breast cancer. Int J Cancer. 2009;124(5):1178–82.
123. Castellano L, et al. The estrogen receptor-alpha-induced microRNA signature regulates itself and its transcriptional response. Proc Natl Acad Sci USA. 2009;106(37):15732–7.
124. Huang GL, et al. Clinical significance of miR-21 expression in breast cancer: SYBR-Green I-based real-time RT-PCR study of invasive ductal carcinoma. Oncol Rep. 2009;21(3):673–9.
125. Frankel LB, et al. Programmed cell death 4 (PDCD4) is an important functional target of the microRNA miR-21 in breast cancer cells. J Biol Chem. 2008;283(2):1026–33.
126. Song B, et al. MicroRNA-21 regulates breast cancer invasion partly by targeting tissue inhibitor of metalloproteinase 3 expression. J Exp Clin Cancer Res. 2010;29:29.
127. Connolly EC, et al. Overexpression of miR-21 promotes an in vitro metastatic phenotype by targeting the tumor suppressor RHOB. Mol Cancer Res. 2010;8(5):691–700.
128. Si ML, et al. miR-21-mediated tumor growth. Oncogene. 2007;26(19):2799–803.
129. Gao J, et al. MiR-26a inhibits proliferation and migration of breast cancer through repression of MCL-1. PLoS ONE. 2013;8(6):e65138.
130. Zhang B, et al. Pathologically decreased miR-26a antagonizes apoptosis and facilitates carcinogenesis by targeting MTDH and EZH2 in breast cancer. Carcinogenesis. 2011;32(1):2–9.
131. Tang W, et al. MiR-27 as a prognostic marker for breast cancer progression and patient survival. PLoS ONE. 2012;7(12):e51702.
132. Guttilla IK, White BA. Coordinate regulation of FOXO1 by miR-27a, miR-96, and miR-182 in breast cancer cells. J Biol Chem. 2009;284(35):23204–16.
133. Tsuchiya Y, et al. MicroRNA regulates the expression of human cytochrome P450 1B1. Cancer Res. 2006;66(18):9090–8.
134. Gebeshuber CA, Zatloukal K, Martinez J. miR-29a suppresses tristetraprolin, which is a regulator of epithelial polarity and metastasis. EMBO Rep. 2009;10(4):400–5.
135. Gerson KD, et al. Integrin beta4 regulates SPARC protein to promote invasion. J Biol Chem. 2012;287(13):9835–44.
136. Sandhu R, et al. Dysregulation of microRNA expression drives aberrant DNA hypermethylation in basal-like breast cancer. Int J Oncol. 2014;44(2):563–72.
137. Wu F, et al. MicroRNA-mediated regulation of Ubc9 expression in cancer cells. Clin Cancer Res. 2009;15(5):1550–7.
138. Yu F, et al. Mir-30 reduction maintains self-renewal and inhibits apoptosis in breast tumor-initiating cells. Oncogene. 2010;29(29):4194–204.
139. Ouzounova M, et al. MicroRNA miR-30 family regulates non-attachment growth of breast cancer cells. BMC Genom. 2013;14:139.
140. Rajabi H, et al. Mucin 1 oncoprotein expression is suppressed by the miR-125b oncomir. Genes Cancer. 2010;1(1):62–8.
141. Zhu N, et al. Endothelial-specific intron-derived miR-126 is down-regulated in human breast cancer and targets both VEGFA and PIK3R2. Mol Cell Biochem. 2011;351(1–2):157–64.

142. Zhang J, et al. The cell growth suppressor, mir-126, targets IRS-1. Biochem Biophys Res Commun. 2008;377(1):136–40.
143. Sachdeva M, Mo YY. MicroRNA-145 suppresses cell invasion and metastasis by directly targeting mucin 1. Cancer Res. 2010;70(1):378–87.
144. Spizzo R, et al. miR-145 participates with TP53 in a death-promoting regulatory loop and targets estrogen receptor-alpha in human breast cancer cells. Cell Death Differ. 2010;17(2):246–54.
145. Bhaumik D, et al. Expression of microRNA-146 suppresses NF-kappaB activity with reduction of metastatic potential in breast cancer cells. Oncogene. 2008;27(42):5643–7.
146. Garcia AI, et al. Down-regulation of BRCA1 expression by miR-146a and miR-146b-5p in triple negative sporadic breast cancers. EMBO Mol Med. 2011;3(5):279–90.
147. Shen J, et al. A functional polymorphism in the miR-146a gene and age of familial breast/ovarian cancer diagnosis. Carcinogenesis. 2008;29(10):1963–6.
148. Kong W, et al. MicroRNA-155 is regulated by the transforming growth factor beta/Smad pathway and contributes to epithelial cell plasticity by targeting RhoA. Mol Cell Biol. 2008;28(22):6773–84.
149. Imam JS, et al. MicroRNA-185 suppresses tumor growth and progression by targeting the Six1 oncogene in human cancers. Oncogene. 2010;29(35):4971–9.
150. Sempere LF, et al. Altered MicroRNA expression confined to specific epithelial cell subpopulations in breast cancer. Cancer Res. 2007;67(24):11612–20.
151. Wu H, Zhu S, Mo YY. Suppression of cell growth and invasion by miR-205 in breast cancer. Cell Res. 2009;19(4):439–48.
152. Kondo N, et al. miR-206 expression is down-regulated in estrogen receptor alpha-positive human breast cancer. Cancer Res. 2008;68(13):5004–8.
153. Adams BD, Furneaux H, White BA. The micro-ribonucleic acid (miRNA) miR-206 targets the human estrogen receptor-alpha (ERalpha) and represses ERalpha messenger RNA and protein expression in breast cancer cell lines. Mol Endocrinol. 2007;21(5):1132–47.
154. Adams BD, Cowee DM, White BA. The role of miR-206 in the epidermal growth factor (EGF) induced repression of estrogen receptor-alpha (ERalpha) signaling and a luminal phenotype in MCF-7 breast cancer cells. Mol Endocrinol. 2009;23(8):1215–30.
155. Radojicic J, et al. MicroRNA expression analysis in triple-negative (ER, PR and Her2/neu) breast cancer. Cell Cycle. 2011;10(3):507–17.
156. Zhang Z, et al. MicroRNA miR-210 modulates cellular response to hypoxia through the MYC antagonist MNT. Cell Cycle. 2009;8(17):2756–68.
157. Crosby ME, et al. MicroRNA regulation of DNA repair gene expression in hypoxic stress. Cancer Res. 2009;69(3):1221–9.
158. Rothe F, et al. Global microRNA expression profiling identifies MiR-210 associated with tumor proliferation, invasion and poor clinical outcome in breast cancer. PLoS ONE. 2011;6(6):e20980.
159. Hui AB, et al. Robust global micro-RNA profiling with formalin-fixed paraffin-embedded breast cancer tissues. Lab Invest. 2009;89(5):597–606.
160. Stinson S, et al. TRPS1 targeting by miR-221/222 promotes the epithelial-to-mesenchymal transition in breast cancer. Sci Signal. 2011;4(177):ra41.
161. Liang Z, et al. Involvement of miR-326 in chemotherapy resistance of breast cancer through modulating expression of multidrug resistance-associated protein 1. Biochem Pharmacol. 2010;79(6):817–24.
162. Negrini M, Calin GA. Breast cancer metastasis: a microRNA story. Breast Cancer Res. 2008;10(2):203.
163. Huang Q, et al. The microRNAs miR-373 and miR-520c promote tumour invasion and metastasis. Nat Cell Biol. 2008;10(2):202–10.
164. Yan GR, et al. Global identification of miR-373-regulated genes in breast cancer by quantitative proteomics. Proteomics. 2011;11(5):912–20.

165. Giricz O, et al. Hsa-miR-375 is differentially expressed during breast lobular neoplasia and promotes loss of mammary acinar polarity. J Pathol. 2012;226(1):108–19.
166. Ward A, et al. Re-expression of microRNA-375 reverses both tamoxifen resistance and accompanying EMT-like properties in breast cancer. Oncogene. 2013;32(9):1173–82.
167. de Simonini PSR, et al. Epigenetically deregulated microRNA-375 is involved in a positive feedback loop with estrogen receptor alpha in breast cancer cells. Cancer Res. 2010;70(22):9175–84.
168. Keklikoglou I, et al. MicroRNA-520/373 family functions as a tumor suppressor in estrogen receptor negative breast cancer by targeting NF-kappaB and TGF-beta signaling pathways. Oncogene. 2012;31(37):4150–63.
169. Heneghan HM, et al. Circulating microRNAs as novel minimally invasive biomarkers for breast cancer. Ann Surg. 2010;251(3):499–505.
170. Roth C, et al. Circulating microRNAs as blood-based markers for patients with primary and metastatic breast cancer. Breast Cancer Res. 2010;12(6):R90.
171. Zhao FL, et al. Serum overexpression of microRNA-10b in patients with bone metastatic primary breast cancer. J Int Med Res. 2012;40(3):859–66.
172. Anfossi S, et al. High serum miR-19a levels are associated with inflammatory breast cancer and are predictive of favorable clinical outcome in patients with metastatic HER2(+) inflammatory breast cancer. PLoS ONE. 2014;9(1):e83113.
173. Wu X, et al. De novo sequencing of circulating miRNAs identifies novel markers predicting clinical outcome of locally advanced breast cancer. J Transl Med. 2012;10:42.
174. Zhu W, et al. Circulating microRNAs in breast cancer and healthy subjects. BMC Res Notes. 2009;2:89.
175. Guo LJ, Zhang QY. Decreased serum miR-181a is a potential new tool for breast cancer screening. Int J Mol Med. 2012;30(3):680–6.
176. Heneghan HM, et al. Systemic miRNA-195 differentiates breast cancer from other malignancies and is a potential biomarker for detecting noninvasive and early stage disease. Oncologist. 2010;15(7):673–82.
177. Schwarzenbach H, et al. Diagnostic potential of PTEN-targeting miR-214 in the blood of breast cancer patients. Breast Cancer Res Treat. 2012;134(3):933–41.

Chapter 14
Molecular Pathology of Fibroepithelial Neoplasms of the Breast

Michelle Yang, Dina Kandil and Ashraf Khan

Introduction

Fibroepithelial neoplasms (FEN) of the breast are biphasic tumors characterized by proliferation of both epithelial and stromal components. Fibroadenoma (FA) and phyllodes tumor (PT) account for over 90 % of all FEN. FA is a benign tumor that occurs in young women usually in the third or fourth decade, although it can be seen in older patients as well. Rarely, FA may progress to invasive and in situ carcinoma with a reported incidence of 0.1–0.3 % [1]. It has also been suggested that a small percentage of FA are monoclonal and can progress to PT [2]. In contrast, PT is a much rare neoplasm accounting for approximately 2.5 % of FEN of the breast and occurs in older patients usually after the fourth decade. Unlike FA, PT can recur locally and up to 25 % have the potential to metastasize to distant organs. In the current WHO classification, PT is categorized into three grades, which include benign, borderline, and malignant PT to predict their prognosis and clinical behavior based primarily on the histomorphology of the stromal component.

FA and PT share some overlapping histologic features but have significant differences in their clinical behavior, therefore differentiating various grades of PT and phyllodes tumor from FA directly affects the appropriate management and outcome for these patients. Core needle biopsy (CNB) or fine needle aspiration (FNA) is often performed for preoperative management in patients with breast

M. Yang · D. Kandil · A. Khan (✉)
Department of Pathology, University of Massachusetts Medical School,
UMassMemorial Medical Center, Three Biotech, One Innovation Drive,
Worcester, MA 01605, USA
e-mail: Ashraf.Khan@umassmemorial.org

© Springer Science+Business Media New York 2015
A. Khan et al. (eds.), *Precision Molecular Pathology of Breast Cancer*,
Molecular Pathology Library 10, DOI 10.1007/978-1-4939-2886-6_14

lesions. Although CNB can provide high negative and positive predictive values, accurate classification of FEN of the breast on a CNB may at times be challenging due to the heterogeneity and overlapping features in these lesions [3–5]. FNA appears to have higher false-negative rate probably due to the lack of characteristic architectural features that assist in the differentiation of PT from FA. In addition, FA can show increased cellularity mimicking PT, and PT may have areas similar to FA. Many studies have suggested the need for biomarkers especially Ki67 immunoreactivity in addition to the histologic features for more accurate preoperative evaluation and classification of FEN [6, 7]. However, there is no single "magic" biomarker yet to differentiate PT from FA [3]. In our practice a cellular fibroepithelial lesion on CNB that is difficult to be classified as FA or PT is best completely excised for further evaluation and accurate classification. Understanding their molecular pathways and developing more specific and sensitive biomarkers is of great interest to both basic scientists and clinicians. In this chapter, we give an overview of the molecular pathways involved in tumorigenesis and progression of FEN. We have also reviewed biomarkers investigated in the differential diagnosis of these tumors.

Molecular Pathways Related to Fibroepithelial Tumors

FA was initially found to be polyclonal and hyperplastic lesion, whereas PT showed clonal or neoplastic stromal cells and polyclonal epithelial component [8]. PCR-based clonal analysis in later studies revealed that some FA may also be monoclonal in origin, although majority were believed to be polyclonal [9]. Therefore, FA is not only closely related to PT morphologically, but monoclonal FA may progress to PT due to some but unknown molecular changes. In addition, carcinoma in situ or invasive carcinoma rarely arises within FA, suggesting that FA may progress in an epithelial direction as well [10]. FA and PT appear to represent the two ends of the spectrum of the FEN.

Insulin-Like Growth Factor (IGF) Signaling Pathway

Insulin-like growth factor signaling pathway involves two polypeptide hormones (IGF1 and IGF2), two transmembrane receptors (IGF1R and IGF2R), several IGF-binding proteins (IGFBP1-6), and many downstream effectors such as PI3K and MAPK pathways [11]. In general, IGF not only plays an important role in regulating normal fetal cell growth and differentiation including mammary gland development and involution [12, 13], but it also regulates cell proliferation and apoptosis during tumorigenesis. Targeting IGF1, IGFBP and IGF1 receptor system for breast cancer treatment is under investigation [14]. IGF bioavailability can also be regulated by IGFBP proteases. IGFBP form a complex with IGF and may function as a latent reservoir of IGF. In breast tissues, IGF1 is thought to be produced in the stroma in response to growth hormone and synergizes with estrogen to promote terminal end duct formation and mammary duct growth. IGF2 overexpression in mice can induce mammary gland tumor growth after multiple pregnancies. Both IGF1 and IGF2 can bind to IGF1 receptor, which is upregulated in the epithelia, and activate downstream intracellular signaling pathways to promote cell proliferation and inhibit apoptosis. Increased IGF signaling has been found in various human tumors including breast cancer.

Interestingly, both IGF1 and IGF2 are overexpressed in the stroma of FEN [15]. In PT, they are particularly found in the densely cellular stromal regions away from the ductal epithelium, although IGF1 expression appeared weak in malignant PT. In the same study, no IGF were expressed in the epithelial component or normal breast tissue [15]. It is believed that the epithelial–stromal interaction is required for normal development, differentiation and functioning of the breast [16, 17]. Disruption of this interaction may contribute to the development and progression of neoplasia. It remains unclear how stromal IGF interacts with epithelial IGFR1 in biphasic fibroepithelial tumors. Additionally, moderate or strong IGF1 expression was associated with moderate/strong β-catenin nuclear localization, suggesting a crosstalk between the IGF-signaling pathway and other signaling transduction pathways in the development of the PT.

Wnt-β-Catenin Signaling Pathway

Wnt-β-catenin signaling pathway also plays an important role in normal mammary gland development and tumorigenesis [18]. Wnt proteins are secreted glycoproteins regulating cell polarity and adhesion, apoptosis and tumorigenesis through direct and indirect interactions with other cell signaling pathways [19]. Deregulation of the Wnt signaling pathway has been implicated in many cancers and causes cytoplasmic β-catenin stabilization, nuclear translocation, and activation of Wnt target genes including oncogenes c-myc, c-jun, Fra, and cyclin D1. Interestingly, in PT abnormal stromal β-catenin nuclear translocation was found in 72 % of the tumors in a study by Sawyer et al. [15]. Meanwhile, aberrant nuclear localization of β-catenin was not associated with CTNNB1 (gene encoding β-catenin) mutations or loss of heterozygosity of tumor suppressor gene APC, but associated with increased Wnt5a expression in the epithelium and to less extent with Wnt2 overexpression in the stroma in PT [20]. The crosstalk of β-catenin with IGF-signaling pathway is also evidenced by a moderate to strong association between β-catenin nuclear staining and IGF1 overexpression in the stroma of the PT as mentioned above.

Epidermal Growth Factor Receptor (EGFR) Signaling Pathway

Epidermal growth factor receptor (EGFR) is a family of transmembrane receptor tyrosine kinases regulating cell proliferation, survival, migration, and differentiation. Four members have been identified, including ERBB1/EGFR, ERBB2 (HER2/neu), ERBB3 (HER3), and ERBB4 [21]. These transmembrane receptors are activated by cognate ligand to form homo- or heterodimers and transduce extracellular signals into cells and play important physiological roles including normal mammary development. Abnormal EGFR signaling is involved in many types of cancers including breast, lung, pancreas, and colorectal cancers [21]. Interestingly, a complex expression pattern of the EGFR family members in breast tumors has been observed. For example, ERBB2 and ERBB3 proteins were often expressed in carcinomas but not in the benign tumors. EGFR showed limited expression in the breast carcinoma, whereas both PT and FA showed EGFR expression. Kersting et al. showed that EGFR was overexpressed in the stromal cells in 12.5 % benign, 10 % borderline, and 63 % malignant PT, with less frequency of gene amplifications [22]. Zelada-Hedman et al. reported that EGFR expression was observed in all FA, which is contradictory to the lack of EGFR overexpression reported by Kersting et al. [23]. These findings suggest that the EGFR may play an important role in the development and progression of FEN.

Insulin-like Growth Factor-2 Binding Proteins (IGF2BPs)

Insulin-like growth factor-2 binding proteins (IGF2BPs, or IMP1, 2, and 3) are a family of proteins related to the IGF-signaling pathway but have distinct role from the previously discussed insulin-like growth factor binding proteins (IGFBPs). They were identified based on their ability to bind to the 5′-UTR of IGF2 mRNA and enhance IGF2 translation [24, 25]. Except for IMP2 protein, IMP1 and IMP3 proteins were only expressed during embryogenesis to promote cell growth and migration and not expressed in normal adult tissues. Mechanistically, unlike IGFBPs that directly bind IGFs, IGF2BPs (particularly IMP3) were positive regulators for the stability and translation of IGF2 mRNA [25, 26]. IMP3 knockdown by siRNA in K562 human leukemia cell line can inhibit the translation of IGF2 leader-3 mRNA without affecting the mRNA level of IGF2 [27]. IMP1 and IMP3 protein level exerted profound effects on cellular adhesion and formation of invadopodia by stabilizing CD44 mRNA, suggesting that re-expression of IMPs in cancer cells may promote tumor invasion and metastasis [28]. Consistent with the notion that re-expression of IMP3 in cancers is important for cancer progression and invasion, knockdown of IMP3 by siRNA is associated with decreased IGF2 protein expression, increased apoptosis, reduced cell migration and invasion in several cell lines including cervical carcinoma cell line HeLa and breast cancer cell line MDA-231 [29, 30]. In the past decade, many studies have demonstrated that IMP3 expression can be used in diagnosis of malignancy and is associated with a poor prognosis in various types of cancer [31]. In breast cancer, our previous study showed that IMP3 may serve as a marker for triple-negative breast cancer and is associated with more aggressive phenotype [32]. Interestingly, more recent data shows that EGFR signaling can induce IMP3 expression, suggesting a complex regulatory pathway of IGF signaling in breast tumorigenesis and progression [30, 33].

The molecular mechanisms by which IMP3 is re-expressed in cancer cells remain unclear. In breast cancer cells, estrogen receptor beta (ERβ) appears to function as a transcriptional repressor of IMP3 [30]. It is conceivable that epigenetic mechanisms for the IMP3 promoter might also play a role for its transcriptional reactivation given that IMP3 promoter possesses CpG island that is potentially a target for DNA demethylases and/or histone modification enzymes. Interestingly, IGFBP3 (not to be confused with IGF2BP3 or IMP3), one member of IGFBP family with an opposite effect to cell growth compared to IMP3, also has a CpG island at its promoter. IGFBP3 expression can be re-induced by DNA demethylation agent 5-AZA-2′-deoxycytidine treatment in hepatoblastoma cell line and consequently restoring IGFBP3 expression in these cells resulted in reduced colony formation, migration, and invasion [34].

Other Signaling Pathways

Using next-generation sequencing, Jardim et al. identified three aberrant genes including activating mutation of NRAS, inactivating mutation of RB1, and TP53 loss in metastatic malignant PT. In addition, phosphorylated AKT (p-AKT), PDGFR, EGFR, TLE3, mTOR, and SPARC expressions were increased with tumor grade by immunohistochemistry. These data suggested possible involvement and crosstalk of PI3K and MAPK signaling pathways in PT and more complex regulations in tumor progression [35].

Molecular Biomarkers Investigated in Fibroepithelial Tumors

Currently, the differentiation of the PT from FA is primarily based on the architecture, stromal cellularity, stromal cell nuclear pleomorphism, mitoses, and Ki67 proliferation index of the stromal cells. Misdiagnosis of these two entities in CNB may occur due to the histopathologic heterogeneity in PT or presence of some overlapping features between the FEN [6, 36]. On the other hand, grading of the PT can be more difficult in CNB due to limited samples. Many immunohistological markers have been investigated to compare their expression in FA and

PT and their association with tumor grade for the latter. Majority of these markers are related to the signaling pathways involved in tumorigenesis and progression of fibroepithelial tumors discussed above. To the best of our knowledge, there is to this date no single "magic" marker to distinguish PT from FA, or to accurately classify PT into benign, borderline, and malignant categories. However, a number of biomarkers have been investigated and some of them may be useful in the differential diagnosis of fibroepithelial tumors.

Ki67 and Cell Proliferation Markers

The nuclear protein Ki67 is a cell proliferation marker expressed only in cycling cells. As a result, quantitative assessment of Ki67 nuclear staining on tumor samples provides a good estimate of the proliferation index of individual tumors. Ki67 index is defined as the percentage of cells with positive nuclear stains by MIB-1 antibody, which recognizes Ki67 antigen in the nucleus. Consistent with other studies, our unpublished data also showed that Ki67 index increased in borderline and especially malignant PT. Ki67 proliferation index has been significantly correlated with disease-free and with overall survival [37]. Evaluation of the proliferative activity of the PT by Ki67 index is one of the current WHO criteria for grading of PT. It seems Ki67 index is considered useful in classification of fibroepithelial lesions but a practical problem that exists is that there is no well-established threshold for Ki67 index for categorizing various grades of PT. The other issue is how the percentage of Ki67 immunoreactivity in tumor cells is estimated by quantitative or semi-quantitative methods. Given its utility and promise as a biomarker, large multicenter study with long-term clinical follow-up and utilizing computer-based image analysis systems to estimate the percentage of Ki67 positive cells may be valuable. Other cell proliferation markers that have been used include DNA Topoisomerase IIα and anaphase-promoting complex 7, whose expression has been shown to correlate well with Ki67 expression [38, 39].

CD117 (c-kit)

CD117 is a transmembrane protein of the type III receptor tyrosine kinase family. It is crucial in regulating cell survival, proliferation, and differentiation. It is recognized as a proto-oncogene with frequent activating mutations and/or overexpression in several types of neoplasms, including gastrointestinal stromal tumors, seminomas, melanomas, and hematopoietic malignancies. Although increased CD117 expression in PT has also been reported in several studies [40–42], there is no association of CD117 expression and the tumor grade and furthermore, KIT activating mutations have not been found in PT in other studies [43–45]. Platelet-derived growth factor receptor alpha (PDGFRA) is also a cell membrane tyrosine kinase receptor of the platelet-derived growth factor family and activating mutations of PDGFRA have been associated with gastrointestinal stromal tumors and a variety of other cancers. However, no overexpression or mutation of PDGFRA has been observed in PT so far. In one study, none of the 41 PT expressed CD117 [46]. Based on current data, the application of CD117 in differentiating FA from PT or in the grading of the latter remains to be investigated.

p53

The prototype tumor suppressor p53 is essential for cell cycle control, DNA damage repair, and apoptosis. Defective p53 may lead to abnormal cell proliferation and decreased cell death, resulting in tumorigenesis. It is therefore not a surprise that deregulation of p53 protein is observed in approximately 50 % of all human tumors. Under normal cellular conditions, p53 is rapidly degraded by the proteasome in a process mediated by MDM2 and *jun* kinase. After cellular stresses, such as exposure to DNA-damaging agents, the half-life of the p53 protein is significantly increased, and p53 accumulates in the nucleus of affected cells. In PT, several studies have shown strong but variable degree of nuclear p53 staining in the stromal cells of malignant PT and p53 positivity was associated with an increased Ki67 index [41, 47–50]. No p53 nuclear staining was observed in benign tumors or FA. p53 immunohistochemistry may be helpful in the grading of PT, but not for the differentiation of FA from benign PT, and the sensitivity is variable.

CD10

Contradictory results of CD10 positivity have been reported. One study by Zamecnik et al. showed frequent CD10 positivity in both FA and PT (60 and 67 %, respectively) [51]. Thus, they believed that this antibody could not assist in the differential diagnosis between FA and PT. This finding is in contrast with other studies in which CD10 was preferentially expressed in borderline and especially malignant PT but not in FA or benign PT, and its expression was associated with tumor grade [52–54]. Moritani and colleagues showed that CD10 appears to highlight the myoepithelial cells in many benign breast lesions including FA and PT [55]. Based on these data, CD10 immunohistochemistry seems to be only helpful in differentiating benign from borderline or malignant PT but not from FA.

Cytokeratins

Chia and colleagues investigated a larger cohort of PTs using a wide panel of commonly used keratins including MNF116, 34βE12, CK7, CK14, Cam5.2 and AE1/3. Contrary to other studies, they observed some expression of keratins

MNF116, 34bE12, CK7, CK14, AE1/3, and Cam5.2 in stromal cells of 11.9, 22, 28.4, 1.8, 8.3 and 1.8 % of PTs, respectively [56]. However, keratin positivity was focal and patchy and found in only 1–5 % of stromal cells in these cases and the explanation for keratin expression is uncertain. In an earlier study by Dunne et al., who applied a panel of keratins (AE1/AE3, 34βE12, CK5 and CK14, Cam5.2, CK7 and CK19, EMA) for which all were negative in stromal components of 26 PTs [57]. There has been another study by Auger et al. showing the presence of stromal keratin expression in malignant PT [58]. In our recent study using a panel of cytokeratins including AE1/AE3, Cytokeratin-OSCAR, CAM 5.2, CK903, CK5/6, we did not find stromal cell immunoreactivity in any case of PT (unpublished data). Overall, the stromal keratin positivity in PT remains inconclusive but given some reported cross reactivity between keratins and stromal cells in malignant PT, differentiation from spindle cell metaplastic carcinoma may be difficult on needle core biopsies, where the entire lesion with its architecture is not seen.

Beta-Catenin and E-cadherin

Many genes are involved in the Wnt-β catenin signaling pathway. The expression of five key markers from the Wnt pathway, including markers β-catenin, E-cadherin, Wnt1, Wnt5a and SFRP4, in the PT were examined by Karim et al. [20]. Results suggested that stromal nuclear β-catenin increased from normal breast tissue to benign PT to borderline PT, and then decreased in malignant PT, although the expression in the latter was still greater than that in normal breast tissue and benign PT. This finding suggested that nuclear stromal accumulation of β-catenin may be involved in the initiation and progression of PT. However, some degree of nuclear β-catenin staining was observed in the stroma of all 30 FAs reported by Sawyer et al. [15]. Furthermore mammary fibromatosis was also associated with nuclear localization of β-catenin and mutation in the β-catenin gene [59]. Therefore β-catenin immunostain has limited role in the differential diagnosis of spindle cell lesions of the breast on needle core biopsies. For E-cadherin, an adhesion molecule forming complex with catenins at epithelial cell–cell junctions and lost during epithelial-to-mesenchymal transition, a positive membrane staining was only seen in the epithelial cells not the stromal cells. Interestingly, decreased E-cadherin expression in the epithelial cell membrane was significantly correlated with increased mean time to recurrence [20].

IGF

The expression of IGF1 and IGF2 in both PT and FA has been studied by Sawyer et al. in 2003 [15]. Many of these tumors showed widespread overexpression of IGF1 and to less extent IGF2 throughout the stroma in both PT and FA. In particular, IGF1 was largely found in the densely cellular stromal regions away from the epithelium. In the normal tissue surrounding the tumors, a very low level of IGF1 and IGF2 expression could be seen in the stroma. No IGF1 or IGF2 expression was seen in the normal or tumor epithelium. Although IGF1 and IGF2 overexpression may be important in the pathogenesis of FEN of the breast, these markers may not be useful in differentiating FA from PT.

EGFR

Several groups have shown EGFR expression in PT and its association with tumor progression [46, 60]. Tse et al. investigated 453 PTs (296 benign, 98 borderline, 59 malignant) for EGFR expression using immunohistochemistry and fluorescence in situ hybridization (FISH) for gene amplification [60]. The results showed a correlation between EGFR expression and tumor margin status, tumor grade, stromal cellularity, mitotic activity, nuclear pleomorphism, and stromal overgrowth. The overall positive rate for EGFR was 16.2 % (48/296), 30.6 % (30/98), and 56 % (33/59) for benign, borderline, and malignant PT respectively. FISH demonstrated EGFR gene amplification in 8 % of EGFR positive cases by immunohistochemistry. In another study by Kersting et al. [22], EGFR positivity was detected in 19 % of all PTs (75 % of malignant tumors) in stromal tumor cells but not in the epithelial component and it was correlated to p53 expression. Like many other biomarkers, the overall low sensitivity can limit their application in daily practice.

P16/Rb

The cell cycle regulators Rb and p16 have been investigated in breast biphasic tumors. Karim et al. reported an increase in p16 and Rb protein by immunohistochemistry in high grade PT [61]. These results were consistent with the report of Kuijper et al. [62]. However, Esposito et al. found there was no significant association between p16 expression and tumor grade in PT [63]. Recent data by Cimino-Mathews et al. showed that there were 2 distinct expression patterns for p16 and Rb in malignant PT including "diffuse p16+/Rb−" or "diffuse Rb+/p16−" in 50 % cases [64]. None of these patterns was observed in borderline, benign PT or FA. Instead, 100 % borderline, 70 % benign, and 100 % FA showed "low p16 +/low Rb+" staining pattern. P16 positivity was not associated high risk human papillomavirus [64].

Epithelial–Mesenchymal Transition (EMT) Related Markers

Epithelial–Mesenchymal Transition (EMT) is a cellular event characterized by a series of molecular and morphological changes in epithelial cells, therefore the epithelial cells gain mesenchymal phenotype and become more motile. EMT was initially characterized in early embryogenesis and later identified as a common phenomenon during cancer progression and invasion. Loss of E-cadherin expression and gain of N-cadherin and transcriptional factors such as Snail, TWIST, ZEB1 and ZEB3 have been well characterized molecular changes during tumor progression. Kwon et al. [65] studied several EMT related markers in a cohort of 207 PTs including 157 benign, 34 borderline, and 16 malignant cases. These markers including TWIST, HMGA2, TGFβ were significantly increased in the stromal component of higher grade PT. In addition, high expression of TWIST was correlated with poor overall survival. However, other studies showed TWIST gene methylation was correlated with tumor grade and both methylation and protein expression were found in breast cancers [66]. These results seem to be contradictory to each other if methylation generally plays a role in gene suppression. Therefore, more investigations are needed to further characterize the use of EMT markers in PT.

Other Proteins Evaluated in PT

Autophagy-related proteins and redox proteins were recently evaluated by Koo group [67, 68]. Autophagy is a lysosomal self-degradation process that is important for balancing sources of energy during development and in response to nutrient stress. Autophagy also plays a housekeeping role in removing misfolded or aggregated proteins, clearing damaged organelles, and eliminating intracellular pathogens. It is an alternative metabolic pathway to conserve energy within tumor cells. Several autophagy proteins including beclin-1, LC3A, LC3B, and p62 were associated with increased stromal cellularity, stromal atypia, mitosis and stromal overgrowth. Particularly, stromal cell nuclear expression of beclin-1 was associated with poor prognosis [68].

Reactive oxygen species (ROS) is known to induce genetic instability, promote angiogenesis and aid proliferating cells to escape apoptosis. ROS signaling is known to be increased in tumor cells. Several redox related proteins were evaluated by immunohistochemistry by Kim et al. [67]. They found an increased expression of catalase, TxNR, TxNIP, and MnSOD redox proteins in stromal cells with the increase in tumor grade in PT. Hypoxia inducing factor (HIF1α) expression was also increased in PT with higher tumor grades, suggesting that excessive stromal growth may induce tissue hypoxia and higher level of ROS-related proteins.

Ang et al. [69] recently identified a group of 29 genes over- or under-expressed in PT by Affymetrix gene chip profiling. Several of these genes showed differential expression in benign, borderline, and malignant PT. HOXB13 was one of the upregulated genes confirmed by immunohistochemistry for protein expression in malignant PT. Nuclear HOXB13 overexpression in stromal cells was correlated with stromal hypercellularity and atypia. However, this study was limited by small number of cases, including 6 benign, 10 borderline, and 5 malignant PT.

IMP3

IMP3 has been recently demonstrated as a novel biomarker in many cancers including lung [70], renal [71], pancreatic [72], cervical adenocarcinoma [29], thyroid [73], and malignant mesotheliomas [74]. In a series of 138 breast cancer cases, our study showed that IMP3 expression was seen in 45 (33 %) cases and 25 of the IMP3+ cases were triple-negative breast carcinoma [32]. There was a significant correlation between IMP3 expression and higher grade, necrosis, triple-negative phenotype, and CK5/6 expression. Cox multivariate analysis showed a hazard ratio of IMP3 expression at 3.14. IMP3 was identified as a novel biomarker for triple-negative (basal-like) invasive mammary carcinoma, and its expression was associated with a more aggressive phenotype and decreased overall survival. Other studies showed that membranous positivity of IMP3 was seen in 81.3 % of primary adenoid cystic carcinomas of breast, a variant of triple-negative breast cancers [75, 76]. In PT of the breast, our recent data showed that IMP3 is preferentially expressed in all malignant PT but not in borderline and benign PT, or benign residual breast tissue [77], suggesting IMP3 may serve as a potential biomarker to identify malignant PT especially in limited material such as CNB.

Chromosomal and Methylation Changes

In a study by Lae et al. [76] results showed that 83 % of the PT had chromosomal imbalance, which segregated into two groups. Benign PT showed one or a few chromosomal changes, compared to numerous chromosomal imbalances in borderline and malignant PT. Among these changes, gain of chromosome 1q and loss of 13q were the hallmark alterations in PT. The role of these chromosomal or genetic changes in the fibroepithelial lesions needs to be further investigated. Huang et al. selectively studied the methylation profile of 11 genes in 15 benign, 28 borderline, 43 malignant PTs, and 26 FAs. They observed significant level of methylation changes in 2 genes including *RASSF1A* (24.4 %) and *TWIST1* (7.1 %) in some PT but none in FA, suggesting that assessment of methylation of *RASSF1A* and *TWIS T1* may aid in the differentiating PT from FA [78]. Kim et al. [79] studied promoter methylation of several genes and found there was a higher methylation status in borderline and malignant PT than in benign tumors, although no significant difference was found between the borderline and malignant ones. However, the specificity has not been addressed and it remains unclear whether FA also have methylation changes. Currently the variable sensitivity of methylation of these genes makes this method impractical.

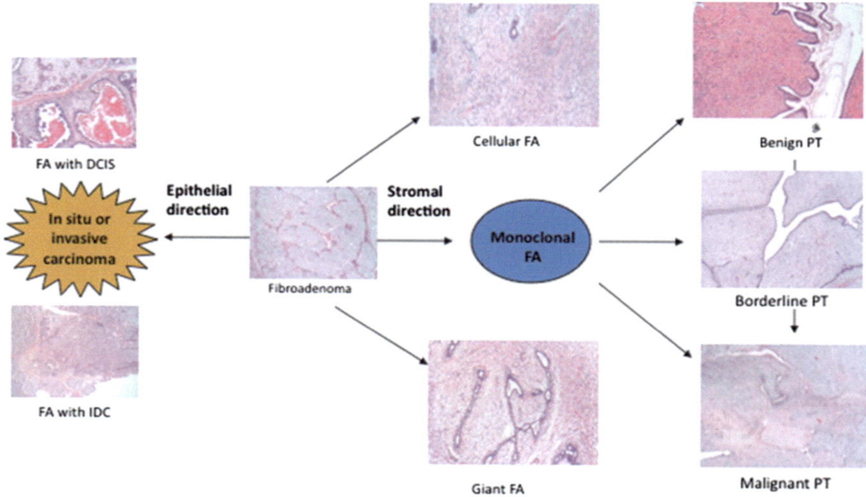

Fig. 14.1 Schematic representation biphasic progression of fibroepithelial tumors

Summary

Fibroepithelial tumors of the breast are a heterogeneous group of biphasic lesions with FA and PT being the most common lesions. Based on the current understanding, we propose a simplified progressive model in which FA and PT may represent the two ends of the spectrum of FEN (Fig. 14.1). Studies have shown that clonal evolution while less common can occur in the stromal cells of FA and the transformation or progression to PT from FA may also occur (Fig. 14.1). On the other hand, when clonal changes occur in the epithelial component, epithelial proliferation into hyperplasia, carcinoma in situ, or invasive carcinoma can also occur (Fig. 14.1). This progressive model might explain why FA are much more common biphasic lesions than PT, and carcinoma only rarely arising within the FA or PT.

PT is further classified into benign, borderline and malignant categories. Due to some overlapping histologic features, differentiation of FA and benign PT and accurate grading of PT may be difficult on small biopsies. Due to significant differences in their clinical behavior, complete excision of such indeterminate lesions on needle biopsies may be needed with appropriate clinical correlation for definitive classification of fibroepithelial tumors. Some immunohistochemical markers have shown promise to aid in this differential diagnosis, especially Ki67 proliferation index. But as of now, there is no "magic marker" with high sensitivity and specificity and morphology on a completely resected tumor remains the gold standard. Large scale or multi-institutional studies with long follow-up may be needed to address these issues in the future.

References

1. Dupont WD, Page DL, Parl FF, Vnencak-Jones CL, Plummer WD Jr, Rados MS, Schuyler PA. Long-term risk of breast cancer in women with fibroadenoma. N Engl J Med. 1994;331(1):10–5.
2. Noguchi S, Yokouchi H, Aihara T, Motomura K, Inaji H, Imaoka S, Koyama H. Progression of fibroadenoma to phyllodes tumor demonstrated by clonal analysis. Cancer. 1995;76(10):1779–85.
3. Giri D. Recurrent challenges in the evaluation of fibroepithelial lesions. Arch Pathol Lab Med. 2009;133(5):713–21.
4. Komenaka IK, El-Tamer M, Pile-Spellman E, Hibshoosh H. Core needle biopsy as a diagnostic tool to differentiate phyllodes tumor from fibroadenoma. Arch Surg. 2003;138(9):987–90.
5. Jacobs TW, Chen YY, Guinee DG Jr, Holden JA, Cha I, Bauermeister DE, Hashimoto B, Wolverton D, Hartzog G. Fibroepithelial lesions with cellular stroma on breast core needle biopsy: are there predictors of outcome on surgical excision? Am J Clin Pathol. 2005;124(3):342–54.
6. Tsang AK, Chan SK, Lam CC, Lui PC, Chau HH, Tan PH, Tse GM. Phyllodes tumours of the breast—differentiating features in core needle biopsy. Histopathology. 2011;59(4):600–8.
7. Jara-Lazaro AR, Akhilesh M, Thike AA, Lui PC, Tse GM, Tan PH. Predictors of phyllodes tumours on core biopsy specimens of fibroepithelial neoplasms. Histopathology. 2010;57(2):220–32.
8. Noguchi S, Motomura K, Inaji H, Imaoka S, Koyama H. Clonal analysis of fibroadenoma and phyllodes tumor of the breast. Cancer Res. 1993;53(17):4071–4.
9. Noguchi S, Aihara T, Koyama H, Motomura K, Inaji H, Imaoka S. Clonal analysis of benign and malignant human breast tumors by means of polymerase chain reaction. Cancer Lett. 1995;90(1):57–63.
10. Kuijper A, Buerger H, Simon R, Schaefer KL, Croonen A, Boecker W, van der Wall E, van Diest PJ. Analysis of the progression of fibroepithelial tumours of the breast by PCR-based clonality assay. J Pathol. 2002;197(5):575–81.
11. Flint DJ, Tonner E, Beattie J, Allan GJ. Role of insulin-like growth factor binding proteins in mammary gland development. J Mammary Gland Biol Neoplasia. 2008;13(4):443–53.
12. Gross JM, Yee D. The type-1 insulin-like growth factor receptor tyrosine kinase and breast cancer: biology and therapeutic relevance. Cancer Metastasis Rev. 2003;22(4):327–36.
13. Allan GJ, Beattie J, Flint DJ. The role of IGFBP-5 in mammary gland development and involution. Domest Anim Endocrinol. 2004;27(3):257–66.
14. Mohanraj L, Oh Y. Targeting IGF-I, IGFBPs and IGF-I receptor system in cancer: the current and future in breast cancer therapy. Recent Pat Anticancer Drug Discov. 2011;6(2):166–77.
15. Sawyer EJ, Hanby AM, Poulsom R, Jeffery R, Gillett CE, Ellis IO, Ellis P, Tomlinson IP. Beta-catenin abnormalities and associated insulin-like growth factor overexpression are important in phyllodes tumours and fibroadenomas of the breast. J Pathol. 2003;200(5):627–32.
16. Sawyer EJ, Hanby AM, Ellis P, Lakhani SR, Ellis IO, Boyle S, Tomlinson IP. Molecular analysis of phyllodes tumors reveals distinct changes in the epithelial and stromal components. Am J Pathol. 2000;156(3):1093–8.
17. Sawhney N, Garrahan N, Douglas-Jones AG, Williams ED. Epithelial–stromal interactions in tumors. A morphologic study of fibroepithelial tumors of the breast. Cancer. 1992;70(8):2115–20.
18. Paul S, Dey A. Wnt signaling and cancer development: therapeutic implication. Neoplasma. 2008;55(3):165–76.
19. Howe LR, Brown AM. Wnt signaling and breast cancer. Cancer Biol Ther. 2004;3(1):36–41.

20. Karim RZ, Gerega SK, Yang YH, Horvath L, Spillane A, Carmalt H, Scolyer RA, Lee CS. Proteins from the Wnt pathway are involved in the pathogenesis and progression of mammary phyllodes tumours. J Clin Pathol. 2009;62(11):1016–20.
21. Mahipal A, Kothari N, Gupta S. Epidermal growth factor receptor inhibitors: coming of age. Cancer Control. 2014;21(1):74–9.
22. Kersting C, Kuijper A, Schmidt H, Packeisen J, Liedtke C, Tidow N, Gustmann C, Hinrichs B, Wulfing P, Tio J, et al. Amplifications of the epidermal growth factor receptor gene (egfr) are common in phyllodes tumors of the breast and are associated with tumor progression. Lab Invest. 2006;86(1):54–61.
23. Zelada-Hedman M, Werer G, Collins P, Backdahl M, Perez I, Franco S, Jimenez J, Cruz J, Torroella M, Nordenskjold M, et al. High expression of the EGFR in fibroadenomas compared to breast carcinomas. Anticancer Res. 1994;14(5A):1679–88.
24. Nielsen FC, Nielsen J, Christiansen J. A family of IGF-II mRNA binding proteins (IMP) involved in RNA trafficking. Scand J Clin Lab Invest Suppl. 2001;234:93–9.
25. Dai N, Rapley J, Angel M, Yanik MF, Blower MD, Avruch J. mTOR phosphorylates IMP2 to promote IGF2 mRNA translation by internal ribosomal entry. Genes Dev. 2011;25(11):1159–72.
26. Liao B, Hu Y, Herrick DJ, Brewer G. The RNA-binding protein IMP-3 is a translational activator of insulin-like growth factor II leader-3 mRNA during proliferation of human K562 leukemia cells. J Biol Chem. 2005;280(18):18517–24.
27. Liao B, Hu Y, Brewer G. RNA-binding protein insulin-like growth factor mRNA-binding protein 3 (IMP-3) promotes cell survival via insulin-like growth factor II signaling after ionizing radiation. J Biol Chem. 2011;286(36):31145–52.
28. Vikesaa J, Hansen TV, Jonson L, Borup R, Wewer UM, Christiansen J, Nielsen FC. RNA-binding IMPs promote cell adhesion and invadopodia formation. EMBO J. 2006;25(7):1456–68.
29. Lu D, Yang X, Jiang NY, Woda BA, Liu Q, Dresser K, Mercurio AM, Rock KL, Jiang Z. IMP3, a new biomarker to predict progression of cervical intraepithelial neoplasia into invasive cancer. Am J Surg Pathol. 2011;35(11):1638–45.
30. Samanta S, Sharma VM, Khan A, Mercurio AM. Regulation of IMP3 by EGFR signaling and repression by ERbeta: implications for triple-negative breast cancer. Oncogene 2012; 1–9 (Epub ahead of print).
31. Findeis-Hosey JJ, Xu H. The use of insulin like-growth factor II messenger RNA binding protein-3 in diagnostic pathology. Hum Pathol. 2011;42(3):303–14.
32. Walter O, Prasad M, Lu S, Quinlan RM, Edmiston KL, Khan A. IMP3 is a novel biomarker for triple negative invasive mammary carcinoma associated with a more aggressive phenotype. Hum Pathol. 2009;40(11):1528–33.
33. Jin T, George Fantus I, Sun J. Wnt and beyond Wnt: multiple mechanisms control the transcriptional property of beta-catenin. Cell Signal. 2008;20(10):1697–704.
34. Regel I, Eichenmuller M, Joppien S, Liebl J, Haberle B, Muller-Hocker J, Vollmar A, von Schweinitz D, Kappler R. IGFBP3 impedes aggressive growth of pediatric liver cancer and is epigenetically silenced in vascular invasive and metastatic tumors. Mol Cancer. 2012;11(1):9.
35. Jardim DL, Conley A, Subbiah V. Comprehensive characterization of malignant phyllodes tumor by whole genomic and proteomic analysis: biological implications for targeted therapy opportunities. Orphanet J Rare Dis. 2013;8:112.
36. Huo L, Gilcrease MZ. Fibroepithelial lesions of the breast with pleomorphic stromal giant cells: a clinicopathologic study of 4 cases and review of the literature. Ann Diagn Pathol. 2009;13(4):226–32.
37. Niezabitowski A, Lackowska B, Rys J, Kruczak A, Kowalska T, Mitus J, Reinfuss M, Markiewicz D. Prognostic evaluation of proliferative activity and DNA content in the phyllodes tumor of the breast: immunohistochemical and flow cytometric study of 118 cases. Breast Cancer Res Treat. 2001;65(1):77–85.
38. Lynch BJ, Guinee DG Jr, Holden JA. Human DNA topoisomerase II-alpha: a new marker of cell proliferation in invasive breast cancer. Hum Pathol. 1997;28(10):1180–8.

39. Kang Y, Kim JH, Lee TH, Kim TS, Jung WH, Chung HC, Park BW, Sheen SS, Han JH. Expression of anaphase-promoting complex7 in fibroadenomas and phyllodes tumors of breast. Hum Pathol. 2009;40(1):98–107.
40. Tse GM, Putti TC, Lui PC, Lo AW, Scolyer RA, Law BK, Karim R, Lee CS. Increased c-kit (CD117) expression in malignant mammary phyllodes tumors. Mod Pathol. 2004;17(7):827–31.
41. Tan PH, Jayabaskar T, Yip G, Tan Y, Hilmy M, Selvarajan S, Bay BH. p53 and c-kit (CD117) protein expression as prognostic indicators in breast phyllodes tumors: a tissue microarray study. Mod Pathol. 2005;18(12):1527–34.
42. Chen CM, Chen CJ, Chang CL, Shyu JS, Hsieh HF, Harn EJ. CD34, CD117, and actin expression in phyllodes tumor of the breast. J Surg Res. 2000;94(2):84–91.
43. Korcheva VB, Levine J, Beadling C, Warrick A, Countryman G, Olson NR, Heinrich MC, Corless CL, Troxell ML. Immunohistochemical and molecular markers in breast phyllodes tumors. Appl Immunohistochem Mol Morphol. 2011;19(2):119–25.
44. Djordjevic B, Hanna WM. Expression of c-kit in fibroepithelial lesions of the breast is a mast cell phenomenon. Mod Pathol. 2008;21(10):1238–45.
45. Bose P, Dunn ST, Yang J, Allen R, El-Khoury C, Tfayli A. c-Kit expression and mutations in phyllodes tumors of the breast. Anticancer Res. 2010;30(11):4731–6.
46. Agelopoulos K, Kersting C, Korsching E, Schmidt H, Kuijper A, August C, Wulfing P, Tio J, Boecker W, van Diest PJ, et al. Egfr amplification specific gene expression in phyllodes tumours of the breast. Cell Oncol. 2007;29(6):443–51.
47. Chan YJ, Chen BF, Chang CL, Yang TL, Fan CC. Expression of p53 protein and Ki-67 antigen in phyllodes tumor of the breast. J Chin Med Assoc. 2004;67(1):3–8.
48. Kuenen-Boumeester V, Henzen-Logmans SC, Timmermans MM, van Staveren IL, van Geel A, Peeterse HJ, Bonnema J, Berns EM. Altered expression of p53 and its regulated proteins in phyllodes tumours of the breast. J Pathol. 1999;189(2):169–75.
49. Tse GM, Putti TC, Kung FY, Scolyer RA, Law BK, Lau TS, Lee CS. Increased p53 protein expression in malignant mammary phyllodes tumors. Mod Pathol. 2002;15(7):734–40.
50. Yonemori K, Hasegawa T, Shimizu C, Shibata T, Matsumoto K, Kouno T, Ando M, Katsumata N, Fujiwara Y. Correlation of p53 and MIB-1 expression with both the systemic recurrence and survival in cases of phyllodes tumors of the breast. Pathol Res Pract. 2006;202(10):705–12.
51. Zamecnik M, Kinkor Z, Chlumska A. CD10+ stromal cells in fibroadenomas and phyllodes tumors of the breast. Virchows Arch. 2006;448(6):871–2.
52. Tse GM, Tsang AK, Putti TC, Scolyer RA, Lui PC, Law BK, Karim RZ, Lee CS. Stromal CD10 expression in mammary fibroadenomas and phyllodes tumours. J Clin Pathol. 2005;58(2):185–9.
53. Tsai WC, Jin JS, Yu JC, Sheu LF. CD10, actin, and vimentin expression in breast phyllodes tumors correlates with tumor grades of the WHO grading system. Int J Surg Pathol. 2006;14(2):127–31.
54. Ibrahim WS. Comparison of stromal CD10 expression in benign, borderline, and malignant phyllodes tumors among Egyptian female patients. Indian J Pathol Microbiol. 2011;54(4):741–4.
55. Moritani S, Kushima R, Sugihara H, Bamba M, Kobayashi TK, Hattori T. Availability of CD10 immunohistochemistry as a marker of breast myoepithelial cells on paraffin sections. Mod Pathol. 2002;15(4):397–405.
56. Chia Y, Thike AA, Cheok PY, Yong-Zheng Chong L, Man-Kit Tse G, Tan PH. Stromal keratin expression in phyllodes tumours of the breast: a comparison with other spindle cell breast lesions. J Clin Pathol. 2012;65(4);339–347.
57. Dunne B, Lee AH, Pinder SE, Bell JA, Ellis IO. An immunohistochemical study of metaplastic spindle cell carcinoma, phyllodes tumor and fibromatosis of the breast. Hum Pathol. 2003;34(10):1009–15.
58. Auger M, Hanna W, Kahn HJ. Cystosarcoma phylloides of the breast and its mimics. An immunohistochemical and ultrastructural study. Arch Pathol Lab Med. 1989;113(11):1231–5.

59. Lacroix-Triki M, Geyer FC, Lambros MB, Savage K, Ellis IO, Lee AH, Reis-Filho JS. Beta-catenin/Wnt signalling pathway in fibromatosis, metaplastic carcinomas and phyllodes tumours of the breast. Mod Pathol. 2010;23(11):1438–48.
60. Tse GM, Lui PC, Vong JS, Lau KM, Putti TC, Karim R, Scolyer RA, Lee CS, Yu AM, Ng DC, et al. Increased epidermal growth factor receptor (EGFR) expression in malignant mammary phyllodes tumors. Breast Cancer Res Treat. 2009;114(3):441–8.
61. Karim RZ, Gerega SK, Yang YH, Spillane A, Carmalt H, Scolyer RA, Lee CS. p16 and pRb immunohistochemical expression increases with increasing tumour grade in mammary phyllodes tumours. Histopathology. 2010;56(7):868–75.
62. Kuijper A, de Vos RA, Lagendijk JH, van der Wall E, van Diest PJ. Progressive deregulation of the cell cycle with higher tumor grade in the stroma of breast phyllodes tumors. Am J Clin Pathol. 2005;123(5):690–8.
63. Esposito NN, Mohan D, Brufsky A, Lin Y, Kapali M, Dabbs DJ. Phyllodes tumor: a clinicopathologic and immunohistochemical study of 30 cases. Arch Pathol Lab Med. 2006;130(10):1516–21.
64. Cimino-Mathews A, Hicks JL, Sharma R, Vang R, Illei PB, De Marzo A, Emens LA, Argani P. A subset of malignant phyllodes tumors harbors alterations in the Rb/p16 pathway. Hum Pathol. 2013;44(11):2494–500.
65. Kwon JE, Jung WH, Koo JS. Molecules involved in epithelial-mesenchymal transition and epithelial-stromal interaction in phyllodes tumors: implications for histologic grade and prognosis. Tumour Biol. 2012;33(3):787–98.
66. Gort EH, Suijkerbuijk KP, Roothaan SM, Raman V, Vooijs M, van der Wall E, van Diest PJ. Methylation of the TWIST1 promoter, TWIST1 mRNA levels, and immunohistochemical expression of TWIST1 in breast cancer. Cancer Epidemiol Biomark Prev. 2008;17(12):3325–30.
67. Kim S, Kim do H, Jung WH, Koo JS. The expression of redox proteins in phyllodes tumor. Breast Cancer Res Treat. 2013;141(3):365–74.
68. Kim SK, Jung WH, Koo JS. Expression of autophagy-related proteins in phyllodes tumor. Int J Clin Exp Pathol. 2013;6(10):2145–56.
69. Ang MK, Ooi AS, Thike AA, Tan P, Zhang Z, Dykema K, Furge K, Teh BT, Tan PH. Molecular classification of breast phyllodes tumors: validation of the histologic grading scheme and insights into malignant progression. Breast Cancer Res Treat. 2011;129(2):319–29.
70. Bellezza G, Cavaliere A, Sidoni A. IMP3 expression in non-small cell lung cancer. Hum Pathol. 2009;40(8):1205–6.
71. Jiang Z, Chu PG, Woda BA, Rock KL, Liu Q, Hsieh CC, Li C, Chen W, Duan HO, McDougal S, et al. Analysis of RNA-binding protein IMP3 to predict metastasis and prognosis of renal-cell carcinoma: a retrospective study. Lancet Oncol. 2006;7(7):556–64.
72. Schaeffer DF, Owen DR, Lim HJ, Buczkowski AK, Chung SW, Scudamore CH, Huntsman DG, Ng SS, Owen DA. Insulin-like growth factor 2 mRNA binding protein 3 (IGF2BP3) overexpression in pancreatic ductal adenocarcinoma correlates with poor survival. BMC Cancer. 2010;10:59.
73. Slosar M, Vohra P, Prasad M, Fischer A, Quinlan R, Khan A. Insulin-like growth factor mRNA binding protein 3 (IMP3) is differentially expressed in benign and malignant follicular patterned thyroid tumors. Endocr Pathol. 2009;20(3):149–57.
74. Shi M,, Fraire AE, Chu P, Cornejo K, Woda BA, Dresser K, Rock KL, Jiang Z. Oncofetal protein IMP3, a new diagnostic biomarker to distinguish malignant mesothelioma from reactive mesothelial proliferation. Am J Surg Pathol. 2011;35(6):878–82.
75. Vranic S, Gurjeva O, Frkovic-Grazio S, Palazzo J, Tawfik O, Gatalica Z. IMP3, a proposed novel basal phenotype marker, is commonly overexpressed in adenoid cystic carcinomas but not in apocrine carcinomas of the breast. Appl Immunohistochem Mol Morphol. 2011;19(5):413–6.

76. Lae M, Vincent-Salomon A, Savignoni A, Huon I, Freneaux P, Sigal-Zafrani B, Aurias A, Sastre-Garau X, Couturier J. Phyllodes tumors of the breast segregate in two groups according to genetic criteria. Mod Pathol. 2007;20(4):435–44.
77. Yang X, Kandil D, Cosar EF, Khan A. Fibroepithelial tumors of the breast: pathologic and immunohistochemical features and molecular mechanisms. Arch Pathol Lab Med. 2014;138(1):25–36.
78. Huang KT, Dobrovic A, Yan M, Karim RZ, Lee CS, Lakhani SR, Fox SB. DNA methylation profiling of phyllodes and fibroadenoma tumours of the breast. Breast Cancer Res Treat. 2010;124(2):555–65.
79. Kim JH, Choi YD, Lee JS, Lee JH, Nam JH, Choi C, Park MH, Yoon JH. Borderline and malignant phyllodes tumors display similar promoter methylation profiles. Virchows Arch. 2009;455(6):469–75.

Chapter 15
Molecular Features of Mesenchymal Tumors of the Breast

Marjan Mirzabeigi, Ashraf Khan and Dina Kandil

Background

Mesenchymal lesions of the breast represent a rare, heterogeneous group of benign and malignant lesions. Most mesenchymal lesions occurring anywhere in the body have also been reported in the breast, the vast majority being of fibroblastic or myofibroblastic origin, reflecting the normal constituents of the breast parenchyma. Other mesenchymal lesions include those of vascular, lipomatous and muscle origin. These lesions resemble their extramammary counterparts, both histologically and immunophenotypically. Additionally, the molecular changes that characterize these extramammary mesenchymal lesions have also been identified in cases that affect the breast. Although the molecular characteristics have been described in most of these lesions, some, such as pseudoangiomatous stromal hyperplasia and hemangiomas, have not been identified. Since detailed discussion of all mesenchymal lesions of the breast is beyond the scope of this chapter, the focus will be on those lesions with identifiable molecular changes with a review of their histological and immunophenotypical profiles. A summary of these lesions and their characteristic immunophenotypic and molecular features is given in Table 15.1.

M. Mirzabeigi · A. Khan · D. Kandil (✉)
Department of Pathology, University of Massachusetts Medical School,
UMassMemorial Medical Center, Three Biotech, One Innovation Drive,
Worcester, MA 01605, USA
e-mail: dina.kandil@umassmemorial.org

A. Khan
e-mail: Ashraf.Khan@umassmemorial.org

© Springer Science+Business Media New York 2015
A. Khan et al. (eds.), *Precision Molecular Pathology of Breast Cancer*,
Molecular Pathology Library 10, DOI 10.1007/978-1-4939-2886-6_15

Table 15.1 Summary of mesenchymal lesions of the breast and their characteristic immunophenotypic and molecular features

Lesion	Immunohistochemistry	Molecular characteristics
Nodular fasciitis	Pos: SMA, MSA, vimentin, calponin and desmin (rare) Neg: CK, S100-protein, CD34, Beta-catenin	Deletion of chromosome 2 and 13, der(15), t(2; 15)(q31; q26), tetraploidy and del (6), gains of 10p and 20q, USP6 rearrangement, t(17; 22)(p13; q13) (MYH 9—USP6 gene fusion)
Myofibroblastoma	Pos: desmin, CD34, SMA, BCL2, CD99, CD10, ER, PR, AR, H-caldesmon (rare) Neg: CK	Partial monosomy of 13q and 16q monoallelic loss of FOXO1 gene, deletion of 13q14 region
Desmoid-type fibromatosis	Pos: Beta-catenin (80 %, nuclear), ER (rare) Neg: CK, CD34	Trisomy 8 and 20, loss of 5q, 5q allelic loss, nonrandom X chromosome inactivation, Beta-*catenin* gene mutations, somatic or germline *APC* gene alterations mutation
Inflammatory myofibroblastic tumor	Pos: ALK (50 %), desmin, SMA, keratin (±)	Rearrangement of the ALK gene. Common fusion partners are TPM3, TPM4, ATIC, RANBP2, CLTC, CARS, PPF1BP1, SEC3111, RANBP2
Lipoma	S-100 protein	
Coventional lipoma		Karyotypic aberrations of 12q, 6p, 13q, t(3; 12) (q27–28; q14–15) resulting in HMGA2-LPP gene fusion, 12q15 rearrangements, and t(3; 6)(q27; p21) resulting in HMGA1-LPP gene rearrangement
Hibernoma		11q13–21 rearrangements
Lipoblastoma		8q11–13 rearrangements
Chondrolipoma		t(11; 16) (q13; p12–13) resulting in C11orf95-MLK gene fusion
Spindle cell/pleomorphic lipomas		Aberration or partial monosomy of 16q, and loss of 13q14
Granular cell tumor	Pos: S-100 protein, CD68, PGP9.5, CEA and vimentin (focal)	Losses of 13q21, 4, 18q, 10, 1p, 22q
		Gains of 1p32-pter, 9q33-qter, 20q, 7
	Neg: CK	Some associations with (germline PTEN mutation, PTPN11 mutation)
		Malignant lesions: Nonspecific complex clonal karyotype, Losses (-5, -6, -13, -15, -17, 17q-, -18 and -21)

(continued)

Table 15.1   (continued)

Lesion	Immunohistochemistry	Molecular characteristics
Peripheral nerve sheath tumor	Pos: S-100 protein, GFAP, EMA (capsule), SOX10 ($\pm$), ALK ($\pm$)	Trisomy 10, loss of 9p21 (harboring INK4A/p16 and INK4A/p14 genes). 22q12 hyperploidy (EWSR1gene). May be associated with NF1 gene and NF2 gene mutations. Alterations of 9p and 22q
	Neg: SMARCB1	
Solitary fibrous tumor	Pos: CD34, BCL-2, vimentin, Beta-catenin, STAT6, GRIA2	Breakpoints in 12q13 resulting in NAB2-STAT6 fusion gene
Angiosarcoma	Pos: CD31, CD34, Factor VIII, MYC and prox-1 (negative in AVL), CK (focal)	Amplifications on chromosome 8q24.21 10p12.33 and 5q35.3, 8q24.21 (MYC, in secondary AS). Co-amplification of FLT4
Liposarcoma	Pos: S-100 protein	
Well-differentiated LS	MDM2/CDK4	Supernumerary ring and giant marker chromosomes with 12q amplification resulting in overexpression of MDM2 and CDK4 genes
De-differentiated LS	MDM2/CDK4	Co-amplification of 1p32, 6q23 and 6q25
Myxoid/round cell LS		t(12; 16)(q13; p11) resulting in FUS-DDIT3 gene fusion. t(12; 22) (q13; q12) resulting in EWSR1-DDIT3 gene fusion
Spindle cell LS		Monosomy 7 alone, or rearrangement of 13q
Rhabdo-myosarcoma	Pos: Myogenin, MyoD1, CK, neuroendocrine markers, PAX5, ALK1, CK ($\pm$focal)	
Embryonal RMS		Loss or uniparental disomy of 11p15.5, gains in chromosomes 2, 8, 11, 12, 13, and 20 resulting in gene overexpression (IGF2, H19, CDKN1C and HOTS)
Alveolar RMS		FOXO1 gene rearrangements including: t(2; 13)(q35; q14) (PAX3-FOXO1), t(1; 13)(p36; q14)(PAX7-FOXO1) and t(8; 13) (p12; q13)
		FOXO1-FGFR1 gene fusion. t(x; 2)(q13; q35), t(2; 2)(q35; p23), t(2; 8)(q35; q13) resulting in PAX3-FOX04, PAX3-NCOA1 and PAX3-NCOA2 respectively. N-MYC amplification (poor prognostic feature)
Spindle cell/sclerosing RMS		8q13 rearrangements resulting in SRF-NCOA2 or TEAD1-NCOA2 gene fusions

(continued)

Table 15.1 (continued)

Lesion	Immunohistochemistry	Molecular characteristics
Osteosarcoma	Pos: ALP, vimentin, SMA, desmin, S-100 protein, SATB2	Diploid to near tetraploidy, Gain in chromosome 1, loss of chromosome 9, 10, 13, and 17. Rearrangement: 1p11,1q21, 11p14, 14p11, 15p11, 17p and 19q13
		Gains and losses in DNA copy numbers
		Amplifications of 6p21, 8q24, and 12q14 and loss of heterozygosity of 10q21.1
		TP53 and Rb genes dysfunction
Leiomyosarcoma	Pos: desmin, SMA, CK, EMA	Loss of 13q (Rb1 gene) and 10q (PTEN)
		Point mutation of PTEN gene. DNA copy number gains (high-grade lesions), and
		DNA copy number loss (low-grade lesions)

Nodular Fasciitis

Nodular fasciitis (NF) is a rare lesion, which classically occurs in the subcutaneous tissue of the extremities and trunk in young adults. Few cases have been reported in the breast [1, 2]. Clinically, it presents as a painful, rapidly growing, well-circumscribed lesion, which can arise within the breast parenchyma or the subcutaneous tissue. Typically, the lesion undergoes spontaneous regression within a 1–2 month period, which contributes to the low rate of cases sampled. Histologically, the lesion is composed of uniform fibroblasts or myofibroblasts arranged in short fascicles with alternating hypo- and hyper-cellular areas creating a "zonation" effect. The stroma is loose and myxoid with a "tissue culture" appearance, and contains inflammatory cells, erythrocytes and thin-walled blood vessels. Brisk mitotic activity and significant cytologic atypia may be seen, raising the suspicion for malignancy. In those problematic cases, a panel of immunohistochemical stains is helpful in making this distinction.

Immunohistochemistry

NF should always be distinguished from malignant spindle cell lesions of the breast. Negative immunoreactivity to keratins helps exclude a metaplastic carcinoma of spindle cell type (carcinosarcoma) and fibromatosis-like variant. In NF, the lesional cells are consistently positive for smooth-muscle actin with "tram track" (sub-membranous pattern of staining of myofibroblasts), vimentin, and rarely for desmin [3]. S100-protein and CD34 are typically negative.

Molecular Characteristics

This lesion was initially considered as a polyclonal reactive process. However, subsequent studies showed cytogenetic abnormalities, pointing to a clonal neo-plastic process. Several case studies are noted in the literature reporting a wide array of chromosomal abnormalities in NF of the breast including, deletion of chromosome 2 and 13, derivative chromosome (15), t(2; 15)(q31; q26), tetraploidy and del (6) [4, 5] as well as gains of 10p and 20q. A more recent study of 48 cases of NF from different sites, highlighted both genomic rearrangements of the USP6 locus and a balanced translocation t(17; 22) (p13; q13) resulting in fusion of MYH 9 promoter region to the entire coding region of USP6, causing an overexpression of USP6 gene in these lesions [6]. USP6 is a proto-oncogene, located on chromosome 17p13, and is part of a large family of de-ubiquitinating enzymes, involved in processes such as intracellular trafficking, protein turnover, inflammatory signaling and cell transformation [7, 8]. Therefore, it acts as a transcription upregulator. MYH9 is a proto-oncogene, located on chromosome 22q12.3-q13, and belongs to non-muscle myosin class II family [9–12] that encodes for a protein involved in cytokinesis, cell motility, and maintenance of cell shapes and plays a role in actin network disassembly of moving cells. These genetic alterations coupled with spontaneous regression, suggest that NF may represent an interesting form of "transient neoplasia".

Myofibroblastoma

Myofibroblastoma is a benign stromal spindle cell neoplasm composed of fibroblasts and myofibroblasts. It occurs in women between the ages of 25 and 87 years. It can also occur in men, occasionally in the setting of gynecomastia [13, 14]. Clinically, the lesion presents as a slow-growing solitary mass. It appears on imaging studies as a well-circumscribed, solid nodule that usually measures three cm or less. Calcifications are not seen. Microscopically, the lesion is well-circumscribed, unencapsulated mass with pushing borders. The classic type is composed of spindle cells that are haphazardly oriented in short fascicles within a collagenous stroma. In the epitheloid variant, the cells are larger with small nucleoli, mimicking an invasive lobular carcinoma. A prominent adipocytic component is usually present, mimicking a spindle cell lipoma. Smooth muscle, cartilaginous or osseous metaplasia may also be focally present. Normally there isn't any entrapment of mammary ducts or lobules, which helps to differentiate it from fibromatosis.

Immunohistochemistry

The lesional cells may be positive for desmin, CD34, smooth-muscle actin, BCL2, CD99 and CD10 [14]. Negative immunoreactivity to keratins helps distinguish epitheloid myofibroblastoma from invasive lobular carcinoma, especially since both express estrogen and progesterone receptors. Androgen receptor is also positive in these lesions. H-caldesmon has been described in rare cases showing smooth-muscle differentiation [15].

Molecular Characteristics

Being a part of the same spectrum as spindle cell lipoma, myofibroblastoma shares the same cytogenetic abnormalities affecting chromosome 13, mainly partial monosomy of 13q with monoallelic loss of FOXO1 gene. Deletion of 13q14 region was also identified by fluorescence in situ hybridization [16–18]. Partial monosomy of 16q has also been reported [16].

Desmoid-Type Fibromatosis

Desmoid-type fibromatosis is a locally infiltrative lesion that arises from the fibroblasts and myofibroblasts of the breast parenchyma or, more commonly, from the pectoral fascia and extending into the breast. The lesion is more common in females and can occur at any age. It is rare and is usually associated with a history of trauma or surgery, including breast implants [19, 20]. The lesion commonly presents as a non-tender, palpable mass with occasional retraction of the overlying skin [20–22], concerning for malignancy. Histologically, the lesion resembles fibromatosis arising elsewhere in the body. It is composed of long, intersecting fascicles of bland spindle cells with infiltrating borders, and entrapment of the normal breast parenchyma. Lymphocytes are often present, especially at the tumor edges (Fig. 15.1a).

Immunohistochemistry

Nuclear beta-catenin expression is a characteristic feature of these lesions (Fig. 15.1b), seen in about 80 % of cases [23]. Although this helps to differentiate mammary fibromatosis from NF, which is negative for beta-catenin, expression may be seen with other lesions including spindle cell carcinoma, phyllodes tumors, and fibrosarcoma [24, 25]. Therefore, additional markers such as keratin panels and CD34 are helpful in this differentiation as they are both negative in

(a) **(b)**

(c)

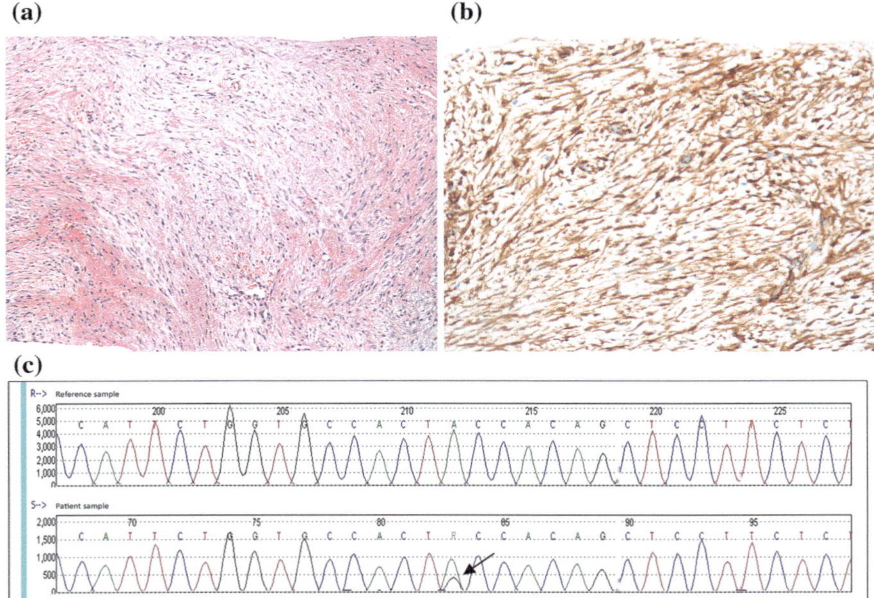

Fig. 15.1 Desmoid-type fibromatosis of the breast. **a** H&E stain, 100X. **b** Positive nuclear staining with B-catenin, 100X. **c** Capillary electropherogram showing a heterozygous mutation (nucleotide c.121A > AG, *black arrow*) involving codon 41 in exon 3 of CTNNB1 gene (encoding for beta-catenin). This results in substitution of amino acid Threonine by Alanine. *Courtesy of Dr. Ediz Cosar, Department of Pathology, UMass Memorial Medical Center*

fibromatosis. A weak expression of estrogen receptor has also been reported in mammary fibromatosis [26].

Molecular Characteristics

Desmoid tumors have been proven to be clonal and, therefore, true neoplastic lesions rather than a reactive process. Early publications reported recurrent, nonrandom chromosomal aberrations such as trisomy 8 and trisomy 20 as well as loss of 5q [27, 28] with a suggestion of an increased risk of recurrence in cases associated with trisomy 8. Another study showed nonrandom X chromosome inactivation in some tumors, with the same inactivation patterns identified in multiple recurrent lesions, suggesting that they were derived from the same cell clone as the primary lesions. The morphologic resemblance of these tumors to deep fibromatosis elsewhere in the body is also evident at the molecular level. Recent publications [23, 24, 29] have demonstrated somatic alterations of the *APC*/β-*catenin* pathway in the majority of breast fibromatoses, similar to those seen in desmoid tumors. These included activating β-*catenin* gene mutations and somatic *APC* gene alterations, either by mutation, 5q allelic loss or both. The occasional occurrence of these tumors in patients with familial adenomatous polyposis also reflects the finding of germline mutations of the *APC* gene in this group of patients.

Beta-catenin, a cadherin binding protein, is encoded by a proto-oncogene, CTNNB1, located on chromosome 3 with dual function of regulating the coordination of cell–cell adhesion and gene transcriptional coactivator, as a part of the canonical Wnt signaling pathway which promotes cellular proliferation and their differentiation. The Wnt proteins bind to receptors on the cell surface called "frizzled proteins," triggering a multi-step process to allow Beta-catenin entry into the cell. Without Wnt signaling, the Beta-catenin would be degraded because of a "destruction complex," a composition of multiple proteins including APC and glycogen synthetase kinase-3beta (GSK-3β), a regulator of the Beta-catenin level, preventing its accumulation within the cells. The APC encoded by a tumor suppressor gene is located on long arm of chromosome 5 is a key component of this complex. Any alterations of the Wnt signaling pathway or *APC* gene mutation will result in an accumulation of β-catenin in the cytoplasm with its eventual entry into the nucleus to form a complex with TCF (T cell factor-1)/LEF (lymphoid enhancing factor-1) factors and thereby acting as a transcription coactivator of cellular oncogene, including cyclin D1, c-JUN and c-myc. Additionally, somatic CTNNB1 gene mutation (Fig. 15.1c) results will alter serine/threonine residues at GSK-3β phosphorylation sites. The same mutations have been identified in fibromatosis outside of the breast. An additional 21-bp deletion spanning codons 42 through 48 has also been reported [29]. All together, these mutations will prevent the destruction complex to degrade Beta-catenin within the cytoplasm, and ultimately entering the nucleus followed by gene transcription activation, which then leads to the stromal cell proliferation seen in mammary fibromatosis [23, 24, 29].

Inflammatory Myofibroblastic Tumor

Inflammatory Myofibroblastic Tumors (IMT) commonly occur in children and young adults, usually in the abdominopelvic region, lung or retroperitoneum. Only a few case reports of IMT in the breast have been published [30, 31]. Clinically, it presents as a painless, well-circumscribed mass, and histologically, the lesion is composed of fascicles of myofibroblasts with minimal cytologic atypia. A prominent mixed inflammatory infiltrate dominated by plasma cells is the hallmark of these tumors. Lymphocytes and neutrophils can also be frequent.

Immunohistochemistry

The cells in IMT stain positively with smooth-muscle actin and occasionally with desmin and/or keratin. A characteristic feature of these tumors is their immunoreactivity for anaplastic lymphoma kinase (ALK) protein. Approximately 50 % of cases stain positively for ALK [31]. Both nuclear and cytoplasmic (primarily) staining can be seen. ALK-positivity is not very specific and can be seen in other lesions such as rhabdomyosarcomas and malignant peripheral nerve sheath tumors [32, 33]. However, it helps to differentiate this inflammatory cell-rich neoplasm from mastitis.

Molecular Characteristics

The ALK gene (2p23) encodes a receptor tyrosine kinase that, under normal conditions, is only present in normal tissue. Clonal alterations involving the ALK gene have been initially described in anaplastic large cell lymphoma (ALCL). However, ALK gene alterations can also be seen in some soft tissue neoplasms. Approximately 50 % of IMT cases exhibit rearrangement of the ALK gene [34, 35]. Several fusion partners have been identified in IMTs, the most common being TPM3 at 1p23. Others include TPM4 at 19p13, ATIC at 2q35, CLTC at 17q23, CARS at 11p15, RANBP2 at 2q13, PPF1BP1 at 12p11, SEC31l1 at 4q21 and RANBP2 at 2q13. The latter may be associated with poor prognosis. All the aforementioned fusion gene rearrangements are reflected as a cytoplasmic immunostaining pattern, with the exception of RANBP2 (a nuclear pore protein) which exhibits a nuclear staining pattern. Interestingly, NMP-ALK, the most common fusion gene seen with ALCL, has not been reported in IMTs, while TPM3-ALK, ATIC-ALK, and CLTC-ALK were identified in both neoplasms, thus, representing rare examples of translocation-derived chimeric tyrosine kinases, driving both mesenchymal and lymphoid neoplasms.

Lipoma

Lipomas of the breast present as painless, solitary masses arising within the subcutaneous tissue of the skin overlying the breast rather than breast parenchyma itself [14]. Microscopically, conventional lipoma is a proliferation of mature adipocytes surrounded by a thin capsule. A conventional lipoma can be difficult to distinguish from the normal breast adipose tissue, especially in a core biopsy specimen where the capsule is not easily identifiable. Lipomas with small vessels containing fibrin thrombi are characteristic of angiolipomas, which contrary to other sites, are painless. Other variants reported in the breast include angiolipoma [36–38], spindle cell/pleomorphic lipoma [39], angiomyolipoma [40], hibernoma [41], adenolipoma [42], fibrolipoma [42], lipoblastoma [43], and chondrolipoma [44].

Immunohistochemistry

With the exception of some variants where the morphologic evidence of a lipomatous origin can be obscured, immunohistochemistry is usually of little, if any, value. The cells show diffuse positivity with S-100 protein.

Molecular Characteristics

Multiple chromosomal abnormalities have been described in lipomas. Karyotypic aberrations affecting 12q, 6p, and 13q have been described in over 80 % of conventional lipomas, while up to 87 % of spindle cell/pleomorphic lipomas have aberration of 16q. A subset of spindle cell lipomas shares the same genetic abnormality with conventional lipomas, which include loss of 13q material, particularly 13q14 [45]. This leads to a diminished expression of multiple genes, including C13orf1, DHRS12, ATP7B, ALG11 and VPS36 and C13orf1.

Multiple studies highlighted a subset of conventional lipomas with a specific t(3; 12)(q27–28; q14–15) chromosomal translocation causing a fusion of high motility group A2 (HMGA2, exons 1–3) gene and the lipoma preferred partner (LPP, exons 9–11) gene [46–51]. The high mobility group proteins are nuclear proteins that bind DNA and function as transcription cofactors, including HMGI-C (encoded by a gene on 12q15) and HMGI-Y (encoded by a gene on 6p21) [46, 52, 53]. Normally both genes are only expressed in embryos but not in adult tissue [54–57]. However, both genes are expressed in some tumors and transformed cell lines [57] including lipomas (by chromosomal segment rearrangement at either 12q15 or at 6p21) and atypical lipomatous tumors (by amplification in the ring and giant marker chromosomes at 12q15) [47, 48, 58]. Subsequent study by Kubo et al. [59] showed a reciprocal LPP-HMGA2 fusion gene in a subset of lipomas involving exons 7 and 8 of LPP gene and exon 4 of HMGA2 gene. While 12q15 rearrangements and t(3; 12) (q27–28; q13–15) seem to be the most common genetic alterations seen in conventional lipomas, in a study by Wang et al., a case of lipoma with t(3; 6)(q27; p21) causing fusion of HMGA1 to the LPP/TPRG1 intergenic region has been reported [60]. Another publication exhibited a genetic link between spindle cell lipoma, cellular angiofibroma, and myofibroblastoma, which consists of either breaks or deletions of a limited region within 13q14, in the vicinity of retinoblastoma (RB1) gene, BRCA2 and lipoma high mobility group proteins (HMGI-C) fusion partner genes (LHPF) or partial monosomy of 16q, as well as chromosomal rearrangements of 13q and 16q [16, 61]. Hibernomas have been reported to frequently harbor 11q13–21 rearrangements, which has subsequently shown to cause homozygous or hemizygous gene loss of two tumor suppressor genes MEN1 and/or AIP that present a low expression in hibernomas but high expression of genes upregulated in brown fat including PPARA, PPARG, PPARGC1A and UCP1 [62, 63].

Lipoblastomas have been reported to harbor 8q11–13 rearrangements or to exhibit excess copies of chromosome 8 which results in overexpression of PLAG1 [62, 64]. Pleomorphic adenoma gene 1 or PLAG1 is a proto-oncogene, which encodes a zinc finger protein with 2 putative nuclear localization signals. It is considered a Transcription factor whose activation results in upregulation of target genes, such as IGFII, leading to uncontrolled cell proliferation and its overexpression has been reported in pleomorphic adenoma of salivary gland as well as lipoblastomas. Chondroid lipomas have also been reported to harbor t(11; 16)(q13; p12–13) resulting in C11orf95 (chromosome 11 open reading frame 95)-MKL2 (myocardin like 2) fusion oncogene [65].

Granular Cell Tumor

Granular cell tumor is a neoplasm of the Schwann cells of the peripheral nerves. Up to 8.5 % of all granular cell tumors occur in the breast [66–68], more frequently in females and over a broad age range. Although benign, the lesion may have a worrisome radiologic appearance with irregular or speculated borders. Moreover, it can cause nipple inversion and skin retraction, further mimicking carcinoma. Grossly, the tumor has a homogenous, tan-white cut surface, and histologically, it is composed of infiltrative clusters and sheets of uniform, round to polygonal cells with indistinct cell borders and round to oval nuclei. The cytoplasm is characteristically filled with fine, periodic acid-Schiff (PAS)/diastase resistant cytoplasmic granules.

Immunohistochemistry

The lesional cells are diffusely and strongly positive for S-100 protein and CD68 [69]. Together with pan-keratin negativity, a panel of these 3 stains is helpful in differentiating this lesion from infiltrating carcinoma, especially lobular and apocrine types. There is also a strong expression of PGP9.5 and focal expression of carcinoembryonic antigen (CEA) and vimentin. The ki-67 proliferation index is typically low.

Molecular Characteristics

Comparative genomic hybridization analysis of GCT occurring within central nervous system has shown a variety of genetic changes. Overall, losses (−13q21, −4, −18q, −10, −1p, −22q) were more frequent than gains (+1p32-pter, +9q33-qter, +20q, and +7) [70]. Multiple lesions have been reported to be associated with some inherited familial syndromes such as Neurofibromatosis, Cowden syndrome (via germline PTEN mutation on chromosome 10), Bannayan-Ruvalcaba-Riley syndrome (via germline PTEN mutation on chromosome 10), Leopard syndrome (via PTPN11 mutation on chromosome 12, implicating the Ras/MAP kinase pathway) and Noonan syndrome (via PTPN11 mutation on chromosome 12, implicating the Ras/MAP kinase pathway) [71–75]. Malignant granular cell tumors (MGCT) appear to exhibit a very complex clonal karyotype. In one case report, which presents a case of MGCT of the ulnar nerve, 21 cells underwent cytogenetic analysis a very complex karyotype was reported as 44 to 47, XY, +X, del(1)(p?), del(5)(p?), add(20)(q13), +22, +mar(cp 11) [76]. In another case report of MGCT of the lateral femoral cutaneous nerve, cytogenetic analysis of seventeen cells in metaphases, showed two clonal karyotype, one complex-44 to 47, XY, +del (1) (p?), del (5) (p?), add (20) (q13), −22, +mar (cp11) and one normal-46, XY [77]. The modal number was near diploid (range, chromosome 44 to 47). In addition, occasional aberrations such as -5, -6, -13, -15, -17, 17q-, -18 and -21 were also detected. In another case report of MGCT, a karyotype of 46, XX, +X,dic (5; 15) has been reported [78]. Therefore, it appears that to this day, despite the complexity of these genetic alterations, no specific recurrent karyotype alteration has been linked to these lesions.

Peripheral Nerve Sheath Tumor

These tumors are derived from the sheath of the peripheral nerves and include Schwannoma and Neurofibroma. These tumors are almost always benign, however, rare cases of malignant peripheral nerve sheath tumor (MPNST) have been reported [79–83]. Histologically, neurofibroma is an unencapsulated lesion, characterized by a fascicular proliferation of spindle cells, with occasional mast cells and focal myxoid changes, while Schwannoma is classically an encapsulated, biphasic lesion with alternating hypercellular (Antoni A) and hypocellular (Antoni B) spindle cell areas out cytologic atypia. Cytologic atypia, mitotic activity and necrosis are features of MPNST.

Immunohistochemistry

The lesion is positive for S-100 protein and GFAP. EMA stains the capsule surrounding Schwannoma. A subset of MPNST stains positive with SOX10 and ALK, and exhibits a loss of normal SMARCB1 nuclear staining [84]. SMARCB1(INI1) is a member of SWI/SNF multi subunit chromatin remodeling complex which plays an important role in regulating transcription [85].

Molecular Characteristics

There are reports of MPNST demonstrating trisomy 10 [86, 87]. Chromosome 10 harbors many oncogenesis including PTEN, which has been implicated in numerous human malignancies. In addition, in the same study, fluorescence in situ hybridization (FISH) analysis revealed loss of locus 9p21 (encoding for proteins INK4A/p16 and INK4A/p14 which regulate cell cycle, ensuring underphosphorylation of Rb gene) in 94 % of the examined cells and 22q12 (containing cancer related gene EWSR1) hyperploidy in 83.1 % of the examined tumor cells. Alterations of 9p and 22q have also been reported with several malignancies, including MPNST [86–88]. In addition, multiple neurofibromas have been reported in association with neurofibromatosis type 1 by deletion or mutation of NF1 tumor suppressor gene located on chromosome 17q, while multiple Schwannomas are reported either in association with type 2 neurofibromatosis, by monosomy or partial loss of NF2 tumor suppressor gene on chromosome 22 or by a germline mutation of INI1/SMARCB1(located on chromosome 22) [89] in familial schwannomatosis with high risk of malignant transformation [90]. Lastly MPNST can result from 17q loss, causing an NF1 (somatic or germline) mutation [91].

Solitary Fibrous Tumor

Solitary fibrous tumor (SFT) rarely occurs in the breast, with only a few case reports [92]. This lesion presents clinically as a slow-growing mass. Histologically, it is composed of spindle cells arranged in short fascicles haphazardly arranged in a myxoid background with sometimes a prominent vascular network (hemangiopericytoma-like) creating the customary "patternless pattern" type of morphology.

Immunohistochemistry

The lesional cells are immunoreactive for CD34, BCL-2, vimentin, Beta-catenin, STAT6 [93, 94] and GRIA2 [95]

Molecular Characteristics

A constant genetic alteration reported with this lesion includes recurrent breakpoints in 12q13 clustering near the NAB2 and STAT6 genes resulting in NAB2-STAT6 fusion gene, which will cause cell proliferation and activation of the expression of EGR-responsive genes [93, 95–97]. More recently gene expression profiling has highlighted a number of upregulated genes in SFT [96–98]. GRIA2 has been identified as one of the most common and highly expressed genes, encoding an AMPA-selective ionotropic glutamate receptor subunit which controls the membrane calcium permeability and appears to be involved in cell proliferation and motility. GRIA2 is normally involved in nervous system development, in some neurodegenerative disorders [99–101] as well as some tumors [100, 102–104]. The exact mechanism of action of GRIA2 has not been fully elucidated. A study by Ishiuchi et al. [105] suggests that GRIA2 is involved in PI3 K-independent activation of the AKT signaling pathway. While the involvement of GRIA2 in oncogenesis seems undeniable, more studies are needed to fully understand its exact mechanism of action.

Angiosarcoma and Atypical Vascular Lesions

Clinically, angiosarcomas (AS) of the breast can be divided into two subtypes. Primary angiosarcoma [106, 107] which arises de novo within the breast parenchyma. Although rare, primary AS represents the second most common mesenchymal malignancy after malignant phyllodes tumors, with an in incidence of 0.05 % of all breast malignancies [108]. Secondary angiosarcoma develops in the skin of the breast, chest wall, or the breast parenchyma, classically in breast cancer patients, who underwent axillary lymph node dissection followed by radiation therapy. The frequency of secondary AS has been notably increasing in the last two decades making it the most common radiation-associated sarcoma in the breast. This increasing number of cases reflects the increasing frequency in this treatment modality [109, 110].

Atypical vascular lesions (AVL) are vascular proliferations that develop in the skin of the breast in women who were treated with lumpectomy and radiation therapy for invasive breast carcinoma. Some believe these lesions may be the precursors to angiosarcoma, especially since a preceding or a synchronous AVL may be encountered in patients with angiosarcoma [111–119]. Clinically, AVL presents as ill-defined brown/erythematous patches or plaques on the skin of the breast within the radiation field, approximately 6 years into treatment. Microscopically, the lesion shows a dissecting, interconnecting vascular network lined by plump endothelial cells with prominent nuclei, but without significant cytologic atypia (Fig. 15.2a) [113, 118, 119]. On the other hand, AS usually presents as a bulky mass with bruise-like changes of the overlying skin. Histologically, a well-differentiated AS consists of anastomosing vascular channels lined by neoplastic endothelial cells with prominent and hyperchromatic nuclei with rare mitosis and lack of solid areas. In addition to the above findings, a poorly differentiated AS exhibits an epithelioid cell morphology, numerous mitotic figures, areas of necrosis as well as areas of solid tumor growth (Fig. 15.3).

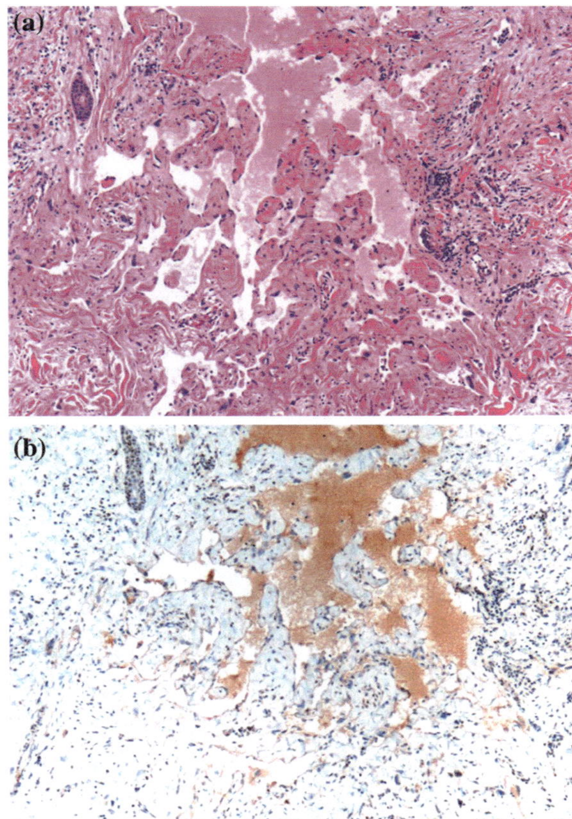

Fig. 15.2 Atypical vascular lesion of the breast. **a** H&E stain, 100X. **b** MYC stain shows negative staining, 100X. *Courtesy of Dr. Kristine Cornejo, Department of Pathology, UMass Memorial Medical Center*

Immunohistochemistry

While poorly differentiated AS is easy to recognize as malignant, a well-differentiated AS may be mistaken for pseudoangiomatous stromal hyperplasia (PASH), hemangiomas, and even with AVL. PASH is a myofibroblastic proliferation disguised in a vascular microscopic appearance. It usually presents as an incidental finding and only rarely as a mass-forming lesion. Its myofibroblastic origin can be unmasked by showing immunoreactivity to actin, desmin, calponin, progesterone receptor as well as CD34, and negativity for endothelial cell markers such as factor VIII and CD31. Hemangiomas usually present as non-palpable lesions identified on mammography. Microscopically, hemangiomas show a proliferation of variably sized, anastomosing vascular channels that infiltrate the interlobular stroma without disrupting the lobular architecture. This is an important feature differentiating it from well-differentiated AS. Differentiating AVL from a well-differentiated AS can be challenging particularly on core needle biopsies,

Fig. 15.3 Post-radiation angiosarcoma of the breast. **a** H&E stain, 400X. **b** Positive nuclear staining for MYC, 400X. **c** Strong and diffuse cytoplasmic staining (3+) for FLT4, 400X. *Courtesy of Dr. Kristine Cornejo, Department of Pathology, UMass Memorial Medical Center*

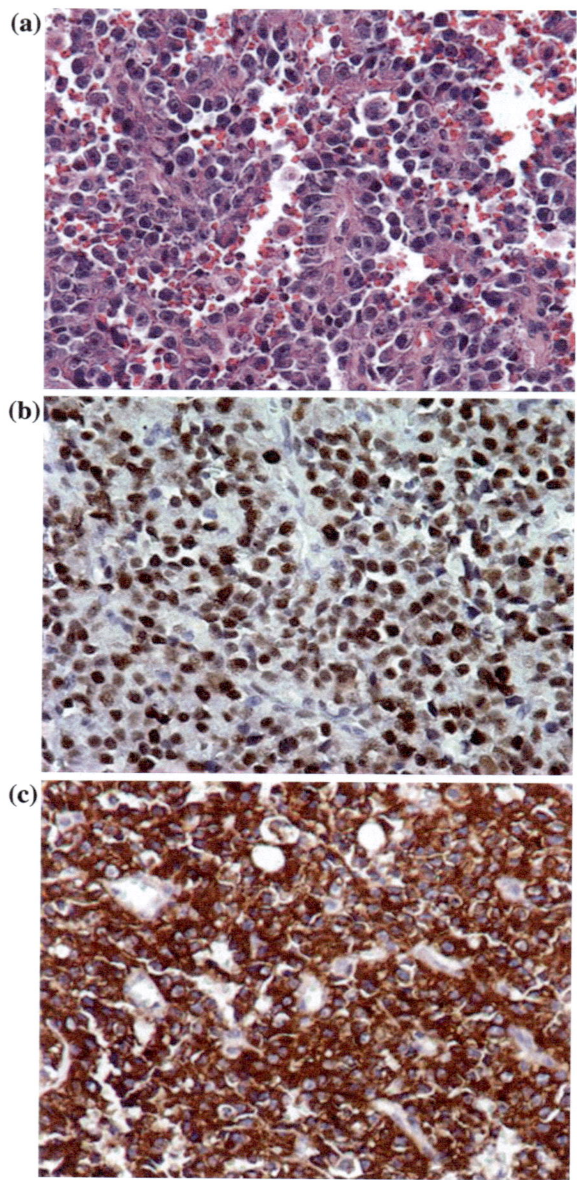

and in samples obtained from the edge of the lesion. Immunoreactivity to MYC and prox-1 has been proposed as potential marker differentiating AVL (negative for MYC and focally positive for prox-1) from AS which is positive for both (Figs. 15.2b and 15.3b) [120]. Finally, cytokeratin may show focal expression in AS, but should not be mistaken for a spindle cell carcinoma.

Molecular Characteristics

In a study done by Antonescu et al., in which 42 samples from 39 patients with AS from diverse sites including breast (primary and secondary lesions) have been examined, these lesions were reported to exhibit an upregulation of vascular specific tyrosine kinases, including TIE1, SNRK, KDR, TEK and FLT1. In addition, 10 % of patients showed KDR mutations and these lesions were all of primary breast site (primary or secondary lesion) [121]. In another study by Manner, et al., in which samples from 28 patients with primary AS and 33 patients with secondary AS were analyzed by array comparative genomic hybridization, the authors showed recurrent genetic alterations in 22 cases, all of which presented with secondary AS. The most frequent of these alterations included high level amplifications of chromosome 8q24.21 (50 %), 10p12.33 (33 %) and 5q35.3 (11 %) [122]. These findings indicate that primary AS and secondary AS are two genetically distinct lesions, despite their clinical and histological resemblance. Few studies have also demonstrated MYC gene (8q24.21) amplification in approximately 55 % of secondary AS [123–125]. In a study comparing AS to AVL [123], MYC amplification by FISH was identified in all AS cases, in contrast to AVL where all samples were negative. Other studies showed co-amplification of FLT4 (encoding VEGFR3) which was only observed in 25 % of cases of secondary AS (Fig. 15.4)

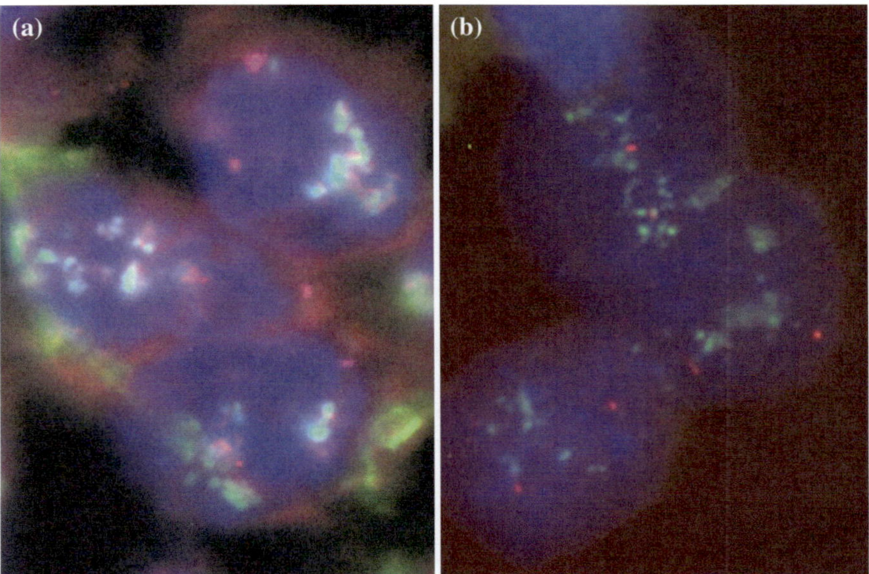

Fig. 15.4 MYC and FLT4 FISH in post-radiation angiosarcoma. **a** Markedly increased intensity and number of FLT4 (*red*) and MYC (*green*) signals compared to CEP8 (*magenta*). **b** Confirmation of FLT4 amplification using different probes showing increased signals of FLT4 (*green*) compared to CEP5 (*magenta*). *Courtesy of Dr. Kristine Cornejo, Department of Pathology, UMass Memorial Medical Center*

[124] and strong and diffuse nuclear staining with prox-1 which was present in secondary AS and was lacking in AVL (Fig. 15.2) [125].

Liposarcoma

Liposarcomas are the most common soft tissue sarcomas; however, primary liposarcoma of the breast is an extremely rare lesion [126–127]. It commonly occurs as a heterologous component in the setting of a malignant phyllodes tumor. Rare post-radiation liposarcoma of the breast are also reported [128]. Liposarcoma usually presents as a slowly growing, sometimes painful mass. Grossly, it is a well-circumscribed mass, but may have an infiltrative edge. Of all subtypes, the well-differentiated liposarcoma/atypical lipomatous tumor is the most common tumor of the primary mammary liposarcomas. Histologically, the hallmark feature is the presence of lipoblasts, which are immature adipocytes with hyperchromatic, scalloped nuclei and cytoplasmic vacuoles.

Immunohistochemistry

As in extramammary liposarcoma; the lesional cells stain positive with S-100 protein. Well-differentiated liposarcoma and de-differentiated liposarcomas are also immunoreactive for MDM2/CDK4 [129, 130].

Molecular Features

Atypical lipomatous tumors as well as the well- and de-differentiated liposarcomas have a supernumerary ring and giant marker chromosomes, containing amplified material from the long arm of chromosome 12, an area which harbors many proto-oncogenes leading to overexpression of MDM2 and CDK4 as well as other genes, including HMGA2, YEASTS4, CPM, and FRS2 [129–135]. Occasionally, 1q21–25 segment is co-amplified, which can cause ATF6 and DUSP12 amplification in a subset of these lesions [136]. In cases of the aggressive de-differentiated liposarcoma, in addition to the previously mentioned genetic alterations, a co-amplification of 1p32, 6q23 and 6q25 sequences can be seen, causing JUN, ASK1 and MAP3 K7IP2 amplification respectively [137, 156]. Distinct genetic alterations including t(12; 16)(q13; p11) have been reported in over 90 % of myxoid/round cell type which results in FUS-DDIT3 gene fusion, and rare cases have t(12; 22)(q13; q12) resulting in EWSR1-DDIT3 gene fusion [138]. The spindle cell type liposarcoma, has been reported to exhibit a monosomy of 7 alone or a rearrangement of 13q, without the usual 12q amplification. These data are supported by the fact that these lesions are also MDM2/CDK4 negative [139–141].

Rhabdomyosarcoma

As in other breast sarcomas, rhabdomyosarcoma occurs more commonly as focal component in older women with malignant phyllodes and metaplastic carcinomas [142, 143]. Conversely, primary rhabdomyosarcomas of the breast are very rare [144], and occur mainly in children and young adults. Although, embryonal rhabdomyosarcoma is the most common soft tissue subtype, primary breast rhabdomyosarcoma is almost often the alveolar type [144] which is histologically characterized by thin fibrous septae lined by small round blue cells in an alveolar growth pattern.

Immunohistochemistry

Alveolar rhabdomyosarcoma should be distinguished from lobular carcinoma with an alveolar growth pattern, especially that pan-cytokeratin may show focal positivity in rhabdomyosarcoma. Immunoreactivity to skeletal cell markers such as myogenin and myoD1 is characteristic [145–147]. Neuroendocrine markers [147], PAX5 [148] and ALK1 can also be positive.

Molecular Characteristics

There are no specific reports on the molecular makeup of primary breast rhabdomyosarcoma. However, the alveolar type is associated with FOXO1 gene (a member of the fork-head family, formerly known as FKHR) translocations. The most common translocation is t(2; 13)(q35; q14) resulting in PAX3-FOXO1 gene fusion. Other translocations include t(1; 13)(p36; q14), t(X; 2)(q13; q35), t(2; 2) (q35; p23), t(2; 8)(q35; q13) and t(8; 13)(p12; q13) resulting respectively in PAX7-FOXO1, PAX3-FOXO4, PAX3-NCOA1, PAX3-NCOA2 and FOXO1-FGFR1 fusion gene formation [149–157]. N-MYC amplification has been proposed as a poor prognostic feature in alveolar rhabdomyosarcoma [158]. The embryonal type has been linked to either a loss or a uniparental disomy of 11p15.5 with gains in chromosomes 2, 8, 11, 12, 13, and 20, which will cause amplification of genes such as IGF2, H19, CDKN1C and HOTS [149–151]. Spindle cell/sclerosing type rhabdomyosarcoma, a recently described subtype, presents 8q13 rearrangements, which will result in SRF-NCOA2 or TEAD1-NCOA2 fusion gene formation [159].

Osteosarcoma

Pure osteosarcoma represents approximately 12 % of all breast sarcomas [160, 161]. As with other sarcomas, it is more commonly encountered as part of meta-plastic carcinoma or malignant phyllodes. Clinically, it presents as an enlarging solitary mass that may be painful. Areas of calcifications may be detected on mammogram. Histologically, the lesion has well-circumscribed margins, and is composed of pleomorphic spindle to ovoid cells with varying degree of osteoid formation. Most histologic variants such as fibroblastic, osteoclastic-rich, osteo-blastic, and telangiectatic type have also been described in osteosarcoma of the breast.

Immunohistochemistry

The lesion is immunoreactive for alkaline phosphatase and vimentin, with vari-able smooth-muscle actin and desmin, S-100 protein (if chondroid differentiation is present). The most recent addition to this panel is SATB2 (Special AT-rich—sequence-Binding protein 2) [162], a nuclear matrix protein which plays a role in osteoblast lineage commitment.

Molecular Features

Osteosarcomas have complex genetic alterations. Early publications reported a high propensity towards aneuploidy in these tumors [163, 164]. Boehm et al. [165] examined the cytogenetic profile of 36 cases of osteosarcoma and found that approximately 69 % of the cases exhibited polyploidy. The most common numer-ical abnormalities were gain in chromosome 1 and loss of chromosomes 9, 10, 13, and 17, while the most common chromosomal structural rearrangements were 1p11–13, 1q11–12, 1q21–22, 11p14–15, 14p11–13, 15p11–13, 17p and 19q13. Comparative genomic hybridization studies showed both gains and losses in DNA copy numbers [166]. Osteosarcoma can be seen in association with certain genetic syndromes, including Bloom syndrome, Rothmund-Thompson syndrome, Werner syndrome, Li-Fraumeni syndrome, and hereditary retinoblastoma [167]. Bloom, Rothmund-Thompson and Werner [168] syndromes are due to genetic defects in the RecQ helicase family. DNA-helicases cause separation of double stranded DNA before replication [169, 170]. Another study reported amplifications of chro-mosomes 6p21, 8q24, and 12q14 loci and loss of heterozygosity of 10q21.1 as the most common genetic alterations noted in osteosarcomas [171]. Additional numer-ical chromosomal abnormalities include loss of chromosomes 9, 10, 13 and 17 as well as gain of chromosome 1 [172]. Osteosarcoma can also be caused by tumor suppressor gene dysfunction, including TP53 and Rb genes. TP53 gene mutation is also identified in approximately 22 % of osteosarcomas [172]. In normal conditions, TP53 gene inactivates G1/S-Cdk and S-Cdk complexes causing an arrest of the cell cycle in G1 [173]. Therefore, TP53 gene mutation results in uncontrolled persistent cell proliferation. This also explains the occasional link of osteosarcoma and Li-Fraumeni syndrome, which is due to a germline mutation of TP53 gene [174]. Similarly, Rb gene normally inhibits the cell cycle by binding to the transcription factor E2F. The Rb gene will exercise its inhibitory effect till the CDK4/cyclin D complex phosphorylates Rb. Mutation in the Rb gene results in a continuous cell cycle [174]. Osteosarcoma can be caused by both somatic or germline mutation of the Rb gene [175].

Leiomyoma and Leiomyosarcoma

Leiomyomas and leiomyosarcomas represent less than 1 % of mammary tumors. Most occur superficially in the skin of the periareolar region in both men and women. However, deeper lesions are almost exclusively seen in women [176]. Both present as slowly growing masses. Superficial lesions are palpable and can be painful or tender, while deep lesions may be clinically nondistinctive. Histologically, the lesions are composed of interlacing fascicles of spindle cells. In leiomyomas, the cells have the characteristic elongated, cigar-shaped nuclei and eosinophilic cytoplasm with minimal/absent cytologic atypia, and rare, if any, mitosis. Leiomyosarcomas, however, are characterized by moderate/marked cytologic atypia, mitosis and tumor cell necrosis [177].

Immunohistochemistry

The lesional cells are immunoreactive for desmin, smooth-muscle actin and as many as 40 % can stain positive with pan-keratin and epithelial membrane antigen antibodies.

Molecular Characteristics

Leiomyosarcomas have been reported to exhibit a very complex and unstable karyotype [178]. These include losses of chromosomes 13q and 10q where the tumor suppressor genes Rb1 and phosphatase and tensin homolog (PTEN) are respectively located [178–186]. Point mutation of PTEN has also been reported in LMS [187–189]. PTEN gene encodes for a protein and phosphatase that inhibits the lipid kinase activity of phosphatidyl inositol 3-kinase (PI3 K). Therefore, PTEN mutations will result in dysregulation of PI3K and hyperactivation of Akt, which will ultimately result in an increased cell proliferation as well as inhibition of apoptosis leading to tumorogenesis. Studies have shown that high-grade sarcomas exhibit higher DNA copy number gains, while low-grade tumors show DNA copy number losses, suggesting that tumor suppressor gene loss may be an early event followed by oncogene activation during malignant transformation [184]. In a study of animal model by Hernando et al. the author reported that while the PTEN suppression appears to be an important and initiating step in the development of LMS, additional steps such as TP53 gene mutation are required for tumorogenesis [190], and suggested that activation of Akt, can cause inactivation of TP53 via stabilization of MDM2.

Mesenchymal lesions of the breast are very uncommon. They resemble their extra-mammary counterparts not only in their morphologic features, but also in their immunophenotypic and molecular phenotypes. Immunohistochemical testing and molecular testing may be needed to establish the diagnosis, and avoid misinterpretation.

Key Points

- Mesenchymal lesions of the breast resemble their extramammary counterparts histologically, immunophenotypically and in their molecular characteristics.
- Pure soft tissue sarcomas of the breast are rare, and usually occur as a heterologous component in the setting of a malignant phyllodes tumor or as part of metaplastic carcinoma.
- Spindle cell lipoma and myofibroblastoma share the same cytogenetic abnormalities affecting chromosome 13.
- Epitheloid myofibroblastoma can mimic invasive lobular carcinoma, especially given its immunoreactivity to estrogen receptor.
- Nuclear beta-catenin expression is a characteristic feature of desmoid-type fibromatosis.
- Approximately 50 % of IMT cases are immunoreactive for ALK.
- More than 80 % of conventional lipomas have aberrations affecting 12q, 6p, and 13q while spindle cell/pleomorphic lipomas are characterized by 16q aberration.
- Despite their clinical and histological resemblance, primary AS and secondary AS are considered two genetically distinct lesions.
- The frequency of secondary AS has been notably increasing in the last two decades making it the most common radiation-associated sarcoma in the breast.
- Primary breast rhabdomyosarcoma is almost often of the alveolar type, which may resemble lobular carcinoma with alveolar growth pattern.

References

1. Green JS, Crozier AE, Walker RA. Case report: nodular fasciitis of the breast. Clin Radiol. 1997;52(12):961–2.
2. Brown V, Carty NJ. A case of nodular fascitis of the breast and review of the literature. Breast. 2005;14(5):384–7.
3. Kayaselcuk F, Demirhan B, Kayaselcuk U, Ozerdem OR, Tuncer I. Vimentin, smooth muscle actin, desmin, S-100 protein, p53, and estrogen receptor expression in elastofibroma and nodular fasciitis. Ann Diagn Pathol. 2002;6(2):94–9.
4. Birdsall SH, Shipley JM, Summersgill BM, Black AJ, Jackson P, Kissin MW, Gusterson BA. Cytogenetic findings in a case of nodular fasciitis of the breast. Cancer Genet Cytogenet. 1995;81(2):166–8.
5. Meng GZ, Zhang HY, Zhang Z, Wei B, Bu H. Myofibroblastic sarcoma vs nodular fasciitis: a comparative study of chromosomal imbalances. Am J Clin Pathol. 2009;131(5):701–9.
6. Erickson-Johnson MR, Chou MM, Evers BR, Roth CW, Seys AR, Jin L, Ye Y, Lau AW, Wang X, Oliveira AM. Nodular fasciitis: a novel model of transient neoplasia induced by MYH9-USP6 gene fusion. Lab Invest: J Tech Methods Pathol. 2011;91(10):1427–33.
7. Oliveira AM, Perez-Atayde AR, Inwards CY, Medeiros F, Derr V, Hsi BL, Gebhardt MC, Rosenberg AE, Fletcher JA. USP6 and CDH11 oncogenes identify the neoplastic cell in primary aneurysmal bone cysts and are absent in so-called secondary aneurysmal bone cysts. Am J Pathol. 2004;165(5):1773–80.
8. Oliveira AM, Perez-Atayde AR, Dal Cin P, Gebhardt MC, Chen CJ, Neff JR, Demetri CD, Rosenberg AE, Bridge JA, Fletcher JA. Aneurysmal bone cyst variant translocations upregulate USP6 transcription by promoter swapping with the ZNF9, COL1A1, TRAP150, and OMD genes. Oncogene. 2005;24(21):3419–26.
9. Wilson CA, Tsuchida MA, Allen GM, Barnhart EL, Applegate KT, Yam PT, Ji L, Keren K, Danuser G, Theriot JA. Myosin II contributes to cell-scale actin network treadmilling through network disassembly. Nature. 2010;465(7296):373–7.
10. Hu A, Wang F, Sellers JR. Mutations in human nonmuscle myosin IIA found in patients with May-Hegglin anomaly and Fechtner syndrome result in impaired enzymatic function. J Biol Chem. 2002;277(48):46512–7.
11. Lamant L, Gascoyne RD, Duplantier MM, Armstrong F, Raghab A, Chhanabhai M, Rajcan-Separovic E, Raghab J, Delsol G, Espinos E. Non-muscle myosin heavy chain (MYH9): a new partner fused to ALK in anaplastic large cell lymphoma. Genes Chromosom Cancer. 2003;37(4):427–32.
12. Heath KE, Campos-Barros A, Toren A, Rozenfeld-Granot G, Carlsson LE, Savige J, Denison JC, Gregory MC, White JG, Barker DF, et al. Nonmuscle myosin heavy chain IIA mutations define a spectrum of autosomal dominant macrothrombocytopenias: May-Hegglin anomaly and Fechtner, Sebastian, Epstein, and Alport-like syndromes. Am J Hum Genet. 2001;69(5):1033–45.
13. Magro G. Mammary myofibroblastoma: a tumor with a wide morphologic spectrum. Arch Pathol Lab Med. 2008;132(11):1813–20.
14. Tavassoli FA, Eusebi V, American Registry of Pathology, Armed Forces Institute of Pathology (U.S.). Tumors of the mammary gland. Washington, D.C.: American Registry of Pathology in collaboration with the Armed Forces Institute of Pathology. 2009.
15. Magro G, Gurrera A, Bisceglia M. H-caldesmon expression in myofibroblastoma of the breast: evidence supporting the distinction from leiomyoma. Histopathology. 2003;42(3):233–8.
16. Pauwels P, Sciot R, Croiset F, Rutten H, Van den Berghe H, Dal Cin P. Myofibroblastoma of the breast: genetic link with spindle cell lipoma. J Pathol. 2000;191(3):282–5.
17. Magro G, Righi A, Casorzo L, Antonietta T, Salvatorelli L, Kacerovska D, Kazakov D, Michal M. Mammary and vaginal myofibroblastomas are genetically related lesions:

fluorescence in situ hybridization analysis shows deletion of 13q14 region. Hum Pathol. 2012;43(11):1887–93.

18. Maggiani F, Debiec-Rychter M, Verbeeck G, Sciot R. Extramammary myofibroblastoma is genetically related to spindle cell lipoma. Virchows Archiv: Int J Pathol. 2006;449(2):244–7.

19. Jamshed S, Farhan MI, Marshall MB, Nahabedian MY, Liu MC. Fibromatosis of the breast after mammary prosthesis implantation. Clin Adv Hematol Oncol H&O. 2008;6(9):687–94.

20. Neuman HB, Brogi E, Ebrahim A, Brennan MF, Van Zee KJ. Desmoid tumors (fibromatoses) of the breast: a 25-year experience. Ann Surg Oncol. 2008;15(1):274–80.

21. Rosen PP, Ernsberger D. Mammary fibromatosis. A benign spindle-cell tumor with significant risk for local recurrence. Cancer. 1989;63(7):1363–9.

22. Wargotz ES, Norris HJ, Austin RM, Enzinger FM. Fibromatosis of the breast. A clinical and pathological study of 28 cases. Am J Surg Pathol. 1987;11(1):38–45.

23. Abraham SC, Reynolds C, Lee JH, Montgomery EA, Baisden BL, Krasinskas AM, Wu TT. Fibromatosis of the breast and mutations involving the APC/beta-catenin pathway. Hum Pathol. 2002;33(1):39–46.

24. Lacroix-Triki M, Geyer FC, Lambros MB, Savage K, Ellis IO, Lee AH, Reis-Filho JS. beta-catenin/Wnt signalling pathway in fibromatosis, metaplastic carcinomas and phyllodes tumours of the breast. Mod Pathol: Official J U S Can Acad Pathol Inc. 2010;23(11):1438–48.

25. Ng TL, Gown AM, Barry TS, Cheang MC, Chan AK, Turbin DA, Hsu FD, West RB, Nielsen TO. Nuclear beta-catenin in mesenchymal tumors. Mod Pathol: Official J U S Can Acad Pathol Inc. 2005;18(1):68–74.

26. Devouassoux-Shisheboran M, Schammel MD, Man YG, Tavassoli FA. Fibromatosis of the breast: age-correlated morphofunctional features of 33 cases. Arch Pathol Lab Med. 2000;124(2):276–80.

27. Fletcher JA, Naeem R, Xiao S, Corson JM. Chromosome aberrations in desmoid tumors. Trisomy 8 may be a predictor of recurrence. Cancer Genet Cytogenet. 1995;79(2):139–43.

28. De Wever I, Dal Cin P, Fletcher CD, Mandahl N, Mertens F, Mitelman F, Rosai J, Rydholm A, Sciot R, Tallini G, et al. Cytogenetic, clinical, and morphologic correlations in 78 cases of fibromatosis: a report from the CHAMP Study Group. CHromosomes And Morphology. Mod Pathol: Official J U S Can Acad Pathol Inc. 2000;13(10):1080–5.

29. Kim T, Jung EA, Song JY, Roh JH, Choi JS, Kwon JE, Kang SY, Cho EY, Shin JH, Nam SJ, et al. Prevalence of the CTNNB1 mutation genotype in surgically resected fibromatosis of the breast. Histopathology. 2012;60(2):347–56.

30. Haj M, Weiss M, Loberant N, Cohen I. Inflammatory pseudotumor of the breast: case report and literature review. Breast J. 2003;9(5):423–5.

31. Khanafshar E, Phillipson J, Schammel DP, Minobe L, Cymerman J, Weidner N. Inflammatory myofibroblastic tumor of the breast. Ann Diagn Pathol. 2005;9(3):123–9.

32. Yoshida A, Shibata T, Wakai S, Ushiku T, Tsuta K, Fukayama M, Makimoto A, Furuta K, Tsuda H. Anaplastic lymphoma kinase status in rhabdomyosarcomas. Mod Pathol: Official J U S Can Acad Pathol Inc. 2013;26(6):772–81.

33. Cessna MH, Zhou H, Sanger WG, Perkins SL, Tripp S, Pickering D, Daines C, Coffin CM. Expression of ALK1 and p80 in inflammatory myofibroblastic tumor and its mesenchymal mimics: a study of 135 cases. Mod Pathol: Official J U S Can Acad Pathol Inc. 2002;15(9):931–8.

34. Gleason BC, Hornick JL. Inflammatory myofibroblastic tumours: where are we now? J Clin Pathol. 2008;61(4):428-37.

35. Li J, Yin WH, Takeuchi K, Guan H, Huang YH, Chan JK. Inflammatory myofibroblastic tumor with RANBP2 and ALK gene rearrangement: a report of two cases and literature review. Diagn Pathol. 2013;8:147.

36. Kahng HC, Chin NW, Opitz LM, Pahuja M, Goldberg SL. Cellular angiolipoma of the breast: immunohistochemical study and review of the literature. Breast J. 2002;8(1):47–9.

37. Kryvenko ON, Chitale DA, VanEgmond EM, Gupta NS, Schultz D, Lee MW. Angiolipoma of the female breast: clinicomorphological correlation of 52 cases. Int J Surg Pathol. 2011;19(1):35–43.
38. Yu GH, Fishman SJ, Brooks JS. Cellular angiolipoma of the breast. Mod Pathol: Official J U S Can Acad Pathol Inc. 1993;6(4):497–9.
39. Chan KW, Ghadially FN, Alagaratnam TT. Benign spindle cell tumour of breast—a variant of spindled cell lipoma or fibroma of breast? Pathology. 1984;16(3):331–6.
40. Damiani S, Chiodera P, Guaragni M, Eusebi V. Mammary angiomyolipoma. Virchows Archiv: Int J Pathol. 2002;440(5):551–2.
41. Padilla-Rodriguez AL. Pure hibernoma of the breast: insights about its origins. Ann Diagn Pathol. 2012;16(4):288–91.
42. Riveros M, Cubilla A, Perotta F, Solalinde V. Hamartoma of the breast. J Surg Oncol. 1989;42(3):197–200.
43. Zani A, Cozzi DA, Uccini S, Cozzi F. Unusual breast enlargement in an infant: a case of breast lipoblastoma. Pediatr Surg Int. 2007;23(4):361–3.
44. Banev SG, Filipovski VA. Chondrolipoma of the breast—case report and a review of literature. Breast. 2006;15(3):425–6.
45. Bartuma H, Nord KH, Macchia G, Isaksson M, Nilsson J, Domanski HA, Mandahl N, Mertens F. Gene expression and single nucleotide polymorphism array analyses of spindle cell lipomas and conventional lipomas with 13q14 deletion. Genes Chromosom Cancer. 2011;50(8):619–32.
46. Ashar HR, Fejzo MS, Tkachenko A, Zhou X, Fletcher JA, Weremowicz S, Morton CC, Chada K. Disruption of the architectural factor HMGI-C: DNA-binding AT hook motifs fused in lipomas to distinct transcriptional regulatory domains. Cell. 1995;82(1):57–65.
47. Schoenmakers EF, Wanschura S, Mols R, Bullerdiek J, Van den Berghe H, Van de Ven WJ. Recurrent rearrangements in the high mobility group protein gene, HMGI-C, in benign mesenchymal tumours. Nat Genet. 1995;10(4):436–44.
48. Petit MM, Mols R, Schoenmakers EF, Mandahl N, Van de Ven WJ. LPP, the preferred fusion partner gene of HMGIC in lipomas, is a novel member of the LIM protein gene family. Genomics. 1996;36(1):118–29.
49. Matsui Y, Hasegawa T, Kubo T, Goto T, Yukata K, Endo K, Bando Y, Yasui N. Intrapatellar tendon lipoma with chondro-osseous differentiation: detection of HMGA2-LPP fusion gene transcript. J Clin Pathol. 2006;59(4):434–6.
50. Kubo T, Matsui Y, Goto T, Yukata K, Endo K, Sato R, Tsutsui T, Yasui N. MRI characteristics of parosteal lipomas associated with the HMGA2-LPP fusion gene. Anticancer Res. 2006;26(3B):2253–7.
51. Ida CM, Wang X, Erickson-Johnson MR, Wenger DE, Blute ML, Nascimento AG, Oliveira AM. Primary retroperitoneal lipoma: a soft tissue pathology heresy?: report of a case with classic histologic, cytogenetics, and molecular genetic features. Am J Surg Pathol. 2008;32(6):951–4.
52. Manfioletti G, Giancotti V, Bandiera A, Buratti E, Sautiere P, Cary P, Crane-Robinson C, Coles B, Goodwin GH. cDNA cloning of the HMGI-C phosphoprotein, a nuclear protein associated with neoplastic and undifferentiated phenotypes. Nucleic Acids Res. 1991;19(24):6793–7.
53. Chau KY, Patel UA, Lee KL, Lam HY, Crane-Robinson C. The gene for the human architectural transcription factor HMGI-C consists of five exons each coding for a distinct functional element. Nucleic Acids Res. 1995;23(21):4262–6.
54. Giancotti V, Bandiera A, Buratti E, Fusco A, Marzari R, Coles B, Goodwin GH. Comparison of multiple forms of the high mobility group I proteins in rodent and human cells. Identification of the human high mobility group I-C protein. Eur J Biochem/FEBS. 1991;198(1):211–6.

55. Giancotti V, Bandiera A, Ciani L, Santoro D, Crane-Robinson C, Goodwin GH, Boiocchi M, Dolcetti R, Casetta B. High-mobility-group (HMG) proteins and histone H1 subtypes expression in normal and tumor tissues of mouse. Eur J Biochem/FEBS. 1993;213(2):825–32.
56. Rogalla P, Drechsler K, Frey G, Hennig Y, Helmke B, Bonk U, Bullerdiek J. HMGI-C expression patterns in human tissues. Implications for the genesis of frequent mesenchymal tumors. Am J Pathol. 1996;149(3):775–9.
57. Zhou X, Benson KF, Ashar HR, Chada K. Mutation responsible for the mouse pygmy phenotype in the developmentally regulated factor HMGI-C. Nature. 1995;376(6543):771–4.
58. Mitelman F, Johansson B, Mertens F. Catalog of chromosome aberrations in cancer. 5th ed. New York: Wiley-Liss; 1994.
59. Kubo T, Matsui Y, Naka N, Araki N, Goto T, Yukata K, Endo K, Yasui N, Myoui A, Kawabata H, et al. Expression of HMGA2-LPP and LPP-HMGA2 fusion genes in lipoma: identification of a novel type of LPP-HMGA2 transcript in four cases. Anticancer Res. 2009;29(6):2357–60.
60. Wang X, Zamolyi RQ, Zhang H, Pannain VL, Medeiros F, Erickson-Johnson M, Jenkins RB, Oliveira AM. Fusion of HMGA1 to the LPP/TPRG1 intergenic region in a lipoma identified by mapping paraffin-embedded tissues. Cancer Genet Cytogenet. 2010;196(1):64–7.
61. Dahlen A, Debiec-Rychter M, Pedeutour F, Domanski HA, Hoglund M, Bauer HC, Rydholm A, Sciot R, Mandahl N, Mertens F. Clustering of deletions on chromosome 13 in benign and low-malignant lipomatous tumors. Int J Cancer (Journal International du Cancer). 2003;103(5):616–23.
62. Fletcher CD, Akerman M, Dal Cin P, de Wever I, Mandahl N, Mertens F, Mitelman F, Rosai J, Rydholm A, Sciot R, et al. Correlation between clinicopathological features and karyotype in lipomatous tumors. A report of 178 cases from the Chromosomes and Morphology (CHAMP) Collaborative Study Group. Am J Pathol. 1996;148(2):623–30.
63. Nord KH, Magnusson L, Isaksson M, Nilsson J, Lilljebjorn H, Domanski HA, Kindblom LG, Mandahl N, Mertens F. Concomitant deletions of tumor suppressor genes MEN1 and AIP are essential for the pathogenesis of the brown fat tumor hibernoma. Proc Natl Acad Sci U S A. 2010;107(49):21122–7.
64. Brandal P, Bjerkehagen B, Heim S. Rearrangement of chromosomal region 8q11–13 in lipomatous tumours: correlation with lipoblastoma morphology. J Pathol. 2006;208(3):388–94.
65. Huang D, Sumegi J, Dal Cin P, Reith JD, Yasuda T, Nelson M, Muirhead D, Bridge JA. C11orf95-MKL2 is the resulting fusion oncogene of t(11;16)(q13;p13) in chondroid lipoma. Genes Chromosom Cancer. 2010;49(9):810–8.
66. Adeniran A, Al-Ahmadie H, Mahoney MC, Robinson-Smith TM. Granular cell tumor of the breast: a series of 17 cases and review of the literature. Breast J. 2004;10(6):528–31.
67. Brown AC, Audisio RA, Regitnig P. Granular cell tumour of the breast. Surg Oncol. 2011;20(2):97–105.
68. Lack EE, Worsham GF, Callihan MD, Crawford BE, Klappenbach S, Rowden G, Chun B. Granular cell tumor: a clinicopathologic study of 110 patients. J Surg Oncol. 1980;13(4):301–16.
69. Le BH, Boyer PJ, Lewis JE, Kapadia SB. Granular cell tumor: immunohistochemical assessment of inhibin-alpha, protein gene product 9.5, S100 protein, CD68, and Ki-67 proliferative index with clinical correlation. Arch Pathol Lab Med. 2004;128(7):771–5.
70. Rickert CH, Paulus W. Genetic characterisation of granular cell tumours. Acta Neuropathol. 2002;103(4):309–12.
71. Martin RW 3rd, Neldner KH, Boyd AS, Coates PW. Multiple cutaneous granular cell tumors and neurofibromatosis in childhood. A case report and review of the literature. Arch Dermatol. 1990;126(8):1051–6.
72. Marchese C, Montera M, Torrini M, Goldoni F, Mareni C, Forni M, Locatelli L. Granular cell tumor in a PHTS patient with a novel germline PTEN mutation. Am J Med Genet Part A. 2003;120A(2):286–8.

73. Schrader KA, Nelson TN, De Luca A, Huntsman DG, McGillivray BC. Multiple granular cell tumors are an associated feature of LEOPARD syndrome caused by mutation in PTPN11. Clin Genet. 2009;75(2):185–9.
74. Ramaswamy PV, Storm CA, Filiano JJ, Dinulos JG. Multiple granular cell tumors in a child with Noonan syndrome. Pediatr Dermatol. 2010;27(2):209–11.
75. Sidwell RU, Rouse P, Owen RA, Green JS. Granular cell tumor of the scrotum in a child with Noonan syndrome. Pediatr Dermatol. 2008;25(3):341–3.
76. Papachristou DJ, Palekar A, Surti U, Cieply K, McGough RL, Rao UN. Malignant granular cell tumor of the ulnar nerve with novel cytogenetic and molecular genetic findings. Cancer Genet Cytogenet. 2009;191(1):46–50.
77. Di Tommaso L, Magrini E, Consales A, Poppi M, Pasquinelli G, Dorji T, Benedetti G, Baccarini P. Malignant granular cell tumor of the lateral femoral cutaneous nerve: report of a case with cytogenetic analysis. Hum Pathol. 2002;33(12):1237–40.
78. Nasser H, Danforth RD Jr, Sunbuli M, Dimitrijevic O. Malignant granular cell tumor: case report with a novel karyotype and review of the literature. Ann Diagn Pathol. 2010;14(4):273–8.
79. Dhingra KK, Mandal S, Roy S, Khurana N. Malignant peripheral nerve sheath tumor of the breast: case report. World J Surg Oncol. 2007;5:142.
80. Fangfang L, Danhua S, Songlin L, Yanfeng Z. An unusual breast malignant peripheral nerve sheath tumour and review of the literature. J Clin Pathol. 2010;63(7):663–4.
81. Medina-Franco H, Gamboa-Dominguez A, de La Medina AR. Malignant peripheral nerve sheath tumor of the breast. Breast J. 2003;9(4):332.
82. Thanapaisal C, Koonmee S, Siritunyaporn S. Malignant peripheral nerve sheath tumor of breast in patient without Von Recklinghausen's neurofibromatosis: a case report. J Med Assoc Thailand = Chotmaihet Thangphaet. 2006;89(3):377–9.
83. Wang H, Ge J, Chen L, Xie P, Chen F, Chen Y. Melanocytic malignant peripheral nerve sheath tumor of the male breast. Breast Care. 2009;4(4):260–2.
84. Carter JM, O'Hara C, Dundas G, Gilchrist D, Collins MS, Eaton K, Judkins AR, Biegel JA, Folpe AL. Epithelioid malignant peripheral nerve sheath tumor arising in a schwannoma, in a patient with "neuroblastoma-like" schwannomatosis and a novel germline SMARCB1 mutation. Am J Surg Pathol. 2012;36(1):154–60.
85. Hollmann TJ, Hornick JL. INI1-deficient tumors: diagnostic features and molecular genetics. Am J Surg Pathol. 2011;35(10):e47–63.
86. Mertens F, Dal Cin P, De Wever I, Fletcher CD, Mandahl N, Mitelman F, Rosai J, Rydholm A, Sciot R, Tallini G. Cytogenetic characterization of peripheral nerve sheath tumours: a report of the CHAMP study group. J Pathol. 2000;190(1):31–8.
87. Cancer Genome Anatomy Project (CGAP). http://cgap.nci.nih.gov/cgap.html.
88. Rao UN, Surti U, Hoffner L, Yaw K. Cytogenetic and histologic correlation of peripheral nerve sheath tumors of soft tissue. Cancer Genet Cytogenet. 1996;88(1):17–25.
89. Hulsebos TJ, Plomp AS, Wolterman RA, Robanus-Maandag EC, Baas F, Wesseling P. Germline mutation of INI1/SMARCB1 in familial schwannomatosis. Am J Hum Genet. 2007;80(4):805–10.
90. Brooks DG. The neurofibromatoses: hereditary predisposition to multiple peripheral nerve tumors. Neurosurg Clin N Am. 2004;15(2):145–55.
91. Lothe RA, Slettan A, Saeter G, Brogger A, Borresen AL, Nesland JM. Alterations at chromosome 17 loci in peripheral nerve sheath tumors. J Neuropathol Exp Neurol. 1995;54(1):65–73.
92. Falconieri G, Lamovec J, Mirra M, Pizzolitto S. Solitary fibrous tumor of the mammary gland: a potential pitfall in breast pathology. Ann Diagn Pathol. 2004;8(3):121–5.
93. Doyle LA, Vivero M, Fletcher CD, Mertens F, Hornick JL. Nuclear expression of STAT6 distinguishes solitary fibrous tumor from histologic mimics. Modern Pathol: Official J U S Can Acad Pathol Inc. 2014;27(3):390–5.

94. Vivero M, Doyle LA, Fletcher CD, Mertens F, Hornick JL. GRIA2 is a novel diagnostic marker for solitary fibrous tumour identified through gene expression profiling. Histopathology 2014.

95. Chmielecki J, Crago AM, Rosenberg M, O'Connor R, Walker SR, Ambrogio L, Auclair D, McKenna A, Heinrich MC, Frank DA, et al. Whole-exome sequencing identifies a recurrent NAB2-STAT6 fusion in solitary fibrous tumors. Nat Genet. 2013;45(2):131–2.

96. Mohajeri A, Tayebwa J, Collin A, Nilsson J, Magnusson L, von Steyern FV, Brosjo O, Domanski HA, Larsson O, Sciot R, et al. Comprehensive genetic analysis identifies a pathognomonic NAB2/STAT6 fusion gene, nonrandom secondary genomic imbalances, and a characteristic gene expression profile in solitary fibrous tumor. Genes Chromosom Cancer. 2013;52(10):873–86.

97. Robinson DR, Wu YM, Kalyana-Sundaram S, Cao X, Lonigro RJ, Sung YS, Chen CL, Zhang L, Wang R, Su F, et al. Identification of recurrent NAB2-STAT6 gene fusions in solitary fibrous tumor by integrative sequencing. Nat Genet. 2013;45(2):180–5.

98. Hajdu M, Singer S, Maki RG, Schwartz GK, Keohan ML, Antonescu CR. IGF2 overexpression in solitary fibrous tumours is independent of anatomical location and is related to loss of imprinting. J Pathol. 2010;221(3):300–7.

99. Day NC, Shaw PJ, McCormack AL, Craig PJ, Smith W, Beattie R, Williams TL, Ellis SB, Ince PG, Harpold MM, et al. Distribution of alpha 1A, alpha 1B and alpha 1E voltage-dependent calcium channel subunits in the human hippocampus and parahippocampal gyrus. Neuroscience. 1996;71(4):1013–24.

100. Chang HJ, Yoo BC, Lim SB, Jeong SY, Kim WH, Park JG. Metabotropic glutamate receptor 4 expression in colorectal carcinoma and its prognostic significance. Clin Cancer Res: Official J Am Assoc Cancer Res. 2005;11(9):3288–95.

101. Tanaka H, Grooms SY, Bennett MV, Zukin RS. The AMPAR subunit GluR2: still front and center-stage. Brain Res. 2000;886(1–2):190–207.

102. Rzeski W, Ikonomidou C, Turski L. Glutamate antagonists limit tumor growth. Biochem Pharmacol. 2002;64(8):1195–200.

103. Hechtman JF, Xiao GQ, Unger PD, Kinoshita Y, Godbold JH, Burstein DE. Anti-glutamate receptor 2 as a new potential diagnostic probe for prostatic adenocarcinoma: a pilot immunohistochemical study. Appl Immunohistochem Mol Morphol: AIMM/Official Publ Soc Appl Immunohistochem. 2012;20(4):344–9.

104. Tsibris JC, Maas S, Segars JH, Nicosia SV, Enkemann SA, O'Brien WF, Spellacy WN. New potential regulators of uterine leiomyomata from DNA arrays: the ionotropic glutamate receptor GluR2. Biochem Biophys Res Commun. 2003;312(1):249–54.

105. Ishiuchi S, Yoshida Y, Sugawara K, Aihara M, Ohtani T, Watanabe T, Saito N, Tsuzuki K, Okado H, Miwa A, et al. Ca^{2+}-permeable AMPA receptors regulate growth of human glioblastoma via Akt activation. J Neurosci: Official J Soc Neurosci. 2007;27(30):7987–8001.

106. Nascimento AF, Raut CP, Fletcher CD. Primary angiosarcoma of the breast: clinicopathologic analysis of 49 cases, suggesting that grade is not prognostic. Am J Surg Pathol. 2008;32(12):1896–904.

107. Rosen PP, Kimmel M, Ernsberger D. Mammary angiosarcoma. The prognostic significance of tumor differentiation. Cancer. 1988;62(10):2145–51.

108. Adem C, Reynolds C, Ingle JN, Nascimento AG. Primary breast sarcoma: clinicopathologic series from the Mayo Clinic and review of the literature. Br J Cancer. 2004;91(2):237–41.

109. Fayette J, Martin E, Piperno-Neumann S, Le Cesne A, Robert C, Bonvalot S, Ranchere D, Pouillart P, Coindre JM, Blay JY. Angiosarcomas, a heterogeneous group of sarcomas with specific behavior depending on primary site: a retrospective study of 161 cases. Ann Oncol: Official J Eur Soc Med Oncol/ESMO. 2007;18(12):2030–6.

110. Mery CM, George S, Bertagnolli MM, Raut CP. Secondary sarcomas after radiotherapy for breast cancer: sustained risk and poor survival. Cancer. 2009;115(18):4055–63.

111. Brenn T, Fletcher CD. Postradiation vascular proliferations: an increasing problem. Histopathology. 2006;48(1):106–14.

112. Brodie C, Provenzano E. Vascular proliferations of the breast. Histopathology. 2008;52(1):30–44.
113. Fineberg S, Rosen PP. Cutaneous angiosarcoma and atypical vascular lesions of the skin and breast after radiation therapy for breast carcinoma. Am J Clin Pathol. 1994;102(6):757–63.
114. Mandrell J, Mehta S, McClure S. Atypical vascular lesion of the breast. J Am Acad Dermatol. 2010;63(2):337–40.
115. Patton KT, Deyrup AT, Weiss SW. Atypical vascular lesions after surgery and radiation of the breast: a clinicopathologic study of 32 cases analyzing histologic heterogeneity and association with angiosarcoma. Am J Surg Pathol. 2008;32(6):943–50.
116. Uchin JM, Billings SD. Radiotherapy-associated atypical vascular lesions of the breast. J Cutan Pathol. 2009;36(1):87–8.
117. Weaver J, Billings SD. Postradiation cutaneous vascular tumors of the breast: a review. Semin Diagn Pathol. 2009;26(3):141–9.
118. Brenn T, Fletcher CD. Radiation-associated cutaneous atypical vascular lesions and angiosarcoma: clinicopathologic analysis of 42 cases. Am J Surg Pathol. 2005;29(8):983–96.
119. Requena L, Kutzner H, Mentzel T, Duran R, Rodriguez-Peralto JL. Benign vascular proliferations in irradiated skin. Am J Surg Pathol. 2002;26(3):328–37.
120. Ginter PS, Mosquera JM, MacDonald TY, D'Alfonso TM, Rubin MA, Shin SJ. Diagnostic utility of MYC amplification and anti-MYC immunohistochemistry in atypical vascular lesions, primary or radiation-induced mammary angiosarcomas, and primary angiosarcomas of other sites. Hum Pathol. 2014;45(4):709–16.
121. Antonescu CR, Yoshida A, Guo T, Chang NE, Zhang L, Agaram NP, Qin LX, Brennan MF, Singer S, Maki RG. KDR activating mutations in human angiosarcomas are sensitive to specific kinase inhibitors. Cancer Res. 2009;69(18):7175–9.
122. Manner J, Radlwimmer B, Hohenberger P, Mossinger K, Kuffer S, Sauer C, Belharazem D, Zettl A, Coindre JM, Hallermann C, et al. MYC high level gene amplification is a distinctive feature of angiosarcomas after irradiation or chronic lymphedema. Am J Pathol. 2010;176(1):34–9.
123. Fernandez AP, Sun Y, Tubbs RR, Goldblum JR, Billings SD. FISH for MYC amplification and anti-MYC immunohistochemistry: useful diagnostic tools in the assessment of secondary angiosarcoma and atypical vascular proliferations. J Cutan Pathol. 2012;39(2):234–42.
124. Guo T, Zhang L, Chang NE, Singer S, Maki RG, Antonescu CR. Consistent MYC and FLT4 gene amplification in radiation-induced angiosarcoma but not in other radiation-associated atypical vascular lesions. Genes Chromosom Cancer. 2011;50(1):25–33.
125. Mentzel T, Schildhaus HU, Palmedo G, Buttner R, Kutzner H. Postradiation cutaneous angiosarcoma after treatment of breast carcinoma is characterized by MYC amplification in contrast to atypical vascular lesions after radiotherapy and control cases: clinicopathological, immunohistochemical and molecular analysis of 66 cases. Mod Pathol: Official J U S Can Acad Pathol Inc. 2012;25(1):75–85.
126. Blanchard DK, Reynolds CA, Grant CS, Donohue JH. Primary nonphylloides breast sarcomas. Am J Surg. 2003;186(4):359–61.
127. Terrier P, Terrier-Lacombe MJ, Mouriesse H, Friedman S, Spielmann M, Contesso G. Primary breast sarcoma: a review of 33 cases with immunohistochemistry and prognostic factors. Breast Cancer Res Treat. 1989;13(1):39–48.
128. Arbabi L, Warhol MJ. Pleomorphic liposarcoma following radiotherapy for breast carcinoma. Cancer. 1982;49(5):878–80.
129. Binh MB, Sastre-Garau X, Guillou L, de Pinieux G, Terrier P, Lagace R, Aurias A, Hostein I, Coindre JM. MDM2 and CDK4 immunostainings are useful adjuncts in diagnosing well-differentiated and dedifferentiated liposarcoma subtypes: a comparative analysis of 559 soft tissue neoplasms with genetic data. Am J Surg Pathol. 2005;29(10):1340–7.
130. Thway K, Flora R, Shah C, Olmos D, Fisher C. Diagnostic utility of p16, CDK4, and MDM2 as an immunohistochemical panel in distinguishing well-differentiated and dedifferentiated liposarcomas from other adipocytic tumors. Am J Surg Pathol. 2012;36(3):462–9.

131. Coindre JM, Pedeutour F, Aurias A. Well-differentiated and dedifferentiated liposarcomas. Virchows Archiv: Int J Pathol. 2010;456(2):167–79.
132. Dei Tos AP, Doglioni C, Piccinin S, Sciot R, Furlanetto A, Boiocchi M, Dal Cin P, Maestro R, Fletcher CD, Tallini G. Coordinated expression and amplification of the MDM2, CDK4, and HMGI-C genes in atypical lipomatous tumours. J Pathol. 2000;190(5):531–6.
133. Coindre JM, Hostein I, Maire G, Derre J, Guillou L, Leroux A, Ghnassia JP, Collin F, Pedeutour F, Aurias A. Inflammatory malignant fibrous histiocytomas and dedifferentiated liposarcomas: histological review, genomic profile, and MDM2 and CDK4 status favour a single entity. J Pathol. 2004;203(3):822–30.
134. Sirvent N, Coindre JM, Maire G, Hostein I, Keslair F, Guillou L, Ranchere-Vince D, Terrier P, Pedeutour F. Detection of MDM2-CDK4 amplification by fluorescence in situ hybridization in 200 paraffin-embedded tumor samples: utility in diagnosing adipocytic lesions and comparison with immunohistochemistry and real-time PCR. Am J Surg Pathol. 2007;31(10):1476–89.
135. Sandberg AA. Updates on the cytogenetics and molecular genetics of bone and soft tissue tumors: liposarcoma. Cancer Genet Cytogenet. 2004;155(1):1–24.
136. Heidenblad M, Hallor KH, Staaf J, Jonsson G, Borg A, Hoglund M, Mertens F, Mandahl N. Genomic profiling of bone and soft tissue tumors with supernumerary ring chromosomes using tiling resolution bacterial artificial chromosome microarrays. Oncogene. 2006;25(53):7106–16.
137. Mariani O, Brennetot C, Coindre JM, Gruel N, Ganem C, Delattre O, Stern MH, Aurias A. JUN oncogene amplification and overexpression block adipocytic differentiation in highly aggressive sarcomas. Cancer Cell. 2007;11(4):361–74.
138. Engstrom K, Willen H, Kabjorn-Gustafsson C, Andersson C, Olsson M, Goransson M, Jarnum S, Olofsson A, Warnhammar E, Aman P. The myxoid/round cell liposarcoma fusion oncogene FUS-DDIT3 and the normal DDIT3 induce a liposarcoma phenotype in transfected human fibrosarcoma cells. Am J Pathol. 2006;168(5):1642–53.
139. Italiano A, Chambonniere ML, Attias R, Chibon F, Coindre JM, Pedeutour F. Monosomy 7 and absence of 12q amplification in two cases of spindle cell liposarcomas. Cancer Genet Cytogenet. 2008;184(2):99–104.
140. Mentzel T, Palmedo G, Kuhnen C. Well-differentiated spindle cell liposarcoma ('atypical spindle cell lipomatous tumor') does not belong to the spectrum of atypical lipomatous tumor but has a close relationship to spindle cell lipoma: clinicopathologic, immunohistochemical, and molecular analysis of six cases. Mod Pathol: Official J U S Can Acad Pathol Inc. 2010;23(5):729–36.
141. Mentzel T, Reisshauer S, Rutten A, Hantschke M, Soares de Almeida LM, Kutzner H. Cutaneous clear cell myomelanocytic tumour: a new member of the growing family of perivascular epithelioid cell tumours (PEComas). Clinicopathological and immunohistochemical analysis of seven cases. Histopathology. 2005;46(5):498–504.
142. Barnes L, Pietruszka M. Rhabdomyosarcoma arising within a cystosarcoma phyllodes. Case report and review of the literature. Am J Surg Pathol. 1978;2(4):423–9.
143. Foschini MP, Dina RE, Eusebi V. Sarcomatoid neoplasms of the breast: proposed definitions for biphasic and monophasic sarcomatoid mammary carcinomas. Semin Diagn Pathol. 1993;10(2):128–36.
144. Hays DM, Donaldson SS, Shimada H, Crist WM, Newton WA Jr, Andrassy RJ, Wiener E, Green J, Triche T, Maurer HM. Primary and metastatic rhabdomyosarcoma in the breast: neoplasms of adolescent females, a report from the Intergroup Rhabdomyosarcoma Study. Med Pediatr Oncol. 1997;29(3):181–9.
145. Cessna MH, Zhou H, Perkins SL, Tripp SR, Layfield L, Daines C, Coffin CM. Are myogenin and myoD1 expression specific for rhabdomyosarcoma? A study of 150 cases, with emphasis on spindle cell mimics. Am J Surg Pathol. 2001;25(9):1150–7.
146. Morotti RA, Nicol KK, Parham DM, Teot LA, Moore J, Hayes J, Meyer W, Qualman SJ. Children's Oncology G: an immunohistochemical algorithm to facilitate diagnosis and

subtyping of rhabdomyosarcoma: the Children's Oncology Group experience. Am J Surg Pathol. 2006;30(8):962–8.

147. Bahrami A, Gown AM, Baird GS, Hicks MJ, Folpe AL. Aberrant expression of epithelial and neuroendocrine markers in alveolar rhabdomyosarcoma: a potentially serious diagnostic pitfall. Mod Pathol: Official J U S Can Acad Pathol Inc. 2008;21(7):795–806.

148. Sullivan LM, Atkins KA, LeGallo RD. PAX immunoreactivity identifies alveolar rhabdomyosarcoma. Am J Surg Pathol. 2009;33(5):775–80.

149. Gallego Melcon S, de Toledo Sanchez, Codina J. Molecular biology of rhabdomyosarcoma. Clin Transl Oncol: Official Publ Fed Span Oncol Soc Natl Cancer Inst Mex. 2007;9(7):415–9.

150. Davicioni E, Anderson MJ, Finckenstein FG, Lynch JC, Qualman SJ, Shimada H, Schofield DE, Buckley JD, Meyer WH, Sorensen PH, et al. Molecular classification of rhabdomyosarcoma–genotypic and phenotypic determinants of diagnosis: a report from the Children's Oncology Group. Am J Pathol. 2009;174(2):550–64.

151. Parham DM, Ellison DA. Rhabdomyosarcomas in adults and children: an update. Arch Pathol Lab Med. 2006;130(10):1454–65.

152. Linardic CM. PAX3-FOXO1 fusion gene in rhabdomyosarcoma. Cancer Lett. 2008;270(1):10–8.

153. Skapek SX, Anderson J, Barr FG, Bridge JA, Gastier-Foster JM, Parham DM, Rudzinski ER, Triche T, Hawkins DS. PAX-FOXO1 fusion status drives unfavorable outcome for children with rhabdomyosarcoma: a children's oncology group report. Pediatr Blood Cancer. 2013;60(9):1411–7.

154. Barr FG, Qualman SJ, Macris MH, Melnyk N, Lawlor ER, Strzelecki DM, Triche TJ, Bridge JA, Sorensen PH. Genetic heterogeneity in the alveolar rhabdomyosarcoma subset without typical gene fusions. Cancer Res. 2002;62(16):4704–10.

155. Liu J, Guzman MA, Pezanowski D, Patel D, Hauptman J, Keisling M, Hou SJ, Papenhausen PR, Pascasio JM, Punnett HH, et al. FOXO1-FGFR1 fusion and amplification in a solid variant of alveolar rhabdomyosarcoma. Mod Pathol: Official J U S Can Acad Pathol Inc. 2011;24(10):1327–35.

156. Sumegi J, Streblow R, Frayer RW, Dal Cin P, Rosenberg A, Meloni-Ehrig A, Bridge JA. Recurrent t(2; 2) and t(2; 8) translocations in rhabdomyosarcoma without the canonical PAX-FOXO1 fuse PAX3 to members of the nuclear receptor transcriptional coactivator family. Genes Chromosom Cancer. 2010;49(3):224–36.

157. Wachtel M, Dettling M, Koscielniak E, Stegmaier S, Treuner J, Simon-Klingenstein K, Buhlmann P, Niggli FK, Schafer BW. Gene expression signatures identify rhabdomyosarcoma subtypes and detect a novel t(2; 2)(q35; p23) translocation fusing PAX3 to NCOA1. Cancer Res. 2004;64(16):5539–45.

158. Mitani K, Kurosawa H, Suzuki A, Hayashi Y, Hanada R, Yamamoto K, Komatsu A, Kobayashi N, Nakagome Y, Yamada M. Amplification of N-myc in a rhabdomyosarcoma. Jpn J Cancer Res: Gann. 1986;77(11):1062–5.

159. Mosquera JM, Sboner A, Zhang L, Kitabayashi N, Chen CL, Sung YS, Wexler LH, LaQuaglia MP, Edelman M, Sreekantaiah C, et al. Recurrent NCOA2 gene rearrangements in congenital/infantile spindle cell rhabdomyosarcoma. Genes Chromosom Cancer. 2013;52(6):538–50.

160. Silver SA, Tavassoli FA. Primary osteogenic sarcoma of the breast: a clinicopathologic analysis of 50 cases. Am J Surg Pathol. 1998;22(8):925–33.

161. Jacob S, Japa D. Primary osteogenic sarcoma of the breast. Indian J Pathol Microbiol. 2010;53(4):785–6.

162. Conner JR, Hornick JL. SATB2 is a novel marker of osteoblastic differentiation in bone and soft tissue tumours. Histopathology. 2013;63(1):36–49.

163. Hiddemann W, Roessner A, Wormann B, Mellin W, Klockenkemper B, Bosing T, Buchner T, Grundmann E. Tumor heterogeneity in osteosarcoma as identified by flow cytometry. Cancer. 1987;59(2):324–8.

164. Stark A, Kreicbergs A, Nilsonne U, Silfversward C. The age of osteosarcoma patients is increasing. An epidemiological study of osteosarcoma in Sweden 1971 to 1984. J Bone Joint Surg Br. 1971;72(1):89–93.
165. Boehm AK, Neff JR, Squire JA, Bayani J, Nelson M, Bridge JA. Cytogenetic findings in 36 osteosarcoma specimens and a review of the literature. Pediatr Pathol Mol Med. 2000;19(5):359–76.
166. Tarkkanen M, Elomaa I, Blomqvist C, Kivioja AH, Kellokumpu-Lehtinen P, Bohling T, Valle J, Knuutila S. DNA sequence copy number increase at 8q: a potential new prognostic marker in high-grade osteosarcoma. Int J Cancer (Journal International du Cancer). 1999;84(2):114–21.
167. Tan ML, Choong PF, Dass CR. Osteosarcoma: Conventional treatment vs. gene therapy. Cancer Biol Ther. 2009;8(2):106–17.
168. Greenspan A, Jundt G, Remagen W, Greenspan A. Differential diagnosis in orthopaedic oncology. 2nd ed. Philadelphia: Lippincott Williams & Wilkins; 2007.
169. German J, Crippa LP, Bloom D. Bloom's syndrome. III. Analysis of the chromosome aberration characteristic of this disorder. Chromosoma. 1974;48(4):361–6.
170. Fukuchi K, Martin GM, Monnat RJ Jr. Mutator phenotype of Werner syndrome is characterized by extensive deletions. Proc Natl Acad Sci U S A. 1989;86(15):5893–7.
171. Smida J, Baumhoer D, Rosemann M, Walch A, Bielack S, Poremba C, Remberger K, Korsching E, Scheurlen W, Dierkes C, et al. Genomic alterations and allelic imbalances are strong prognostic predictors in osteosarcoma. Clin Cancer Res: Official J Am Assoc Cancer Res. 2010;16(16):4256–67.
172. Ta HT, Dass CR, Choong PF, Dunstan DE. Osteosarcoma treatment: state of the art. Cancer Metastasis Reviews. 2009;28(1–2):247–63.
173. Alberts B, Wilson JH, Hunt T. Molecular biology of the cell. 5th ed. New York: Garland Science; 2008.
174. Hauben EI, Arends J, Vandenbroucke JP, van Asperen CJ, van Marck E, Hogendoorn PC. Multiple primary malignancies in osteosarcoma patients. Incidence and predictive value of osteosarcoma subtype for cancer syndromes related with osteosarcoma. Eur J Hum Genet: EJHG. 2003;11(8):611–8.
175. McIntyre JF, Smith-Sorensen B, Friend SH, Kassell J, Borresen AL, Yan YX, Russo C, Sato J, Barbier N, Miser J, et al. Germline mutations of the p53 tumor suppressor gene in children with osteosarcoma. J Clinical Oncol: Official J Am Soc Clin Oncol. 1994;12(5):925–30.
176. Ende L, Mercado C, Axelrod D, Darvishian F, Levine P, Cangiarella J. Intraparenchymal leiomyoma of the breast: a case report and review of the literature. Ann Clin Lab Sci. 2007;37(3):268–73.
177. Rane SU, Batra C, Saikia UN. Primary leiomyosarcoma of breast in an adolescent girl: a case report and review of the literature. Case Rep Pathol. 2012;2012:491984.
178. Yang J, Du X, Chen K, Ylipaa A, Lazar AJ, Trent J, Lev D, Pollock R, Hao X, Hunt K, et al. Genetic aberrations in soft tissue leiomyosarcoma. Cancer Lett. 2009;275(1):1–8.
179. El-Rifai W, Sarlomo-Rikala M, Knuutila S, Miettinen M. DNA copy number changes in development and progression in leiomyosarcomas of soft tissues. Am J Pathol. 1998;153(3):985–90.
180. Otano-Joos M, Mechtersheimer G, Ohl S, Wilgenbus KK, Scheurlen W, Lehnert T, Willeke F, Otto HF, Lichter P, Joos S. Detection of chromosomal imbalances in leiomyosarcoma by comparative genomic hybridization and interphase cytogenetics. Cytogenet Cell Genet. 2000;90(1–2):86–92.
181. Wang R, Lu YJ, Fisher C, Bridge JA, Shipley J. Characterization of chromosome aberrations associated with soft-tissue leiomyosarcomas by twenty-four-color karyotyping and comparative genomic hybridization analysis. Genes Chromosom Cancer. 2001;31(1):54–64.
182. Lee J, Li S, Torbenson M, Liu QZ, Lind S, Mulvihill JJ, Bane B, Wang J. Leiomyosarcoma of the breast: a pathologic and comparative genomic hybridization study of two cases. Cancer Genet Cytogenet. 2004;149(1):53–7.

183. Hu J, Rao UN, Jasani S, Khanna V, Yaw K, Surti U. Loss of DNA copy number of 10q is associated with aggressive behavior of leiomyosarcomas: a comparative genomic hybridization study. Cancer Genet Cytogenet. 2005;161(1):20–7.
184. Larramendy ML, Kaur S, Svarvar C, Bohling T, Knuutila S. Gene copy number profiling of soft-tissue leiomyosarcomas by array-comparative genomic hybridization. Cancer Genet Cytogenet. 2006;169(2):94–101.
185. Giacinti C, Giordano A. RB and cell cycle progression. Oncogene. 2006;25(38):5220–7.
186. Meza-Zepeda LA, Kresse SH, Barragan-Polania AH, Bjerkehagen B, Ohnstad HO, Namlos HM, Wang J, Kristiansen BE, Myklebost O. Array comparative genomic hybridization reveals distinct DNA copy number differences between gastrointestinal stromal tumors and leiomyosarcomas. Cancer Res. 2006;66(18):8984–93.
187. Amant F, de la Rey M, Dorfling CM, van der Walt L, Dreyer G, Dreyer L, Vergote I, Lindeque BG, Van Rensburg EJ. PTEN mutations in uterine sarcomas. Gynecol Oncol. 2002;85(1):165–9.
188. Saito T, Oda Y, Kawaguchi K, Takahira T, Yamamoto H, Tamiya S, Tanaka K, Matsuda S, Sakamoto A, Iwamoto Y, et al. PTEN/MMAC1 gene mutation is a rare event in soft tissue sarcomas without specific balanced translocations. Int J Cancer (Journal International du Cancer). 2003;104(2):175–8.
189. Kawaguchi K, Oda Y, Saito T, Takahira T, Yamamoto H, Tamiya S, Iwamoto Y, Tsuneyoshi M. Genetic and epigenetic alterations of the PTEN gene in soft tissue sarcomas. Hum Pathol. 2005;36(4):357–63.
190. Hernando E, Charytonowicz E, Dudas ME, Menendez S, Matushansky I, Mills J, Socci ND, Behrendt N, Ma L, Maki RG, et al. The AKT-mTOR pathway plays a critical role in the development of leiomyosarcomas. Nat Med. 2007;13(6):748–53.

Chapter 16
Molecular Pathology of Breast Cancer Metastasis

Mohammed A. Aleskandarany, Ian O. Ellis and Emad A. Rakha

Introduction

Breast cancer development and progression follow the known seven fundamental changes in cellular physiology, which together determine the malignant phenotype known as the 'Hallmarks of Cancer'. These hallmarks are: self-sufficiency in growth signals, insensitivity to growth inhibitory signals, limitless replicative potential, evasion of apoptosis, defective DNA repair, sustained angiogenesis, and the *ability to invade and metastasise* [1, 2]. Although malignant solid tumours, including breast cancer, arise from clonal expansion of a single transformed cell, the transformed mass of cells becomes enriched with some variants/clones more able to evade host defences and is likely to be more aggressive [3].

Metastasis, the ability to invade and metastasise, is formation of tumour implants discontinuous with the primary tumour. This occurs through colonisation of remote or distant organs by malignant cells having the privilege to invade and metastasise.

Metastasis is the crucial unequivocal difference between a tumour being benign, locally malignant or malignant. In stricter terms, the capacity of at least some of a tumour cell population to detach, migrate and colonise remote tissues is a "sure" distinctive feature of malignant tumours from benign and locally malignant. However, not all detached invasive malignant cells succeed in completing the stressful journey from their primary location to colonise the remote organ. Some cancer patients may remain metastasis-free for long times, and even some of them may never develop metastatic deposits [4, 5]. The morbidity and mortality

M.A. Aleskandarany · I.O. Ellis · E.A. Rakha (✉)
Department of Histopathology, Division of Cancer and Stem Cells, School of Medicine,
The University of Nottingham and Nottingham University Hospitals NHS Trust,
Nottingham City Hospital, Nottingham, NG5 1PB, UK
e-mail: Emad.Rakha@nottingham.ac.uk

© Springer Science+Business Media New York 2015
A. Khan et al. (eds.), *Precision Molecular Pathology of Breast Cancer*,
Molecular Pathology Library 10, DOI 10.1007/978-1-4939-2886-6_16

in breast cancer patients are mainly attributable to development of loco-regional or systemic spread of cancer or recurrences of both [6, 7]. Metastases are the cause of 90 % of human cancer deaths [8].

It is noteworthy that breast cancer evolves from a pre-invasive lesion or carcinoma in situ; in which cells display all cytological features of malignancy without invasion of the basement membrane, to an overtly invasive stage. The latter is considered one step removed from invasive cancer; and with time, cells penetrate the basement membrane, infiltrate the sub-epithelial stroma and hereby could metastasise to remote organs [9, 10].

The process of metastasis is collectively known as the metastatic cascade, during which a number of sequential steps have to be completed by cancer cells in order to successfully establish a metastatic focus at a distant location. This process requires the integration of complex arrays of specific molecular pathways. These, from theoretical standpoint, could be divided into the following categories:

Prerequisites for Metastasis

For malignant cells to metastasise, they must fulfil certain tumourigenic functions that are considered as fundamental prerequisites for metastasis. These include: unlimited cellular proliferation, evasion of cell intrinsic and environmental constraints, attraction of a blood supply; angiogenesis, and gaining the capacity to detach, migrate and move away from their original locations. Although such functions are acquired early during tumour initiation and local development and are considered amongst the hallmarks of cancer, they must remain dynamically active throughout malignant progression. The acquisition of these functions is cumulatively gained through tumour-initiating mutations, genetic alterations that occur secondarily to genomic instability and epigenetic changes. With progressive tumour growth, tumour must selectively overcome environmental stresses including cytotoxic immunity, diminished oxygen supply and an acidic environment resulting from enhanced cellular metabolism. Therefore, having these features of aggressiveness is considered prerequisites for metastasis, without which cells would not possess the capacity to proceed into the next metastatic phases [11, 12].

Metastatic Initiation and Dissemination

Dissemination commences when aggressive tumour cells become locally invasive and readily get access into the bloodstream through the newly formed vasculature, which is typically pathologically leaky due to its wide fenestrations, leading to easier entry into the circulation [13]. Moreover, such intravasation is enhanced by an epithelial-to-mesenchymal transition programme, proposed genetic reprogramming of carcinoma cells that confers superadded motility to these cells [14]. In other terms, malignant cells are continually shed from the parent primary tumour mass and circulate within the blood stream. The rate of malignant cell shedding generally increases with increased tumour size [15].

Epithelial Mesenchymal Transition

Mammary epithelial cells are functionally and phenotypically different from the supporting mesenchymal cells. The former form highly specialised surface joined together by specialised junctions and rest on well-organised basal lamina. In addition to basal contact between epithelial cells and basal lamina, epithelial cells have apical-basolateral polarisation that is tightly controlled through localised distribution of adhesion molecules and cellular cytoskeleton [16, 17]. Mesenchymal cells, on the other hand, do not exhibit such architectural organisation, contact each other only focally and lack an underlying basal lamina, which might facilitate their propensity to migrate [18].

The term epithelial–mesenchymal transition (EMT) describes a sequence of events during which epithelial cells lose many of their epithelial characteristics and gradually gain those typical of mesenchymal cells [19]. EMT phenomenon involves complex changes in cell architecture and behaviour and encompasses a wide spectrum of inter-cellular and intra-cellular changes, which are probably controlled by diverse extracellular signals [20]. Loss of epithelial characteristics and gain of mesenchymal characteristics confer invasive and migratory capacity to the malignant cells. However, it is widely conceived that EMT is proposed to be a transient reversible process [14]. Nevertheless, it is noteworthy that EMT does not necessarily denote a lineage switch; but rather a series of complex changes manifesting through phenotypic and functional alterations of malignant cells [21, 22].

EMT has been described with much emphasis in tissue culture and animal models using cancer cell lines [23, 24]. The manifestation of EMT in tissue cultures prompted some authorities to describe EMT as a mere cell culture phenomenon that lacks direct clinical evidence or clear molecular markers in breast cancer [25]. For instance, under specific culture conditions, epithelial cells can transform into fibroblast-like cells, whereby cells could not attain epithelial type polarity; aided by the culture conditions that facilitate discohesiveness. Moreover, cytokeratins commonly used as molecular identifiers of carcinoma cells are often downregulated, while vimentin is upregulated; leading ultimately to difficult characterisation of cultured epithelial cells undergoing EMT from the surrounding stromal cells [26–28].

Whether EMT is a prerequisite of tumour progression or not is a controversial matter. For instance, EMT has been considered as a key role-player in cancer dissemination from local to remote sites [29]. On the other hand, others report that EMT is one possible mechanism behind the process of local invasiveness and progression of cancer [24, 30]; others [31] still doubt its occurrence in real cancers. In addition, breast cancer progression without EMT has been reported [32]. However,

Giampieri and colleagues in their recent works demonstrated the impact of transient TGFß signalling; an EMT trigger, in switching cancer cells from cohesive "collective" to "single cell" motility, which is essential for blood-borne metastasis [33].

Recent insights into molecular EMT-controlling mechanisms indicate that several complex signalling pathways are involved in the initiation and execution of EMT in the contexts of development and cancer progression. These molecular mechanisms significantly overlap with those controlling cellular adhesion, motility, invasion, survival and differentiation [20, 34]. A number of specific molecular pathways and transcription factors have been reported as "EMT triggers" including TGFß [35], Twist1/2 [36], PI3 K/Akt pathway [37], CTEN [38], Snail, Slug, and Zeb1 [39]. When expressed in a variety of cell types, these factors act as transcriptional repressors of E-cadherin and alter the expression of a diverse number of genes denoting *in vitro* EMT with subsequent promotion of cancer invasion and metastasis [38, 40].

Not only is E-cadherin downregulation considered as the sole characteristic molecular phenotypic change of carcinoma cells reported to accompany breast cancer metastasis through EMT programme but upregulation of N-cadherin or "cadherin switching" has been reported to enhance cellular motility of mammary epithelial cell lines [41]. Moreover, N-cadherin expression was reported to be more influential than E-cadherin loss in determining the EMT phenotype and hence progression [42]. The latter notion that E-cadherin loss alone is not sufficient for breast cancer metastatic dissemination is supported by the known character of invasive lobular carcinoma which is typically characterised by loss of E-cadherin expression [43].

Therefore, these integrative molecular changes challenge some prevailing views that propose repression of E-cadherin or deregulation of a single molecular pathway to be sufficient to explain the tendency of certain cancer types to disseminate over others [38, 44].

Furthermore, the privileged occurrence of EMT in some particular breast cancer molecular subtypes has been reported [45]. Different breast cancer molecular subtypes express differential levels of cadherin family members; E-cadherin, N-cadherin and P-cadherin, and upregulation of mesenchymal markers (e.g. SMA); with N-cadherin gain having the highest influence in determining the EMT phenotype [46].

The Tumour Microenvironment and Metastasis

The tumour microenvironment in invasive breast carcinoma normally represents mechano-biological interface between malignant cells and the components of the surrounding stroma [47]. There are different types and subtypes of cells contributing as pro-metastatic or anti-metastatic regulators.

Fibroblasts are spindly, non-epithelial, non-endothelial and non-inflammatory stromal cells. Their main biological functions in normal tissues are the regulation of epithelial cells differentiation, wound healing, secretion of variety collagens types and they are the main producers of ECM proteases [48]. The close presence of malignant cells and the stromal fibroblast in the same local microenvironment will lead to epigenetic alteration of the latter, where some of the genes regulating cellular proliferation of normal fibroblasts may be affected [49]. This paracrine signalling loop may mutate or silence well-known tumour suppressor genes such as P53 and PTEN within cancer associated fibroblasts (CAFs) [50]. CAFs are obligated by their intrinsic genetics and the epigenetic effects of the adjacent malignant cells to secrete growth factors, chemokines, cytokine, and ECM remodelling enzymes [48]. It also may supress the function of immune T cells [51]. Moreover, CAFs and inflammatory cells promote the upregulation of the transcriptional factors genes SNAIL, SLUG, and ZEB1, factors reported as EMT triggers [39]. Probably one of the fascinating examples of synergism between CAFs and breast cancer cells is podoplanin; a glycoprotein encoded by the PDPN gene and expressed in lymphatic vessels, malignant cells and CAFs. It functions as a booster of cellular motility and reducer of cellular adhesion. Overexpression of podoplanin is significantly correlated with breast cancer aggressiveness. Interestingly, podoplanin overexpression in the invasive front of breast carcinoma is the back-up plan of invasion and metastasis if the pathways of EMT are inhibited or hindered, through remodelling the cytoskeletal structures and forming invasive protrusions: the filopodia [52]. Therefore, this phenomenon illustrates the potent synergism between paracrine signalling from CAFs and epigenetics from malignant cells to invade lymphatic vessels.

Different phenotypes of lymphocytes and myeloid cells are present in the tumour microenvironment. The presence of T lymphocytes is reported to be associated with good prognosis in the case of Cytotoxic CD8+ memory T cells and CD4+ T helper 1 cells [53]. Cytotoxic CD8+ memory T cells are able to eradicate malignant cells at the invasive front of the tumour. This tumour-cell cytotoxicity is supported by CD4+ T helper 1 cell cytokines; Interleukin-2 (IL-2) and Interferon gamma (IFN-γ), which play crucial roles in the differentiation of naive T cells into memory T cells. The latter cells can fight tumour formation with cytostatic and cytotoxic mechanisms [54]. In contrast to Cytotoxic CD8+ memory T cells, Natural Killer (NK) and Natural Killer T (NKT) cells infiltrate the tumour stroma with no major effects on malignant cells [53].

Although infiltrating CD4+ cells had good prognosis implications, not all the CD4+ cells subtypes possess same influence. For instance, T regulatory cells (Tregs) have immune-inhibitory characteristics with subsequent protection of malignant cells from cytotoxic CD8+ T cells' elimination [55]. This opposition of the immune function could be attributed to the suppression of the cellular recognition of the malignant cells due to the expression of CD152 receptor protein (also known as cytotoxic lymphocyte associated protein-4, CTLA4) that reverses the activation of the immune response and transmits inhibition signals. Moreover, the immune dysregulatory actions of transcriptional factors forkhead box P3 (FOXP3) and others are other explanations [56, 57].

The other type of lymphocytes of the adaptive immune system is B lymphocytes. Generally speaking, B lymphocytes have good prognostic implications if they infiltrate the tumour microenvironment owing to production of specific antibodies against the tumour cell antigens [58]. However, the vast majority of those immunity cells tend to localise further in the stroma or even at lymphoid structures contiguous to the microenvironment, contrasting cytotoxic CD8+ T cells that are often proximate to the malignant cells [59]. Likewise the inhibitory effect of Tregs, regulatory B cells (Bregs) impairs the tumour specific immune response. Furthermore, it induces a special immune evasion mechanism on behalf of the malignant cells [60].

In contrast to the tumour infiltrating lymphocytes, tumour associated macrophages (TAMs) are strongly linked with breast cancer poor prognosis. TAMs are well-known to produce Interleukin-10 and angiogenic factors [61], and they aggregate nearby necrotic and hypoxic areas of the tumour microenvironment [62]. Hence, and under this hypoxic environment, growth factors that promote blood and lymph neovascularization are upregulated and secreted by the malignant cells. Vascular Endothelial Growth Factor-A (VEGFA) is essential requirement for hemangiogenesis, and it is a chemoattractant for macrophages [63]. The attracted and recruited macrophages will aid the invasion and metastasis process through a dual-direction reaction loop of paracrine signalling with the malignant epithelial cells. Therefore, the intravasation of malignant cells into BV or LV and their migration through endothelium will be facilitated [64]. Moreover, this may lead to suppression of cytotoxic T cells and increase the propagation of pro-metastatic phenotypes of TAMs [65]. Therefore, the use of immunomodulation drug therapy aims to interfere with the tumour-induced immunosuppression mechanisms, and it is more likely to be beneficial than using non-specific cytotoxic drugs [66].

Invasion of the Extracellular Matrix (ECM)

The ECM is the complex structural entity surrounding and supporting mammary epithelial cells and is physically defined into the basement membrane and the interstitial tissue. Three major classes of macromolecules are physically associated to form the ECM; structural proteins, assembled into fibrous components, such as collagens and elastins, a diverse group of adhesive specialised glycoproteins, including fibrillin, fibronectin and laminin and a gel of proteoglycans and hyaluronan [67]. Four different families of collagen are characterised, where type I, II and III are the most abundant and form fibrils of similar structure. Type IV collagen forms a two-dimensional reticulum and is a major component of the basement membranes, and in such a case it is synthesised by epithelial and endothelial cells [68]. The ECM not only provides physico-mechanical and structural support for the mammary epithelium yet it encodes a large variety of specific signals which dynamically influence breast cancer cell growth, invasion and migration [69, 70].

Following detachment from the primary tumour cell mass, the breast carcinoma cells first adhere to the matrix components. Receptor-mediated attachment of the malignant cells to laminins and fibronectin is critically important for invasion and metastasis [71–73]. Within the interstitial ECM, breast carcinoma cells must create their passageway for migration through active proteolytic degradation of the ECM components. Such enzymatic degradation is carried out by proteases at the invading edge of the tumour [74]. Different classes of proteases have been evidenced as pro-metastatic proteins including the serine [75], cysteine [76], aspartic [77] and the matrix metalloproteinases (MMPs) [78]. The latter is a broad family of zinc-dependant endopeptidases comprising 23 members in humans. To date, at least fourteen MMPs are implicated in breast cancer development and progression [79]. MMPs are produced both by the malignant cells and the peritumoural stromal [80]. The action of proteases is tightly regulated by antiproteases which increase in response to elevated protease level. It is the balance between proteases and antiproteases at the invading/cutting edge of the tumour which promotes or halts tumour cell propagation [79, 81]. Proteolysis of ECM facilitates breast cancer cell invasion through their propulsion, or simply, locomotion. Migration is an active process and is affected by multiple factors, both autocrine and tumour-cell derived motility factors, and cleavage products of matrix components derived from collagen and proteoglycans [82, 83]. Cells migrate through the ECM by extending membrane protrusions; filopodia and lamellipodia, at their leading edges. Their formation is driven by the reorganisation and polymerisation of actin filaments. The propagation of tumour cells is a complex highly integrated process controlled by complex signalling cascades within the cells and cell-stromal crosstalk [83, 84].

Lympho-Vascular Invasion

Lymphatic Vascular Invasion (LVI) is one of the crucial steps in the metastatic cascade. Presence of LVI, as detected by histopathological examination in invasive breast cancer, is a marker of metastatic potential, a predictive factor of metastasis into the lymphatic system and is associated with poor outcome [85]. In a previous study of 3812 invasive breast cancer we have demonstrated that LVI is strongly associated with outcome in the entire series and in different subgroups. LVI was an independent predictor of outcome and provided survival disadvantage equivalent to that provided by 1 or 2 involved lymph nodes and to that provided by 1 size category [85]. Using a panel of endothelial markers in more than 1000 invasive breast cancer we [86] have demonstrated that VI was present 22 and in 97 % of cases it was LVI. Blood vascular invasion (BVI) was detected in 3 % of cases [86]. The current clinicopathological studies that investigated the role of LVI in breast carcinoma focused on the capacity, the size, and the location of the vessel involved; whether intratumoural, peritumoural, or both [85, 87]. Immunohistochemical detection of LVI and BVI improves their detection rate and prognostic/predictive values in primary invasive breast cancer [86, 88, 89].

The multiple chemotaxis and cytotaxis interactions due to the EMT and their consequences in the tumour microenvironment will dramatically alter the adjacent lymphatics [90]. The angiogenesis and lymphangiogenesis are strongly related with tumour aggressiveness. The presence of BV and LV within the solid tumours is an eminent sign of the stimulation of embryogenesis of the endothelium by the malignant cells. Complex cellular events, including proliferation, sprouting, migration and tube formation are involved in the process of lymphangiogenesis. These functions depend on vascular endothelial growth factor receptor 2 (VEGFR2) and VEGFR3 signalling controlled by VEGFC or VEGFD [91]. These signalling events are more or less the counterparts of the molecular regulation of angiogenesis by VEGFA signalling via VEGFR2 [92].

The intratumoural vessels usually get collapsed under the increased mass of the growing tumour [93]. On the other hand, the peritumoural vessels, and under the influence of the VEGFC and VEGFD, are highly proliferative. The enlarged peritumoural vessels have been detected with substantial diameter that lead to an increase of the contacting surface area between malignant cells and LV, which indicates higher propensity of the LVI incidence [94]. Indeed, the chemotactic and cytotactic effects are crucial in tumour metastasis; nevertheless, the transcellular lymphatic drainage that is caused by the elevated interstitial flow of lymphatic fluids may polarise the malignant cells toward the nearest LV through the autologous secretion of C-C Chemokine Receptor 7 (CCR7). This expression of the specific receptor and its specific ligand portrays the physio-chemical autocrine mechanisms possessed by some clones of the malignant cells [95]. The latter is an example illustrating the capacity of some malignant cell to intensify the chemokinetics of metastatic progression via directing themselves to the preferential metastasis target.

Recently, the significant association between the breast cancer molecular subtype and LVI and LN metastasis has been documented through the clinical trial performed by American College of Surgeons Oncology Group (ACOSOG) [96]. Triple negative or basal-like molecular subtype showed the least association with LVI and axillary LN metastasis although it is strongly related with poor prognosis and high propensity to recur locally. Conversely, the Estrogen Receptor and Progesterone Receptor and HER2 positive molecular subtypes showed the highest incidence of LVI. Triple negative malignant cells are more mitotic [97], and less likely to express claudin protein than the positive ER, PR, and HER2/*neu* molecular subtypes. Furthermore, the triple negative molecular subtype expresses proteins that are crucial to transform the malignant epithelial cell to the mesenchymal form; hence, are potently invasive and metastatic [98]. These results are reinforced by the recent report from the Danish Breast Cancer Cooperative Group reporting reduced risk of axillary lymph node involvement at the time of diagnosis in triple negative breast cancer compared to patients with other subtypes [99]. Therefore, tumour invasiveness and the routes through which breast cancer disseminates to regional lymph nodes or distant metastatic sites are different among to the known breast cancer molecular subtypes.

Following invasion into the local stromal and intravasation, the malignant cells must manage to survive within the luminal cavities of the LV or capillaries [100]. To survive the stresses during their journey, malignant breast cancer cells require intrinsic functions, as for instance evading detachment-triggered cell death through AKT signalling pathway activation via neurotrophic tyrosine kinase, receptor type

2 (NTRK2, TrkB) [101]. Moreover, cells must withstand the associated extrinsic shear forces and platelet aggregates [102]. They also need to overcome and escape phagocytosis by circulating macrophages. A subset of circulating luminal breast cancer cells has been reported to express CD47 molecule that helps tumour cells evade macrophage phagocytosis [103].

Metastatic Colonisation

The dissemination of tumour cells to a specific distant organ is influenced by circulation patterns and the mechanical lodging of tumour cells in capillary beds. Metastatic cells enter the parenchyma of the target organ by breaching the capillaries in which they are embedded, either by remodelling vascular networks allowing transmigration across the capillary wall or as a result of disruption of capillary integrity by the mechanical forces of expanding tumour emboli [15]. Adhesion molecules, including different selectins (E, P, and L selectins) [104, 105] and integrins [106], mediate the attachment of tumour cells to capillary endothelium. Specific subtypes of integrin, especially yet not exclusively $\alpha 6\beta 4$, $\alpha v\beta 3$ and $\alpha 3\beta 1$, have been linked to breast cancer aggressiveness, shortened patients' survival and higher tendency of breast cancer cells to colonise bones [107, 108]. Integrins through cooperation with other factors, as for instance EGFR and HER2, increases not only tumour initiation and proliferation but also migration both in the primary location and in distant organ colonisation [109, 110].

Breast cancer cells are known to metastasise to all body organs; however, the common sites for metastatic spread are bone, lung and liver and brain [111]. Metastatic colonisation of a particular organ is a non-random process depending upon sophisticated interactions between breast cancer cells and stromal microenvironment at the target organ. Evidence for these interactions came from animal models, in vivo imaging and functional genomics which led to the discovery of molecular mediators of organ-specific tropism [112]. The chemokine receptor CXCR4 overexpression by breast cancer cells increases the expression of $\alpha v\beta 3$ integrin, therefore increasing in vitro cellular adhesion and invasion 87, 88 and experimental metastasis in vivo 117. Moreover, the extravasation and homing of breast cancer cells into lung, bone and regional lymph nodes is facilitated by their high expression of CXCR4 and CCR7. These target tissues have abundant expression of the specific ligands CXCL12/SDF-1 and CCL21 of CXCR4 and CCR7 [113, 114]. Upon their entry into the target organ parenchyma, metastatic tumour cells are challenged by a distinctive microenvironment which they must withstand, adapt and eventually overtake this new microenvironment. The recruited bone-marrow-derived progenitor cells through providing a permissive niche for metastasis prepare the soil for metastatic cell regrowth [115]. In case of bone metastasis, breast cancer cells produce PTHrP, IL-11, IL-8, IL-6, and RANKL, factors which stimulate osteolysis turning bone more permissive to their growth [116, 117]. Moreover, organ-specific components of the tumour microenvironments synergistically assist active colonisation, as for instance the activation of bone-resorbing osteoclasts by metastatic breast cancer cells during osteolytic metastasis [118], and the release of active TGFB from bone matrix during osteolysis [119].

Following extravasation into a secondary organ, metastatic breast cancer cells undergo one of three possible fates. They may undergo deaths by apoptosis, remain dormant for variable periods of dormancy whether singly or as micromet-astatic deposits, or immediately proliferate, thus manifesting as overt metastatic recurrences [120]. The triggering event of eventual re-activation and outgrowth of dormant metastatic cells remains unknown [121]. The length of dormancy periods has been determined by balancing cell proliferation and apoptosis [122, 123].

Metastasis: An Inherent Early Feature of Cancer

It has long been thought that the ability of some cellular clones within the primary tumour to metastasise to remote tissues is an attribute that is lately acquired in the cascade of multistep carcinogenesis [124]. However, a foundation of evidence is currently accumulating supporting an integrative model implying that metastasis is an early acquired cancer trait. This paradigm shift in understanding of cancer dis-semination comes from clinical observations and is reinforced by gene expression profiling studies [8]. A common diagnostic phenomenon supporting this model is the frequent detection of "micrometastatic" nodules in patients with small early stage breast cancers. Moreover, it has been reported that pairs of human primary breast carcinomas and their distant metastases, which developed years later are highly similar at their transcriptome level [8]. Similarly, extensive similarities at the transcriptome level among the distinct stages of breast cancer progression have been reported. These stages include pre-malignant, pre-invasive/in situ, and invasive breast cancer, suggesting that gene expression alterations conferring the potential for invasive growth are already present in the pre-invasive stages [125–127]. These molecular similarities and the early inherent metastatic capac-ity formed the basis of using the primary tumour to study different genetic and proteomic derangements as a tool to unravel molecular changes underlying and determining the metastatic phenotype, aggressive behaviour and poor prognosis.

Breast Cancer Molecular Subtype and Distant Metastasis

Luminal A tumours, luminal B and HER2+ tumours are associated with higher rates of metastasis to brain, liver, and lung. On the other hand, basal-like tumours have more brain and lung metastases, and lower rates of liver and bone metasta-ses. TN nonbasal tumours follow a pattern similar to basal-like tumours yet metas-tasise more to the liver [128, 129]. Moreover, at the time of primary diagnosis, triple negative breast cancer patients have reduced risks of axillary lymph node involvement compared to other molecular subtypes, independently of other risk factors [99]. These differences in metastatic patterns may indicate haematogenous spread of triple negative breast cancer in contrast to other subtypes which preferably spread via the lymphatic routes [130, 131].

Gene Expression Signatures and Distant Metastasis

Analysis of gene expression in a genome-wide fashion introduced by DNA-microarray technology was able to determine gene expression patterns that can predict the clinical behaviour in breast cancer, especially the occurrence of distant recurrence [132]. Multiple gene signatures have been determined and externally validated including the 70-gene expression signature used in the MammaPrint® [133, 134], the 76-gene signature [135], the genomic grade index (GGI) [136] and the 21-gene profile used in the Oncotype Dx® [137, 138]. Currently, two prognostic platforms based on expression signatures are commercially available: the OncotypeDx measured on paraffin-embedded samples and approved by ASCO, and the Mammaprint, approved by the American FDA [139]. The gene lists within these signatures include genes involved in the cell cycle/proliferation, invasion angiogenesis, in addition to the genes almost exclusively expressed by the stromal cells surrounding the mammary epithelial cells [140–142]. The latter notions underscore the integrative model of metastasis involving cooperative roles played by both the tumour cells and the surrounding microenvironment.

Conclusion

Metastasis is a complex multistep process involving complex molecular and genetic changes in the malignant cells that enable them to interact with surrounding structures including basement membranes structure, extracellular matrix, stromal cells, immune cells, endothelial cells and specialised cells at the metastatic sites. In addition, malignant metastatic cells acquire the ability to survive and grow within different environment including lymphatic or vascular spaces and distant metastatic sites. VI is an important step in the metastatic process. The vast majority of VI in breast cancer is LVI.

References

1. Hanahan D, Weinberg RA. The hallmarks of cancer. Cell. 2000;100(1):57–70.
2. Sledge GW, Miller KD. Exploiting the hallmarks of cancer: the future conquest of breast cancer. Eur J Cancer. 2003;39(12):1668–75.
3. Beckmann MW, Niederacher D, Schnürch HG, Gusterson BA, Bender HG. Multistep carcinogenesis of breast cancer and tumour heterogeneity. J Mol Med. 1997;75(6):429–39.

4. Fidler IJ. The pathogenesis of cancer metastasis: the 'seed and soil' hypothesis revisited. Nat Rev Cancer. 2003;3(6):453–8.
5. Weinberg RA. Mechanisms of malignant progression. Carcinogenesis. 2008;29(6):1092–1095. PubMed PMID: 18453542. Epub 2008/05/06. eng.
6. Rabbani SA, Mazar AP. Evaluating distant metastases in breast cancer: from biology to outcomes. Cancer Metastasis Rev. 2007;26(3–4):663–674. PubMed PMID: 17823779. Epub 2007/09/08. eng.
7. Nicolini A, Giardino R, Carpi A, Ferrari P, Anselmi L, Colosimo S, et al. Metastatic breast cancer: an updating. Biomed Pharmacother. 2006;60(9):548–556. PubMed PMID: 16950593. Epub 2006/09/05. eng.
8. Weigelt B, Peterse JL, van 't Veer LJ. Breast cancer metastasis: markers and models. Nat Rev Cancer. 2005;5(8):591–602. PubMed PMID: 16056258. Epub 2005/08/02. eng.
9. Duffy MJ, McGowan PM, Gallagher WM. Cancer invasion and metastasis: changing views. J Pathol. 2008;214(3):283–293. PubMed PMID: 18095256. Epub 2007/12/21. eng.
10. Virnig BA, Tuttle TM, Shamliyan T, Kane RL. Ductal carcinoma in situ of the breast: a systematic review of incidence, treatment, and outcomes. J Natl Cancer Inst. 2010;102(3):170–8.
11. Christofori G. New signals from the invasive front. Nature. 2006;441(7092):444–450. PubMed PMID: 16724056. Epub 2006/05/26. eng.
12. Gupta GP, Massague J. Cancer metastasis: building a framework. Cell. 2006;127(4):679–695. PubMed PMID: 17110329. Epub 2006/11/18. eng.
13. Shchors K, Evan G. Tumor angiogenesis: cause or consequence of cancer? Cancer Res. 2007;67(15):7059–7061. PubMed PMID: 17671171. Epub 2007/08/03. eng.
14. Thiery JP. Epithelial-mesenchymal transitions in tumour progression. Nat Rev Cancer. 2002;2(6):442–454. PubMed PMID: 12189386. Epub 2002/08/22. eng.
15. Nguyen DX, Massague J. Genetic determinants of cancer metastasis. Nat Rev Genet. 2007;8(5):341–52.
16. Schmidt S, Friedl P. Interstitial cell migration: integrin-dependent and alternative adhesion mechanisms. Cell Tissue Res. 2010;339(1):83–92. PubMed PMID: 19921267. Epub 2009/11/19. eng.
17. Knust E. Regulation of epithelial cell shape and polarity by cell-cell adhesion (Review). Mol Membr Biol. 2002;19(2):113–120. PubMed PMID: 12126229. Epub 2002/07/20. eng.
18. Friedl P. Prespecification and plasticity: shifting mechanisms of cell migration. Curr Opin Cell Biol. 2004;16(1):14–23. PubMed PMID: 15037300. Epub 2004/03/24. eng.
19. Thiery JP, Sleeman JP. Complex networks orchestrate epithelial-mesenchymal transitions. Nat Rev Mol Cell Biol. 2006;7(2):131–142. PubMed PMID: 16493418. Epub 2006/02/24. eng.
20. Moustakas A, Heldin CH. Signaling networks guiding epithelial-mesenchymal transitions during embryogenesis and cancer progression. Cancer Sci. 2007;98(10):1512–1520. PubMed PMID: 17645776. Epub 2007/07/25. eng.
21. Thiery JP, Sleeman JP. Complex networks orchestrate epithelial-mesenchymal transitions. 2006 20060222 DCOM- 20060317(1471-0072 (Print)). eng.
22. Iwatsuki M, Mimori K, Yokobori T, Ishi H, Beppu T, Nakamori S, et al. Epithelial-mesenchymal transition in cancer development and its clinical significance. Cancer Sci. 2010;101(2):293–239. PubMed PMID: 19961486. Epub 2009/12/08. eng.
23. Cardiff R. The Pathology of EMT in Mouse Mammary Tumorigenesis. J Mammary Gland Biol Neoplasia. 2010;15(2):225–33.
24. Tomaskovic-Crook E, Thompson EW, Thiery JP. Epithelial to mesenchymal transition and breast cancer. Breast Cancer Res. 2009;11(6):213. PubMed PMID: 19909494. Epub 2009/11/17. eng.
25. Polyak K, Weinberg RA. Transitions between epithelial and mesenchymal states: acquisition of malignant and stem cell traits. Nat Rev Cancer. 2009;9(4):265–273. PubMed PMID: 19262571. Epub 2009/03/06. eng.
26. Barak V, Goike H, Panaretakis KW, Einarsson R. Clinical utility of cytokeratins as tumor markers. Clin Biochem. 2004;37(7):529–540. PubMed PMID: 15234234. Epub 2004/07/06. eng.

27. Moll R, Divo M, Langbein L. The human keratins: biology and pathology. Histochem Cell Biol. 2008;129(6):705–733. PubMed PMID: 18461349. Epub 2008/05/08. eng.

28. Moll R, Franke WW, Schiller DL, Geiger B, Krepler R. The catalog of human cytokeratins: Patterns of expression in normal epithelia, tumors and cultured cells. Cell. 1982;31(1):11–24.

29. Wu Y, Zhou BP. New insights of epithelial-mesenchymal transition in cancer metastasis. Acta Biochim Biophys Sin (Shanghai). 2008;40(7):643–650. PubMed PMID: 18604456. Epub 2008/07/08. eng.

30. Xue C, Plieth D, Venkov C, Xu C, Neilson EG. The gatekeeper effect of epithelial-mesenchymal transition regulates the frequency of breast cancer metastasis. Cancer Res. 2003;63(12):3386–3394. PubMed PMID: 12810675. Epub 2003/06/18. eng.

31. Tarin D. The fallacy of epithelial mesenchymal transition in neoplasia. Cancer Res. 2005;65(14):5996–6001.

32. Wicki A, Lehembre F, Wick N, Hantusch B, Kerjaschki D, Christofori G. Tumor invasion in the absence of epithelial-mesenchymal transition: podoplanin-mediated remodeling of the actin cytoskeleton. Cancer Cell. 2006;9(4):261–272. PubMed PMID: 16616332. Epub 2006/04/18. eng.

33. Giampieri S, Manning C, Hooper S, Jones L, Hill CS, Sahai E. Localized and reversible TGF[beta] signalling switches breast cancer cells from cohesive to single cell motility. Nat Cell Biol. 2009;11(11):1287–96.

34. Tse JC, Kalluri R. Mechanisms of metastasis: epithelial-to-mesenchymal transition and contribution of tumor microenvironment. J Cell Biochem. 2007;101(4):816–29. PubMed PMID: 17243120. Epub 2007/01/24. eng.

35. Wendt MK, Smith JA, Schiemann WP. Transforming growth factor-beta-induced epithelial-mesenchymal transition facilitates epidermal growth factor-dependent breast cancer progression. Oncogene. 2010;29(49):6485–6498. PubMed PMID: 20802523. Epub 2010/08/31. eng.

36. Yang J, Mani SA, Donaher JL, Ramaswamy S, Itzykson RA, Come C, et al. Twist, a master regulator of morphogenesis, plays an essential role in tumor metastasis. Cell. 2004;117(7):927–939. PubMed PMID: 15210113. Epub 2004/06/24. eng.

37. Lamouille S, Derynck R. Emergence of the phosphoinositide 3-kinase-Akt-mammalian target of rapamycin axis in transforming growth factor-beta-induced epithelial-mesenchymal transition. Cells Tissues Organs. 2011;193(1–2):8–22. PubMed PMID: 21041997. Epub 2010/11/03. eng.

38. Albasri A, Seth R, Jackson D, Benhasouna A, Crook S, Nateri AS, et al. C-terminal Tensin-like (CTEN) is an oncogene which alters cell motility possibly through repression of E-cadherin in colorectal cancer. J Pathol. 2009;218(1):57–65.

39. Moyret-Lalle C, Ruiz E, Puisieux A. Epithelial-mesenchymal transition transcription factors and miRNAs: "Plastic surgeons" of breast cancer. World J Clin Oncol. 2014;5(3):311–322. PubMed PMID: 25114847. Pubmed Central PMCID: PMC4127603. Epub 2014/08/13. eng.

40. Peinado H, Portillo F, Cano A. Transcriptional regulation of cadherins during development and carcinogenesis. Int J Dev Biol. 2004;48(5–6):365–375. PubMed PMID: 15349812. Epub 2004/09/07. eng.

41. Hazan RB, Qiao R, Keren R, Badano I, Suyama K. Cadherin switch in tumor progression. Ann N Y Acad Sci. 2004;1014:155–163. PubMed PMID: 15153430. Epub 2004/05/22. eng.

42. Aleskandarany M, Green A, Rakha E, Powe D, Ellis I. Epithelial mesenchymal transition in invasive breast carcinoma: molecular pathways and relation to molecular subtypes. J Pathol. 2010;222(S1):S1–51.

43. Yoder BJ, Wilkinson EJ, Massoll NA. Molecular and morphologic distinctions between infiltrating ductal and lobular carcinoma of the breast. Breast J. 2007;13(2):172–179. PubMed PMID: 17319859.

44. Mahler-Araujo B, Savage K, Parry S, Reis-Filho JS. Reduction of E-cadherin expression is associated with non-lobular breast carcinomas of basal-like and triple negative phenotype. J Clin Pathol. 2008;61(5):615–20.

45. Sarrio D, Rodriguez-Pinilla SM, Hardisson D, Cano A, Moreno-Bueno G, Palacios J. Epithelial-mesenchymal transition in breast cancer relates to the basal-like phenotype. Cancer Res. 2008;68(4):989–997. PubMed PMID: 18281472. Epub 2008/02/19. eng.
46. Aleskandarany MA, Negm OH, Green AR, Ahmed MA, Nolan CC, Tighe PJ, et al. Epithelial mesenchymal transition in early invasive breast cancer: an immunohistochemical and reverse phase protein array study. Breast Cancer Res Treat. 2014;145(2):339–348. PubMed PMID: 24771047. Epub 2014/04/29. eng.
47. Balkwill FR, Capasso M, Hagemann T. The tumor microenvironment at a glance. J Cell Sci. 2012;125(Pt 23):5591–5596. PubMed PMID: 23420197. Epub 2013/02/20. eng.
48. Kalluri R, Zeisberg M. Fibroblasts in cancer. Nat Rev Cancer. 2006 05//print;6(5):392–401.
49. Drake LE, Macleod KF. Tumour suppressor gene function in carcinoma-associated fibroblasts: from tumour cells via EMT and back again? J Pathol. 2014;232(3):283–8.
50. Kurose K, Gilley K, Matsumoto S, Watson PH, Zhou XP, Eng C. Frequent somatic mutations in PTEN and TP53 are mutually exclusive in the stroma of breast carcinomas. Nature Genet. 2002;32(3):355–357. PubMed PMID: 12379854. Epub 2002/10/16. eng.
51. Phan-Lai V, Florczyk SJ, Kievit FM, Wang K, Gad E, Disis ML, et al. Three-dimensional scaffolds to evaluate tumor associated fibroblast-mediated suppression of breast tumor specific T cells. Biomacromolecules. 2013;14(5):1330–1337. PubMed PMID: 23517456. Pubmed Central PMCID: PMC3664178. Epub 2013/03/23. eng.
52. Wicki A, Lehembre F, Wick N, Hantusch B, Kerjaschki D, Christofori G. Tumor invasion in the absence of epithelial-mesenchymal transition: Podoplanin-mediated remodeling of the actin cytoskeleton. Cancer cell. 2006;9(4):261–272.
53. Fridman WH, Pagès F, Sautès-Fridman C, Galon J. The immune contexture in human tumours: impact on clinical outcome. Nat Rev Cancer. 2012;12(4):298–306.
54. Schoenborn JR, Wilson CB. Regulation of interferon-γ during innate and adaptive immune responses. In: Frederick WA, editor. Advances in immunology 96: Academic Press; 2007. p. 41–101.
55. Hsieh CS, Lee HM, Lio CW. Selection of regulatory T cells in the thymus. Nat Rev Immunol. 2012;12(3):157–167. PubMed PMID: 22322317. Epub 2012/02/11. eng.
56. Jaberipour M, Habibagahi M, Hosseini A, Habibabad SR, Talei A, Ghaderi A. Increased CTLA-4 and FOXP3 transcripts in peripheral blood mononuclear cells of patients with breast cancer. Pathol Oncol Res. 2010;16(4):547–551. PubMed PMID: 20306312. Epub 2010/03/23. eng.
57. Campbell DJ, Koch MA. Treg cells: patrolling a dangerous neighborhood. 2011.
58. Mahmoud SM, Lee AH, Paish EC, Macmillan RD, Ellis IO, Green AR. The prognostic significance of B lymphocytes in invasive carcinoma of the breast. Breast Cancer Res Treat. 2012;132(2):545–553. PubMed PMID: 21671016. Epub 2011/06/15. eng.
59. Andre F, Dieci MV, Dubsky P, Sotiriou C, Curigliano G, Denkert C, et al. Molecular pathways: involvement of immune pathways in the therapeutic response and outcome in breast cancer. Clin Cancer Res. 2013;19(1):28–33. PubMed PMID: 23258741. Epub 2012/12/22. eng.
60. Olkhanud PB, Damdinsuren B, Bodogai M, Gress RE, Sen R, Wejksza K, et al. Tumor-evoked regulatory B cells promote breast cancer metastasis by converting resting CD4+ T cells to T-regulatory cells. Cancer Res. 2011;71(10):3505–15.
61. Joimel U, Gest C, Soria J, Pritchard LL, Alexandre J, Laurent M, et al. Stimulation of angiogenesis resulting from cooperation between macrophages and MDA-MB-231 breast cancer cells: proposed molecular mechanism and effect of tetrathiomolybdate. BMC Cancer. 2010;10:375. PubMed PMID: 20637124. Pubmed Central PMCID: PMC2918575. Epub 2010/07/20. eng.
62. Pollard JW. Macrophages define the invasive microenvironment in breast cancer. J Leukoc Biol. 2008;84(3):623–630. PubMed PMID: 18467655. Pubmed Central PMCID: PMC2516896. Epub 2008/05/10. eng.
63. Cursiefen C, Chen L, Borges LP, Jackson D, Cao J, Radziejewski C, et al. VEGF-A stimulates lymphangiogenesis and hemangiogenesis in inflammatory neovascularization via

macrophage recruitment. J Clin Invest. 2004;113(7):1040–1050. PubMed PMID: 15057311. Pubmed Central PMCID: PMC379325. Epub 2004/04/02. eng.

64. Cheung KJ, Ewald AJ. Illuminating breast cancer invasion: diverse roles for cell–cell interactions. Curr Opin Cell Biol. 2014;30(0):99–111.

65. Cekic C, Day YJ, Sag D, Linden J. Myeloid expression of Adenosine A2A receptor suppresses T and NK cell responses in the solid tumor microenvironment. Cancer Res. 2014. PubMed PMID: 25377469. Epub 2014/11/08. Eng.

66. Kozlowska A, Mackiewicz J, Mackiewicz A. Therapeutic gene modified cell based cancer vaccines. Gene. 2013;525(2):200–207. PubMed PMID: 23566846. Epub 2013/04/10. eng.

67. Lochter A, Bissell MJ. Involvement of extracellular matrix constituents in breast cancer. Semin Cancer Biol. 1995;6(3):165–173.

68. Fu H, Moss J, Shore I, Slade MJ, Coombes RC, Coombes RC. Ultrastructural localization of laminin and type IV collagen in normal human breast. 2002 20020530 DCOM-20021107(0191-3123 (Print)). eng.

69. Lu P, Weaver VM, Werb Z. The extracellular matrix: a dynamic niche in cancer progression. J Cell Biol. 2012;196(4):395–406. PubMed PMID: 22351925. Pubmed Central PMCID: PMC3283993. Epub 2012/02/22. eng.

70. Gehler S, Ponik SM, Riching KM, Keely PJ. Bi-directional signaling: extracellular matrix and integrin regulation of breast tumor progression. Critical reviews in eukaryotic gene expression. 2013;23(2):139–57. PubMed PMID: 23582036. Epub 2013/04/16. eng.

71. Pouliot N, Kusuma N. Laminin-511: a multi-functional adhesion protein regulating cell migration, tumor invasion and metastasis. Cell Adhes Migr. 2013;7(1):142–149. PubMed PMID: 23076212. Pubmed Central PMCID: PMC3544778. Epub 2012/10/19. eng.

72. Gritsenko PG, Ilina O, Friedl P. Interstitial guidance of cancer invasion. J Pathol. 2012;226(2):185–199. PubMed PMID: 22006671. Epub 2011/10/19. eng.

73. Oskarsson T. Extracellular matrix components in breast cancer progression and metastasis. Breast (Edinburgh, Scotland). 2013;22 Suppl 2:S66–72. PubMed PMID: 24074795. Epub 2013/10/01. eng.

74. Rothberg JM, Sameni M, Moin K, Sloane BF. Live-cell imaging of tumor proteolysis: impact of cellular and non-cellular microenvironment. Biochim et Biophys Acta. 2012;1824(1):123–132. PubMed PMID: 21854877. Pubmed Central PMCID: PMC3232330. Epub 2011/08/23. eng.

75. Tang L, Han X. The urokinase plasminogen activator system in breast cancer invasion and metastasis. Biomed Pharmacother. 2013;67(2):179–182. PubMed PMID: 23201006. Epub 2012/12/04. eng.

76. Agrawal AK, Ekonjo GB, Teterycz E, Zyoeko D, Grzebieniak Z, Milan M, et al. Cysteine peptidases and their inhibitors in breast and genital cancer. Folia Histochem et Cytobiologica/Pol Acad Sci Pol Histochem Cytochemical Soc. 2010;48(3):323–327. PubMed PMID: 21071333. Epub 2010/11/13. eng.

77. Dian D, Heublein S, Wiest I, Barthell L, Friese K, Jeschke U. Significance of the tumor protease cathepsin D for the biology of breast cancer. Histol Histopathology. 2014;29(4):433–438. PubMed PMID: 24265119. Epub 2013/11/23. eng.

78. Lebeau A, Nerlich AG, Sauer U, Lichtinghagen R, Lohrs U. Tissue distribution of major matrix metalloproteinases and their transcripts in human breast carcinomas. Anticancer Res. 1999;19(5B):4257–4264. PubMed PMID: 10628384. Epub 2000/01/11. eng.

79. Roy DM, Walsh LA. Candidate prognostic markers in breast cancer: focus on extracellular proteases and their inhibitors. Breast Cancer (Dove Med Press). 2014;6:81–91. PubMed PMID: 25114586. Pubmed Central PMCID: PMC4090043. Epub 2014/08/13. eng.

80. Davies KJ. The complex interaction of matrix metalloproteinases in the migration of cancer cells through breast tissue stroma. Int J Breast Cancer. 2014;2014:839094. PubMed PMID: 24800085. Pubmed Central PMCID: PMC3985306. Epub 2014/05/07. eng.

81. Velinov N, Poptodorov G, Gabrovski N, Gabrovski S. The role of matrixmetalloproteinases in the tumor growth and metastasis. Khirurgiia. 2010 (1):44–49. PubMed PMID: 21972705. Epub 2010/01/01. bul.

82. Friedl P, Wolf K. Proteolytic interstitial cell migration: a five-step process. Cancer Metastasis Rev. 2009;28(1–2):129–135. PubMed PMID: 19153672. Epub 2009/01/21. eng.
83. Stylli SS, Kaye AH, Lock P. Invadopodia: at the cutting edge of tumour invasion. J Clin Neurosci Official J Neurosurg Soc Australas. 2008;15(7):725–737. PubMed PMID: 18468901. Epub 2008/05/13. eng.
84. Davies KJ. Methods of cell propulsion through the local stroma in breast cancer. Int J Breast Cancer. 2014;2014:6.
85. Rakha EA, Martin S, Lee AH, Morgan D, Pharoah PD, Hodi Z, et al. The prognostic significance of lymphovascular invasion in invasive breast carcinoma. Cancer. 2012;118(15):3670–3680. PubMed PMID: 22180017. Epub 2011/12/20. eng.
86. Mohammed RA, Martin SG, Mahmmod AM, Macmillan RD, Green AR, Paish EC, et al. Objective assessment of lymphatic and blood vascular invasion in lymph node-negative breast carcinoma: findings from a large case series with long-term follow-up. J Pathol. 2010 Oct 14. PubMed PMID: 21132836.
87. Gujam FJ, Going JJ, Edwards J, Mohammed ZM, McMillan DC. The role of lymphatic and blood vessel invasion in predicting survival and methods of detection in patients with primary operable breast cancer. Crit Rev Oncol/Hematol. 2014;89(2):231–241. PubMed PMID: 24075309. Epub 2013/10/01. eng.
88. Mohammed RA, Ellis IO, Lee AH, Martin SG. Vascular invasion in breast cancer; an overview of recent prognostic developments and molecular pathophysiological mechanisms. Histopathology. 2009;55(1):1–9.
89. Gujam FJ, Going JJ, Mohammed ZM, Orange C, Edwards J, McMillan DC. Immunohistochemical detection improves the prognostic value of lymphatic and blood vessel invasion in primary ductal breast cancer. BMC Cancer. 2014;14:676. PubMed PMID: 25234410. Pubmed Central PMCID: PMC4177173. Epub 2014/09/23. eng.
90. Stacker SA, Williams SP, Karnezis T, Shayan R, Fox SB, Achen MG. Lymphangiogenesis and lymphatic vessel remodelling in cancer. Nat Rev Cancer. 2014;14(3):159–172.
91. Tammela T, Alitalo K. Lymphangiogenesis: Molecular mechanisms and future promise. Cell. 2010;140(4):460–476. PubMed PMID: 20178740. Epub 2010/02/25. eng.
92. Chung AS, Ferrara N. Developmental and pathological angiogenesis. Annu Rev Cell Dev Biol. 2011;27:563–584. PubMed PMID: 21756109. Epub 2011/07/16. eng.
93. Shayan R, Inder R, Karnezis T, Caesar C, Paavonen K, Ashton MW, et al. Tumor location and nature of lymphatic vessels are key determinants of cancer metastasis. Clin Exp Metastasis. 2013;30(3):345–356. PubMed PMID: 23124573. Epub 2012/11/06. eng.
94. Ji RC. Lymphatic endothelial cells, tumor lymphangiogenesis and metastasis: new insights into intratumoral and peritumoral lymphatics. Cancer Metastasis Rev. 2006;25(4):677–694. PubMed PMID: 17160713. Epub 2006/12/13. eng.
95. Shields JD, Fleury ME, Yong C, Tomei AA, Randolph GJ, Swartz MA. Autologous chemotaxis as a mechanism of tumor cell homing to lymphatics via interstitial flow and autocrine CCR7 signaling. Cancer Cell. 2007;11(6):526–38.
96. Ugras S, Stempel M, Patil S, Morrow M. Estrogen receptor, progesterone receptor, and HER2 status predict lymphovascular invasion and lymph node involvement. Ann Surg Oncol. 2014 2014/11/01;21(12):3780–3786. English.
97. Curtis C, Shah SP, Chin S-F, Turashvili G, Rueda OM, Dunning MJ, et al. The genomic and transcriptomic architecture of 2,000 breast tumours reveals novel subgroups. Nature. 2012;486(7403):346–352.
98. Prat A, Parker JS, Karginova O, Fan C, Livasy C, Herschkowitz JI, et al. Phenotypic and molecular characterization of the claudin-low intrinsic subtype of breast cancer. Breast Cancer Res: BCR. 2010;12(5):R68. PubMed PMID: 20813035. Pubmed Central PMCID: PMC3096954. Epub 2010/09/04. eng.
99. Holm-Rasmussen EV, Jensen MB, Balslev E, Kroman N, Tvedskov TF. Reduced risk of axillary lymphatic spread in triple-negative breast cancer. Breast Cancer Res Treat. 2015;149(1):229–236. PubMed PMID: 25488719. Epub 2014/12/10. eng.

100. Wan L, Pantel K, Kang Y. Tumor metastasis: moving new biological insights into the clinic. Nat Med. 2013;19(11):1450–1464. PubMed PMID: 24202397. Epub 2013/11/10. eng.

101. Douma S, van Laar T, Zevenhoven J, Meuwissen R, van Garderen E, Peeper DS. Suppression of anoikis and induction of metastasis by the neurotrophic receptor TrkB. Nature. 2004;430(7003):1034–1039.

102. Nierodzik ML, Karpatkin S. Thrombin induces tumor growth, metastasis, and angiogenesis: Evidence for a thrombin-regulated dormant tumor phenotype. Cancer Cell. 2006;10(5):355–362. PubMed PMID: 17097558. Epub 2006/11/14. eng.

103. Chao MP, Weissman IL, Majeti R. The CD47-SIRPalpha pathway in cancer immune evasion and potential therapeutic implications. Curr Opin Immunol. 2012;24(2):225–232. PubMed PMID: 22310103. Pubmed Central PMCID: PMC3319521. Epub 2012/02/09. eng.

104. Hiratsuka S, Goel S, Kamoun WS, Maru Y, Fukumura D, Duda DG, et al. Endothelial focal adhesion kinase mediates cancer cell homing to discrete regions of the lungs via E-selectin up-regulation. Proc Natl Acad Sci USA. 2011;108(9):3725–3730. PubMed PMID: 21321210. Pubmed Central PMCID: PMC3048115. Epub 2011/02/16. eng.

105. Bendas G, Borsig L. Cancer cell adhesion and metastasis: selectins, integrins, and the inhibitory potential of heparins. Int J Cell Biol. 2012;2012:676731. PubMed PMID: 22505933. Pubmed Central PMCID: PMC3296185. Epub 2012/04/17. eng.

106. Desgrosellier JS, Cheresh DA. Integrins in cancer: biological implications and therapeutic opportunities. Nat Rev Cancer. 2010;10(1):9–22. PubMed PMID: 20029421. Epub 2009/12/24. eng.

107. Takayama S, Ishii S, Ikeda T, Masamura S, Doi M, Kitajima M. The relationship between bone metastasis from human breast cancer and integrin alpha(v)beta3 expression. Anticancer Res. 2005;25(1A):79–83. PubMed PMID: 15816522. Epub 2005/04/09. eng.

108. Sloan EK, Pouliot N, Stanley KL, Chia J, Moseley JM, Hards DK, et al. Tumor-specific expression of alphavbeta3 integrin promotes spontaneous metastasis of breast cancer to bone. Breast Cancer Res. 2006;8(2):R20. PubMed PMID: 16608535. Pubmed Central PMCID: PMC1557720. Epub 2006/04/13. eng.

109. Guo W, Pylayeva Y, Pepe A, Yoshioka T, Muller WJ, Inghirami G, et al. Beta 4 integrin amplifies ErbB2 signaling to promote mammary tumorigenesis. Cell. 2006;126(3):489–502. PubMed PMID: 16901783. Epub 2006/08/12. eng.

110. Yoon SO, Shin S, Lipscomb EA. A novel mechanism for integrin-mediated ras activation in breast carcinoma cells: the alpha6beta4 integrin regulates ErbB2 translation and trans-activates epidermal growth factor receptor/ErbB2 signaling. Cancer Res. 2006;66(5):2732–2739. PubMed PMID: 16510594. Epub 2006/03/03. eng.

111. Lee YT. Breast carcinoma: pattern of metastasis at autopsy. J Surg Oncol. 1983;23(3):175–180. PubMed PMID: 6345937. Epub 1983/07/01. eng.

112. Lu X, Kang Y. Organotropism of breast cancer metastasis. J Mammary Gland Biol Neoplasia. 2007;12(2–3):153–162. PubMed PMID: 17566854. Epub 2007/06/15. eng.

113. Muller A, Homey B, Soto H, Ge N, Catron D, Buchanan ME, et al. Involvement of chemokine receptors in breast cancer metastasis. Nature. 2001;410(6824):50–56. PubMed PMID: 11242036. Epub 2001/03/10. eng.

114. Mukherjee D, Zhao J. The Role of chemokine receptor CXCR4 in breast cancer metastasis. Am J Cancer Res. 2013;3(1):46–57. PubMed PMID: 23359227 Pubmed Central PMCID: PMC3555200. Epub 2013/01/30. eng.

115. Steeg PS. Tumor metastasis: mechanistic insights and clinical challenges. Nat Med. 2006;12(8):895–904.

116. Kang Y, Siegel PM, Shu W, Drobnjak M, Kakonen SM, Cordon-Cardo C, et al. A multigenic program mediating breast cancer metastasis to bone. Cancer Cell. 2003;3(6):537–549. PubMed PMID: 12842083. Epub 2003/07/05. eng.

117. Guise TA, Mohammad KS, Clines G, Stebbins EG, Wong DH, Higgins LS, et al. Basic Mechanisms Responsible for Osteolytic and Osteoblastic Bone Metastases. Clin Cancer Res. 2006;12(20):6213s–6s.

118. Yin JJ, Pollock CB, Kelly K. Mechanisms of cancer metastasis to the bone. Cell Res. 2005;15(1):57–62.
119. Dallas SL, Rosser JL, Mundy GR, Bonewald LF. Proteolysis of latent transforming growth factor-β (TGF-β)-binding Protein-1 by osteoclasts: a cellular mechanism for release of TGF-β from bone matrix. J Biol Chem. 2002;277(24):21352–60.
120. Brackstone M, Townson J, Chambers A. Tumour dormancy in breast cancer: an update. Breast Cancer Res. 2007;9(3):208. PubMed PMID. doi:10.1186/bcr1677.
121. Wikman H, Vessella R, Pantel K. Cancer micrometastasis and tumour dormancy. APMIS. 2008;116(7–8):754–770. PubMed PMID: 18834417. Epub 2008/10/07. eng.
122. Holmgren L, O'Reilly MS, Folkman J. Dormancy of micrometastases: balanced proliferation and apoptosis in the presence of angiogenesis suppression. Nat Med. 1995;1(2):149–153. PubMed PMID: 7585012. Epub 1995/02/01. eng.
123. Townson JL, Chambers AF. Dormancy of solitary metastatic cells. Cell Cycle. 2006;5(16):1744–1750. PubMed PMID: 16861927. Epub 2006/07/25. eng.
124. Bernards R, Weinberg RA. Metastasis genes: a progression puzzle. Nature. 2002;418(6900):823.
125. Weigelt B, Glas AM, Wessels LF, Witteveen AT, Peterse JL, van't Veer LJ. Gene expression profiles of primary breast tumors maintained in distant metastases. Proc Natl Acad Sci USA. 2003;100(26):15901–15905. PubMed PMID: 14665696.
126. Ma XJ, Salunga R, Tuggle JT, Gaudet J, Enright E, McQuary P, et al. Gene expression profiles of human breast cancer progression. Proc Natl Acad Sci USA. 2003;100(10):5974–9.
127. Weigelt B, van't Veer LJ. Hard-wired genotype in metastatic breast cancer. Cell Cycle. 2004;3(6):756–757. PubMed PMID: 15153810. Epub 2004/05/22. eng.
128. Kennecke H, Yerushalmi R, Woods R, Cheang MC, Voduc D, Speers CH, et al. Metastatic behavior of breast cancer subtypes. J Clin Oncol. 2010;28(20):3271–3277. PubMed PMID: 20498394. Epub 2010/05/26. eng.
129. Rakha EA, Elsheikh SE, Aleskandarany MA, Habashi HO, Green AR, Powe DG, et al. Triple-negative breast cancer: distinguishing between basal and nonbasal subtypes. Clin Cancer Res. 2009;15(7):2302–10.
130. Yaman S, Gumuskaya B, Ozkan C, Aksoy S, Guler G, Altundag K. Lymphatic and capillary invasion patterns in triple negative breast cancer. Am Surg. 2012;78(11):1238–1242. PubMed PMID: 23089442. Epub 2012/10/24. eng.
131. Badve S, Dabbs DJ, Schnitt SJ, Baehner FL, Decker T, Eusebi V, et al. Basal-like and triple-negative breast cancers: a critical review with an emphasis on the implications for pathologists and oncologists. Mod Pathol. 2011;24(2):157–167.
132. Rodenhiser DI, Andrews Jd, Vandenberg TA, Chambers AF. Gene signatures of breast cancer progression and metastasis. Breast Cancer Res. 2011 20111115 DCOM-20140325(1465-542X (Electronic)). eng.
133. van de Vijver MJ, He YD, van't Veer LJ, Dai H, Hart AAM, Voskuil DW, et al. A gene-expression signature as a predictor of survival in breast cancer. N Engl J Med. 2002;347(25):1999–2009. PubMed PMID: ISI:000179874500003.
134. Buyse M, Loi S, van't Veer L, Viale G, Delorenzi M, Glas AM, et al. Validation and clinical utility of a 70-gene prognostic signature for women with node-negative breast cancer. J Natl Cancer Inst. 2006;98(17):1183–1192.
135. Wang Y, Klijn JG, Zhang Y, Sieuwerts AM, Look MP, Yang F, et al. Gene-expression profiles to predict distant metastasis of lymph-node-negative primary breast cancer. Lancet. 2005;365(9460):671–679. PubMed PMID: 15721472.
136. Sotiriou C, Wirapati P, Loi S, Harris A, Fox S, Smeds J, et al. Gene expression profiling in breast cancer: understanding the molecular basis of histologic grade to improve prognosis. J Natl Cancer Inst. 2006;98(4):262–72.
137. Paik S, Shak S, Tang G, Kim C, Baker J, Cronin M, et al. A multigene assay to predict recurrence of tamoxifen-treated, node-negative breast cancer. N Engl J Med. 2004;351(27):2817–26.

138. Sparano JA, Paik S. Development of the 21-gene assay and its application in clinical practice and clinical trials. J Clin Oncol. 2008;26(5):721–8.
139. Ross JS, Hatzis C, Symmans WF, Pusztai L, Hortobagyi GN. Commercialized multigene predictors of clinical outcome for breast cancer. Oncologist. 2008;13(5):477–493. PubMed PMID: 18515733. Epub 2008/06/03. eng.
140. Wirapati P, Sotiriou C, Kunkel S, Farmer P, Pradervand S, Haibe-Kains B, et al. Meta-analysis of gene expression profiles in breast cancer: toward a unified understanding of breast cancer subtyping and prognosis signatures. Breast Cancer Res. 2008;10(4):R65.
141. Haibe-Kains B, Desmedt C, Piette F, Buyse M, Cardoso F, Van't Veer L, et al. Comparison of prognostic gene expression signatures for breast cancer. BMC Genom. 2008;9:394.
142. Mefford D, Mefford J. Stromal genes add prognostic information to proliferation and histo-clinical markers: a basis for the next generation of breast cancer gene signatures. PloS One. 2012;7(6):e37646. PubMed PMID: 22719844. Pubmed Central PMCID: PMC3377707. Epub 2012/06/22. eng.

Chapter 17
The Molecular Pathology of Chemoresistance During the Therapeutic Response in Breast Cancer

James L. Thorne, Andrew M. Hanby and Thomas A. Hughes

Introduction

Chemo-, radio- and/or endocrine therapies are frequently used in combination with surgery to improve patient outcome in breast cancer. Many changes can occur in breast cancer cells in response to these therapies, the most desirable being the induction of apoptosis or death. Unfortunately this is not always the case and other changes may also occur which form part of a resistance phenotype. The response (or lack thereof) to chemotherapy can be quantified histologically [1] but to date there are no systematically reliable molecular markers that augment this analysis post-treatment. Despite this, a number of profiling techniques are being marketed for the likelihood of response in specific tumour subsets such as oncotype [2]. In this review we focus on the specific mechanisms underlying the molecular pathology of chemoresistance rather than these profiling tools.

Diverse responses to chemotherapy between patients reflect the heterogeneity of breast cancer as a group of multiple distinct diseases. A range of molecular responses can be observed for these therapies and this provides a considerable

J.L. Thorne
Department of Mathematical and Physical Sciences (MAPS), School of Food Science
and Nutrition, Woodhouse Lane, University of Leeds, Leeds, West Yorkshire LS2 9JT, UK

A.M. Hanby (✉)
Leeds Institute of Cancer and Pathology (LICAP), St. James University Hospital/
University of Leeds, Beckett Street, Leeds, West Yorkshire LS9 7TF, UK
e-mail: a.m.hanby@leeds.ac.uk

T.A. Hughes
Leeds Institute of Biologial and Clinical Sciences (LIBACS), St. James University Hospital/
University of Leeds, Beckett Street, Leeds, West Yorkshire LS9 7TF, UK

A. Khan et al. (eds.), *Precision Molecular Pathology of Breast Cancer*,
Molecular Pathology Library 10, DOI 10.1007/978-1-4939-2886-6_17

clinical challenge to those endeavouring to tailor the best treatment for individual patients. The biological response and the roles of the Her2 and the hormone nuclear receptors ER and PR have been discussed elsewhere in this book. In this chapter we describe the molecular pathology underlying the response, or lack of it, to conventional chemotherapeutic interventions.

In recent years the continued rise in the use of neoadjuvant chemotherapy (NACT), whereby chemotherapy is given prior to rather than after surgery has provided opportunities to more readily observe response to the regimes used. Researchers and clinicians are able to follow the change in expression of many genes and proteins from before (at core biopsy) and after (at surgical resection) therapy has been administered. In traditional adjuvant chemotherapy, inferences about what molecular pathways may or may not be altered are inherently more speculative due to the lack of available tissue (since this has been removed by surgery). Neoadjuvant therapies are therefore invaluable for researchers to understand mechanisms of resistance.

Mechanisms of Chemoresistance

Mechanisms of chemoresistance have been intensively studied and two broad mechanisms have been proposed. *Acquired* resistance is a reactive process whereby cells become resistant *after* exposure to the agent has caused some level of cellular adaptation to the new environment. Conversely, innate resistance implies that *existing* clonal populations within the tumour already have the required characteristics to survive chemotherapy, and that these are selected for in a Darwinian fashion while their more sensitive counterparts are eliminated by therapy. In actuality these two processes are unlikely to be mutually exclusive and shared phenotypic characteristics such as increased drug efflux and detoxification, evasion of apoptosis and enhanced DNA repair exist. Molecular studies identifying the mechanisms of chemoresistance have been illuminating. It is plausible and likely that heterogeneity between individuals results in differential contributions to resistance from distinct clonal populations. Thus, multiple mechanisms to allow tumour survival after chemotherapeutic insult exist, certainly between individuals but potentially even within individual tumours. It is by definition the clonal populations best equipped to cope or with sufficient plasticity to change, are the ones that are most likely to be the cause of disease recurrence.

A big difference in resistance to chemotherapy is observed between molecular subtypes of breast cancer. The ER negative tumours, which constitute 20–30 % [3] of all cases, are particularly resistant and these patients are more likely to die of their disease and are at increased risk of early recurrence. A ten-year retrospective study indicated that 50 % of hormone receptor negative patients recur within 5 years [4], the majority of these within 2 years [5] and in younger patients rapid recurrence is even more pronounced [6].

The cytotoxins commonly used for the treatment of triple negative breast cancer (TNBC) and the advanced stages of other subtypes are anthracyclines, taxanes and vinca alkaloids. These can all be readily exported from cells by xenobiotic transport pumps and be detoxified. Furthermore, these classes of cytotoxics have even been documented to alter the characteristics and behaviour of the cancer stem-like cell (CSC) population both in primary tumour samples and in cell line models. Cell mediated molecular changes that contribute to resistance are increasingly well documented although therapies targeting them remain underdeveloped.

Detoxification

Enhanced detoxification of chemotherapy agents allows tumours to tolerate higher and higher doses until toxicity in normal tissue is prohibitive. Excellent reviews concerning the process of detoxification can be found (for example [7]) and only a brief description is given here. Metabolism of drugs leads to their detoxification; the anthracycline doxorubicin is metabolized through at least 3 distinct modification routes but approximately 50 % is excreted from the body unaltered. The proportion that is metabolized largely undergoes a two-electron reduction to doxorubicinol via various members of the aldoketoreductase (AKR) family, in a cell type dependent manner. Reflecting this, genetic variation of the *AKR1C3* gene has been linked to doxorubicin pharmacodynamics in breast cancer patients [8]. Anthracyclines may also be modified by the glutathione-S transferase protein and thus labelled for export [9]. Many drugs may be effluxed from the cell before, during and after their metabolism. For example, glutathione (GSH) conjugation alters repertoire of drug transporters that are able to export several compounds including anthracyclines. When doxorubicin is synthetically conjugated to glutathione, it competes with MRP1/ABCC1 specific substrates for export [10]. MRP1 was first identified in cells that had been selected for adriamycin resistance in the presence of a PGP inhibitor [11] and is also overexpressed in cells under selection pressure from epirubicin [12]. Although the ABCC subfamily of ATP-binding cassette proteins are potent GSH-conjugate efflux pumps, the role of MRP1 as a glutathione specific transporter remains unclear. Doxorubicin is exported by this pump both with and without GSH conjugation [13] and whether GSH conjugation of doxorubicin actually occurs in vivo also remains in doubt. Glutathione conjugation of doxorubicin may only be possible under synthetic conditions and not in cell systems [14]. Despite enhanced efflux of doxorubicin from the MRP1 pump when it is conjugated, there is still enhanced cell death associated with this metabolized form of the anthracycline. This appears to be due to potent toxicity to the glutathione-S-transferase pathway [15].

CYP clearance enzymes are induced in the liver by several breast cancer therapy drugs including cisplatin, doxorubicin and etoposide in a p53 dependent manner and is a major route of drug clearance from the body [16]. CYP3A4 is the most abundant CYP is widely induced and inhibited by commonly administered anticancer drugs [17] but studies investigating the induction of CYPs in breast cancer tissue following chemotherapy are lacking. The lack of wild-type p53 in several breast cancer subtypes suggests that CYP induction is not efficient in these cells and may pose a mechanism through which these drugs are more cytotoxic to tumouriogenic p53-null cells than non-transformed cells that retain wild-type protein function. The CYPs also metabolize many other anticancer drugs including cyclophosphamide, 5-FU, etoposide and taxanes, predominantly by CYP3A4 [18]. Paclitaxel induces its own detoxification machinery via the Nuclear Receptor, Pregnane X Receptor (PXR) but docetaxel seems less able to achieve its own detoxification [19]. Doxorubicin reduction by the CYP family member P450R leads to production of the semiquinone radical of doxorubicin which is toxic under hypoxic conditions [20] and P450R levels are predictive of response to doxorubicin [21]. The response to vinca alkaloids is also predicted by P450R levels [22] and it is not surprising therefore that they are also detoxified by CYP3A4. Cell line models overexpressing these two proteins show significant resistance to both vinblastine and vincistrine [22].

Perhaps underlining the importance of detoxification in chemoresistance in breast cancer chemotherapy is a study investigating the molecular changes that occur in a cell line model of ER positive disease [23]. Cyclical chemotherapy was applied to the cells in culture causing multiple population crashes thus modelling clonal selection. Molecular profiling of gene expression revealed detoxification pathways were significantly enriched. The CYP family was activated as were multiple members of the ABC transporter family (described below) and GSTP1, the major glutathione-S transferase factor. Significantly, an eightfold downregulation of ESR1/ER occurred indicating a transition from an ER positive line to a hormone refractive one. Molecular studies such as this clearly have their limitations when attempting to translate conclusions to patients, but they suggest careful therapy choice and dose are required. Full eradication of all tumour cells at first line of therapy is important to prevent regrowth by more aggressive and resistant tumour cells.

ABC Transporters

A major molecular contribution to chemoresistance comes from ATP-binding cassette proteins (ABC), a family of multi-drug resistance proteins. With 49 members, they regulate cellular levels of many compounds including xenobiotics, physiological metabolites and, in the context of cancer treatment, chemotherapeutics. Expression of ABCs can be induced by chemotherapy and several groups have shown ABC expression is linked with poor clinical outcome through mediating chemoresistance [24–27]. However, a consistent pattern of ABC expression has not been associated with recurrence, a fact that may relate in part to the high degree of functional redundancy within the superfamily. Doxorubicin for example is exported by ABCB1, ABCC1, 2, 3, 7 and ABCG2, whilst Daunorubicin and Epirubicin are substrates of at least 4 members of ABC-subfamily ABCC [28].

This issue of redundancy requires attention and can only be addressed through examining the network characteristics of multiple transporters simultaneously. Such coordinated studies examining ABC transporters have been conducted in neuroblastoma [29] and normal hematopoietic stem cells [30] but breast cancer and the context of chemoresistance remain relatively unexplored. Some studies have looked at the response of more than one ABC simultaneously to NAC and have directly compared pre- and post-chemotherapy samples but none have utilized bioinformatics approaches to determine the contribution of redundancy in their systems. In a study examining three of the most relevant ABCs in breast cancer chemoresistance, Kim et al. [25] observed induction of both PGP/ABCB1 and MRP1/ABCC1 in a cohort of patients treated with EC. Only a non-significant trend between induction of protein expression in resection samples and recurrence was observed. Changes in BCRP/ABCG2 expression were also seen but were variable. Crucially, however, expression of BCRP after exposure to epirubicin/cyclophosphamide correlated to disease-free survival. Another study of breast cancer patients undergoing NAC examined the levels of multiple MDR mRNAs. Of those studied, ABCB1, ABCC2 and ABGG1 were found to be significant prognostic markers of disease-free survival [26]. Again, these data were not subject to network analysis and conclusions as to redundancy within this superfamily could not be made.

The taxanes are substrates of several key ABC transporters; both paclitaxel and docetaxel are substrates for ABCB1, ABCC1, 2 and ABCG2 (reviewed in [31]). Taxanes induce expression of ABC transporters in breast tumour tissue and the PXR is documented to mediate this induction [32]. Furthermore, ABCB1 polymorphisms are thought to correlate with disease-free survival in breast cancer patients after taxane therapy [33]. A concern in the clinical setting is that resistance to taxanes caused by induction of these factors may also lead to cross-resistance to anthracyclines.

Predicting which ABC transporters are involved in chemoresistance is difficult due to their substrate overlap but their relevance to chemoresistance remains clear. They are also important in the context of stem-cell biology as they confer some of the defining characteristics of these cells.

Stem Cells

Cancer Stem Cells (CSCs) are increasingly considered a viable source of tumour regrowth after apparent eradication of the primary lesion through surgery and radio or chemotherapy. Through asymmetrical division they self renew and give rise to rapidly proliferating and differentiated daughter cells. The mechanism of their formation is far from established and several hypotheses have been proposed to explain their existence. Firstly, oncogenic transformation of normal multipotent stem cells may allow the usually benign compartment to lose checkpoints and controls for apoptosis, cell division and metabolism, and asymmetrical division ensues giving rise to rapidly dividing tumour cells and new CSCs which retain the oncogenic properties. Alternatively, they may be formed from normal cancer cells that have acquired a substantial genetic and epigenetic mutational load. Such cells re-acquire multipotent characteristics lost during asymmetric division of the original stem cell. Recent studies have indicated that stress signals can reprogram differentiated tumour cells to undergo epithelial–mesenchymal transition and acquiring traits of mesenchymal cells that confer stem-cell like qualities. CSCs have altered metabolic and proliferative potential with enhanced glycolytic flux and lower Ki67 indices. CSCs are a major target for novel therapeutics due to the proposition that they can survive chemotherapy and reinitiate tumours; however, they also have multiple features that render them more chemoresistant than normal cells.

These phenotypes of CSCs make their isolation challenging; quiescence means true expansion in vitro is impossible and their isolation by Fluorescence activated cell sorting (FACS) is capricious. At least five combinations of cell-surface markers have been used for FACS to isolate cells with CSC hallmarks in breast cancer alone [30, 34–37]. ALDH1 for example has been used to identify breast cancer stem cells in combination with other markers and patients with a significant surviving population of ALDH1+ tumour cells after receiving anthracycline in combination with cyclophosphamide have a poor disease-free prognosis [38]. Mechanistically this may be explained by the observation that cyclophosphamide can be detoxified via aldehyde dehydrogenase isoforms ALDH1A1 and ALDH3A1 [39] and elevated ALDH1 gene expression is associated with cyclophosphamide resistance [40].

ABC transporters are also important in CSC biology as they mediate drug resistance in multiple stem-cell types [41] and their expression correlates with several hallmarks of CSCs, they may even confer some of these features. ABCG2/BCRP for example appears to maintain a stem-like state [42], and is a marker of stem cells in multiple organs [30] and could be sufficient for chemoresistance in CSCs [43]. Furthermore, in many tissues, including breast, ABCG2 defines a FACS plot side-population (SP) [44] which exhibits CSC hallmarks such as enhanced self-renewal in colony forming [45] and xenograft assays [37], low proliferation rates and asymmetric division [45, 46]. ABCG2 is regulated by AKT in many cell types including CSCs and this is discussed in detail below.

Of concern is the mounting evidence that chemotherapy may select for cells with CSC qualities. For example, after exposure to doxorubicin the proportion of cancer stem cells (defined as CD44+/CD24−) is increased in breast tumours [38] but surprisingly perhaps not after exposure to epirubicin [47]. Both studies indicated that tumours with a higher proportion of CD44+/CD24− cells were more likely to relapse with distal metastasis. Molecular evidence indicates that CSCs tolerate ROS build up from aerobic glycolysis well and actively maintain low levels [48] which may allow them to escape the damage created by anthracyclines through this mechanism.

Significantly, differentiated tumour cells lacking CSC surface markers may de-differentiate through epithelial–mesenchymal transition (EMT) and reseed tumours [49], particularly in ER− disease [50]. Novel clinical approaches must therefore be developed to tackle all subtypes of CSC and *any* tumour cell surviving chemotherapy capable of de-differentiation [51]. TGFβ signalling, which enhances stem-like properties of breast tumour cells and regulates the EMT [52], is enhanced by paclitaxel during NACT in human breast tumours [53]. Antagonising TGFβ signalling prevents CSC signalling pathways in TNBC cell lines and abrogates tumour regrowth in mouse xenografts after an initial round of paclitaxel treatment [53]. The potential to fortify the stem cell compartment through chemotherapy is clearly an issue and requires further attention by researchers.

Apoptosis

Apoptosis or programmed cell death is the mechanism through which unnecessary cells are disposed of by the body due to normal tissue homeostasis. Potentiated through cell-extrinsic cues such as Fas Ligand or cell-intrinsic pathways such as p53 activation, apoptosis is responsible for maintaining cell numbers and tissue integrity and eradicating cells with excessive mutational loads. The Bcl and Bax/Bad protein families compete for control of mitochondrial membrane integrity which if compromised (from Bax/Bad) results in cytochrome c flooding of the cytoplasm and induction of caspase dependent cell death.

Caspases are themselves regulated by, and mediate the effects of, different chemotherapeutics. Doxorubicin induces caspase-3 activation [54] but its apoptotic effect is also under the control of the caspase-8 inhibitory protein c-FLIP. C-FLIP inhibition either by IFN-γ or experimental modulation results in exacerbated apoptosis in a cell line model of TNBC after exposure to the anthracycline [55]. In the first study of apoptosis comparing pre- and post-NACT, a significant increase in the number of apoptotic nuclei was observed in histopathological examination [56]. Since then numerous studies have indicated the importance of apoptosis in the tumour response to chemotherapy. For example, pathological examination of tumour biopsies at just 48 h post docetaxel/doxorubicin treatment revealed a significant induction of apoptosis markers and down regulation of anti-apoptotic Bcl-2. Tumours with the biggest increases in apoptotic index (AI) and greatest loss of Bcl-2 predicted pathological complete response at surgical resection [57]. The usefulness of Bcl-2 as a marker is not straightforward however; Tiezzi et al. [58] found that AI but not Bcl-2 is correlated with clinical response. Bcl-2 regulation by ER and estrogen also appears significant. When adriamycin is applied to breast cancer cells, the presence of estrogen inhibits the apoptotic potential of the anthracycline. This is mediated by ER control of Bcl-2 expression which when experimentally elevated abrogates this apoptotic effect even in the absence of estrogen [59]. Estradiol has been reported to only regulate Bcl-2 in ER positive but not in ER negative backgrounds [60]. Further underlining the anti-apoptotic role of estrogen signalling in breast cancer is the observation that Selective Estrogen Receptor Modulators (SERM) such as tamoxifen also alter Bcl-2 and other apoptotic and proliferation markers [61].

In an intriguing level of complexity during the interaction between ER and p53 has been explored. Treatment of the p53 wild-type MCF7 cells with doxorubicin results in p53 activation, caspase-3 activation and DNA fragmentation [62]. In non-tumourigenic MCF10A cells also harbouring wild-type p53, apoptosis was not induced after exposure to doxorubicin unless Her2 was overexpressed, thus conferring an extra step in oncogenic transformation to the cells [63]. The observation that ER positive tumours are typically WT for p53 is in stark contrast to ER negative tumours which generally show loss of p53 function [64]. This significant molecular difference manifests with important pathological differences between these two subtypes. Resistance to chemotherapy-induced apoptosis in ER+ tumours in the presence of estrogen is significant and supports the observations that pathological complete response is relatively rare in ER positive tumours compared to ER negative ones. Instead of these tumours undergoing apoptosis it is likely that they instead enter senescence and studies utilizing senescence markers such as beta-galactosidase would be of value to determine if this is indeed the case. The Aromatase Inhibitor, Anastrazole was found to have a significantly greater impact than tamoxifen on reducing the proliferative marker Ki67 in cohort of neoadjuvant endocrine therapy patients [65]. Reduction in proliferation in both anastrozole and tamoxifen groups was seen to correlate with clinical outcomes. Ki67 repressed by FAC is also significantly associated with prognosis in those patients not achieving pCR after NACT [66] further stratifying the molecular response in terms of patient outcomes and prognostic indicators.

At the molecular level ER/p53 interactions have also been investigated. Whilst the SERM tamoxifen, promotes p53 antagonism in a similar manner to estrogen, fulvestrant, a full ER antagonist, completely abolishes bypass of p53-mediated apoptosis in breast cancer cells [64] resulting in significant cell death. ER has also been shown to bind to p53 directly at target gene loci and prevent p53-mediated repression of the survivin (inhibitor of apoptosis) and PGP/ABCB1 genes [67]. Mutant p53 predicts disease resistance to doxorubicin chemotherapy in breast cancer patients [68], but this appears drug- or mutation-dependent as studies linking p53 status with resistance to cyclophosphamide, 5′-FL, methotrexate, prednisone [69], or even tamoxifen [70] did not show any clear evidence of p53 involvement. Not only does estrogen signalling promote cell survival but significant evidence exists to show that ER positive breast cancer cells are fully dependent on ER signalling for survival. Anti-estrogens induce apoptosis in breast tumours as does removal of estrogen from cell lines.

The modulation of ER gene regulatory circuits can be modified by multiple other factors [71–74]. Of particular interest is the observation that doxorubicin and estrogen treated cells show substantial overlap in activation of transcriptional targets [75]. Estrogen signalling prevents full activation of the gene profile that would usually be induced by some chemotherapy agents. This altering of response to chemotherapy by estrogen is another explanation as to why ER positive tumours are less likely to achieve a pCR and also why combinations of anti-estrogens and cytotoxics are highly effective.

Notch Signalling

A major corollary of chemotherapy is the activation of many signalling pathways, some of which can be potently oncogenic. Two of these pathways, Notch and AKT are described here. Notch signalling is a key regulator of cell-fate decisions during differentiation of progenitor cells in development and in self-renewal of adult stem cells, acting mainly to promote proliferation and prevent differentiation [76]. Notch proteins, of which there are 4 (Notch-1 to 4), are transmembrane receptors. They bind as heterodimers to Delta or Jagged ligands that are typically expressed on the surface of neighbouring cells. This receptor/ligand interaction leads to cleavage of Notch by γ-secretase, which releases the Notch intra-cellular domain, Notch^{IC}, from the transmembrane portion. Notch^{IC} translocates to the nucleus where it induces gene transcription by de-repressing the CSL complex (CBF-1/RBP-Jκ, Su(H), Lag-1) which is bound within promoters of target genes.

Evidence supports roles for uncontrolled Notch activity in breast carcinogenesis [77]. Notch over-expression or constitutive activity leads to tumour formation in mouse models [78, 79] while elevated Notch-1 and Jagged-1 expression correlate with poor prognosis in clinical breast cancers [80, 81]. Therefore, Notch has been recognized as a cancer drug target and γ-secretase inhibitors (GSIs) have been developed that prevent Notch activation. These appear promising for breast cancer therapy as they induce cell death in breast cancer cells and may specifically target breast CSCs [82]. However, GSIs are toxic in long-term monotherapy and may be better suited to short-term or combination therapies; breast cancer clinical trials using GSIs are now taking place [83]. Recent data point to a role for Notch in chemotherapy resistance. Notch signalling was identified as a key pathway significantly induced in breast tumours by Gonzalez-Angulo et al. [84]. Also, in breast cancer cell lines Notch has been shown to activate expression of MRP1 [85]. MRP1 expression is inversely correlated to survival of breast cancer patients [86]. It is also of interest to note that Notch-1 has been linked with resistance to other chemotherapy drugs including the taxanes paclitaxel [87] and docetaxel [88]. This resistance appears to occur through strengthening the CSC compartment by increasing the proportion of CD44^{+}/CD24^{-} cells. This is important to bear in mind as oncologists will often switch from anthracyclines to taxanes when inadequate tumour response is observed during the interval MRI scans. Initial treatment with an anthracycline such as Doxorubicin or Epirubicin may therefore induce Notch-1 signalling and generate a tenacious CSC population that is resistant to taxane therapy. Notch-1 dampening by γ-secretase inhibitors prior to the commencement of chemotherapy may therefore play several useful roles in clinic. Such a regimen would both prevent high pre-NAC MRP1 levels associated with poor clinical outcome and sensitize the CD44^{+}/CD24^{-} CSC compartment.

AKT Signalling

AKT regulates several cellular pathways key to tumourigenic progression such as proliferation, apoptosis and glucose metabolism through its kinase activity. In breast cancer cell lines and tumour biopsies AKT regulation has been extensively studied. Its activity is generally elevated in breast cancer tissue and cell lines and this hyperactivity can be exacerbated by cell-intrinsic moieties such as Her2, PI3K [89] or loss of PTEN [90]. Treatment with chemotherapeutic drugs such as cisplatin [91], daunorubicin [92], doxorubicin, trastuzumab, tamoxifen [93] and paclitaxel [94] all activate AKT signalling in breast cancer. Elevated AKT activity has multiple roles in resistance but all utilize its potent ability to phosphorylate targets. Its role in preventing apoptosis is perhaps the most established. AKT targets proapoptotic Bcl-2 family members for phosphorylation thus impairing their ability to destabilize the mitochondrial membrane and limiting cytochrome c release [95–97]. Her2 enhances MDM2 mediated proteosomal degradation of p53 via AKT signalling, [98] thus further impairing apoptosis/senescence in ER positive tumours that contain functional p53.

AKT regulates expression and cellular distribution of several ABC transporters. For example, AKT stimulates NF-kB signalling which in turn induces expression of PGP [99]. PI3K inhibitors prevent the association of BCRP with the plasma membrane, as does transfection of a dominant negative AKT. If exogenous EGFR is applied in the presence of dominant negative AKT, BCRP expression is restored [100]. Loss of AKT in knock-out mice leads to a drastic reduction in the ABCG2/BCRP dependent SP fraction in bone marrow [101] further supporting its regulation of BCRP. Her2 expression in luminal breast cancer patients directly correlates to proportion of cells in the SP fraction and experimental manipulation of AKT abolished the SP fraction in cells isolated from these patients [102]. In other tumour types, PTEN loss results in elevated SP fraction and this can be abrogated through application of the PI3K inhibitor LY294002 [103].

Future Directions

Several areas of research into chemotherapy-induced mechanisms of chemoresistance are incomplete and vital information could be yielded with the proper experimental designs. For example, although many studies have examined the individual ABC transporters, or even 3 at a time, they have not addressed the conundrum that elevated expression of only one of a relevant ABC transporter may be sufficient to confer chemoresistance. In a heterogeneous population it may be that high basal expression of one pump may confer resistance in one individual but stabilization of mRNA (or protein) from an alternative transporter may suffice in another. Encompassing studies examining multiple pumps simultaneously following exposure to chemotherapeutics would begin to address this issue. This approach may also lead to the identification of common regulatory mechanisms that may be targetable through novel drug design.

There is a similar gap in understanding of the regulation of drug detoxification pathways. The increasing use of NAC however allows researchers unique opportunities to measure a baseline level of expression of pre-NAC at core biopsy, compare this with post-NAC in the resected tumour material and correlate these observations to tumour response and clinical outcome. These resources should be utilised to the fullest extent as it will also illuminate the molecular mechanisms at play in adjuvant chemotherapy which remain almost completely unexplored at the molecular level in human subjects.

The variation and clonality within a tumour provides a significant substrate on which selection can act. Indeed, the process of tumour outgrowth has been likened to Darwinian selection, where the clonal population most suited to the environment is more likely to survive and prosper. In aggressive TNBC tumours such a selection pressure may kill the less aggressive clones and allow the strongest competitors to take-over. This is of particular interest with the identification of breast cancer stem cells. Tailoring of drugs to ER negative patients that target the stem-like cell populations is a priority and these patients still have the poorest prognosis and the highest relapse rates.

At a practical, molecular pathology level, despite the multiple pathways detailed above relevant to chemoresistance, there are as yet no novel molecular markers in the pipeline that are likely to be used in routine practice to predict chemoresistance. With the rise in NACT and the facility to observe response directly in serial biopsies, this would seem likely to change.

Key Points

- Chemoresistance may be innate or acquired
- Tumour chemoresistance can arise from enhanced detoxification by CYP proteins and/or efflux by the ABC transporters
- Evolution of tumour resistance occurs in a Darwinian type fashion
- Cancer stems cells can increase in proportion after treatment with chemotherapeutic agents
- Non-CSCs may be able to undergo the epithelial–mesenchymal transition, dedifferentiate and reseed tumour growth, potentially as a response to chemotherapy
- The large family of ABC efflux pumps share many substrates and display functional redundancy
- CYP3A4 is the main metabolizing enzyme of many front line chemotherapy agents
- ABCB1, ABCC1 and ABCG2 are key efflux pumps of chemotherapeutics

References

1. Alvarado-Cabrero I, Alderete-Vazquez G, Quintal-Ramirez M, Patino M, Ruiz E. Incidence of pathologic complete response in women treated with preoperative chemotherapy for locally advanced breast cancer: correlation of histology, hormone receptor status, Her2/Neu, and gross pathologic findings. Ann Diagn Pathol. 2009;13(3):151–7.
2. Pinder SE, Provenzano E, Earl H, Ellis IO. Laboratory handling and histology reporting of breast specimens from patients who have received neoadjuvant chemotherapy. Histopathology. 2007;50(4):409–17.
3. Garcia-Closas M, Couch FJ, Lindstrom S, et al. Genome-wide association studies identify four ER negative-specific breast cancer risk loci. Nat Genet 2013;45(4):392–8, 398e1–2.
4. Dent R, Trudeau M, Pritchard KI, Hanna WM, Kahn HK, Sawka CA, Lickley LA, Rawlinson E, Sun P, Narod SA. Triple-negative breast cancer: clinical features and patterns of recurrence. Clin Cancer Res. 2007;13(15 Pt 1):4429–34.
5. Chang J, Clark GM, Allred DC, Mohsin S, Chamness G, Elledge RM. Survival of patients with metastatic breast carcinoma: importance of prognostic markers of the primary tumor. Cancer. 2003;97(3):545–53.
6. Copson E, Eccles B, Maishman T, Gerty S, Stanton L, Cutress RI, Altman DG, Durcan L, Simmonds P, Lawrence G, Jones L, Bliss J, Eccles D. Prospective observational study of breast cancer treatment outcomes for UK women aged 18–40 years at diagnosis: the POSH study. J Natl Cancer Inst. 2013;105(13):978–88.
7. Xu C, Li CY, Kong AN. Induction of phase I, II and III drug metabolism/transport by xenobiotics. Arch Pharmacal Res. 2005;28(3):249–68.
8. Voon PJ, Yap HL, Ma CY, Lu F, Wong AL, Sapari NS, Soong R, Soh TI, Goh BC, Lee HS, Lee SC. Correlation of aldo-ketoreductase (AKR) 1C3 genetic variant with doxorubicin pharmacodynamics in Asian breast cancer patients. Br J Clin Pharmacol. 2013;75(6):1497–505.
9. Serafino A, Sinibaldi-Vallebona P, Gaudiano G, Koch TH, Rasi G, Garaci E, Ravagnan G. Cytoplasmic localization of anthracycline antitumor drugs conjugated with reduced glutathione: a possible correlation with multidrug resistance mechanisms. Anticancer Res. 1998;18(2A):1159–66.
10. Priebe W, Krawczyk M, Kuo MT, Yamane Y, Savaraj N, Ishikawa T. Doxorubicin- and daunorubicin-glutathione conjugates, but not unconjugated drugs, competitively inhibit leukotriene C-4 transport mediated by MRP/GS-X pump. Biochem Bioph Res Co. 1998;247(3):859–63.
11. Mirski SE, Gerlach JH, Cole SP. Multidrug resistance in a human small cell lung cancer cell line selected in adriamycin. Cancer Res. 1987;47(10):2594–8.
12. Davey RA, Longhurst TJ, Davey MW, Belov L, Harvie RM, Hancox D, Wheeler H. Drug resistance mechanisms and MRP expression in response to epirubicin treatment in a human leukaemia cell line. Leuk Res. 1995;19(4):275–82.
13. Munoz M, Henderson M, Haber M, Norris M. Role of the MRP1/ABCC1 multidrug transporter protein in cancer. IUBMB Life. 2007;59(12):752–7.
14. Gaudiano G, Koch TH, Lo Bello M, Nuccetelli M, Ravagnan G, Serafino A, Sinibaldi-Vallebona P. Lack of glutathione conjugation to adriamycin in human breast cancer MCF-7/DOX cells—inhibition of glutathione S-transferase P1-1 by glutathione conjugates from anthracyclines. Biochem Pharmacol. 2000;60(12):1915–23.
15. Asakura T, Ohkawa K, Takahashi N, Takada K, Inoue T, Yokoyama S. Glutathione-doxorubicin conjugate expresses potent cytotoxicity by suppression of glutathione S-transferase activity: comparison between doxorubicin-sensitive and -resistant rat hepatoma cells. Brit J Cancer. 1997;76(10):1333–7.
16. Goldstein I, Rivlin N, Shoshana OY, Ezra O, Madar S, Goldfinger N, Rotter V. Chemotherapeutic agents induce the expression and activity of their clearing enzyme CYP3A4 by activating p53. Carcinogenesis. 2013;34(1):190–8.

17. Dees EC, Watkins PB. Role of cytochrome P450 phenotyping in cancer treatment. J Clin Oncol. 2005;23(6):1053–5 (official journal of the American Society of Clinical Oncology).
18. Zhang D, Ly VT, Lago M, Tian Y, Gan J, Humphreys WG, Comezoglu SN. CYP3A4-mediated ester cleavage as the major metabolic pathway of the oral taxane 3′-tert-butyl-3′-N-tert-butyloxycarbonyl-4-deacetyl-3′-dephenyl-3′-N-debenzoyl-4-O-methoxycarbonyl-paclitaxel (BMS-275183). Drug Metab Dispos. 2009;37(4):710–8.
19. Harmsen S, Meijerman I, Beijnen JH, Schellens JH. Nuclear receptor mediated induction of cytochrome P450 3A4 by anticancer drugs: a key role for the pregnane X receptor. Cancer Chemother Pharmacol. 2009;64(1):35–43.
20. Riddick DS, Lee C, Ramji S, Chinje EC, Cowen RL, Williams KJ, Patterson AV, Stratford IJ, Morrow CS, Townsend AJ, Jounaidi Y, Chen CS, Su T, Lu H, Schwartz PS, Waxman DJ. Cancer chemotherapy and drug metabolism. Drug Metab Dispos. 2005;33(8):1083–96.
21. Buschini A, Poli P, Rossi C. Saccharomyces cerevisiae as an eukaryotic cell model to assess cytotoxicity and genotoxicity of three anticancer anthraquinones. Mutagenesis. 2003;18(1):25–36.
22. Yao D, Ding S, Burchell B, Wolf CR, Friedberg T. Detoxication of vinca alkaloids by human P450 CYP3A4-mediated metabolism: implications for the development of drug resistance. J Pharmacol Exp Ther. 2000;294(1):387–95.
23. AbuHammad S, Zihlif M. Gene expression alterations in doxorubicin resistant MCF7 breast cancer cell line. Genomics. 2013;101(4):213–20.
24. Choi CH. ABC transporters as multidrug resistance mechanisms and the development of chemosensitizers for their reversal. Cancer Cell Int. 2005;5:30.
25. Kim B, Fatayer H, Hanby AM, Horgan K, Perry SL, Valleley EM, Verghese ET, Williams BJ, Thorne JL, Hughes TA. Neoadjuvant chemotherapy induces expression levels of breast cancer resistance protein that predict disease-free survival in breast cancer. PLoS ONE. 2013;8(5):e62766.
26. Litviakov NV, Garbukov E, Slonimskaia EM, Tsyganov MM, Denisov EV, Vtorushin SV, Khristenko K, Zav'ialova MV, Cherdyntseva NV. Correlation of metastasis-free survival in patients with breast cancer and changes in the direction of expression of multidrug resistance genes during neoadjuvant chemotherapy. Vopr Onkol. 2013;59(3):334–40.
27. Maciejczyk A, Szelachowska J, Ekiert M, Matkowski R, Halon A, Surowiak P. Analysis of BCRP expression in breast cancer patients. Ginekol Pol. 2012;83(9):681–7.
28. Jaeger W. Classical resistance mechanisms. Int J Clin Pharmacol Ther. 2009;47(1):46–8.
29. Porro A, Haber M, Diolaiti D, et al. Direct and coordinate regulation of ATP-binding cassette transporter genes by Myc factors generates specific transcription signatures that significantly affect the chemoresistance phenotype of cancer cells. J Biol Chem. 2010;285(25):19532–43.
30. Fatima S, Zhou S, Sorrentino BP. Abcg2 expression marks tissue-specific stem cells in multiple organs in a mouse progeny tracking model. Stem Cells. 2012;30(2):210–21.
31. Oshiro C, Marsh S, McLeod H, Carrillo MW, Klein T, Altman R. Taxane pathway. Pharmacogenet Genomics. 2009;19(12):979–83.
32. Masuyama H, Suwaki N, Tateishi Y, Nakatsukasa H, Segawa T, Hiramatsu Y. The pregnane X receptor regulates gene expression in a ligand- and promoter-selective fashion. Mol Endocrinol. 2005;19(5):1170–80.
33. Chang H, Rha SY, Jeung HC, Im CK, Ahn JB, Kwon WS, Yoo NC, Roh JK, Chung HC. Association of the ABCB1 gene polymorphisms 2677G> T/A and 3435C> T with clinical outcomes of paclitaxel monotherapy in metastatic breast cancer patients. Ann Oncol. 2009;20(2):272–7 (official journal of the European Society for Medical Oncology/ESMO).
34. Al-Hajj M, Wicha MS, Benito-Hernandez A, Morrison SJ, Clarke MF. Prospective identification of tumorigenic breast cancer cells. Proc Natl Acad Sci U S A. 2003;100(7):3983–8.
35. Croker AK, Goodale D, Chu J, Postenka C, Hedley BD, Hess DA, Allan AL. High aldehyde dehydrogenase and expression of cancer stem cell markers selects for breast cancer cells with enhanced malignant and metastatic ability. J Cell Mol Med. 2009;13(8B):2236–52.

36. Ginestier C, Hur MH, Charafe-Jauffret E, et al. ALDH1 is a marker of normal and malignant human mammary stem cells and a predictor of poor clinical outcome. Cell Stem Cell. 2007;1(5):555–67.
37. Patrawala L, Calhoun T, Schneider-Broussard R, Zhou J, Claypool K, Tang DG. Side population is enriched in tumorigenic, stem-like cancer cells, whereas ABCG2+ and ABCG2− cancer cells are similarly tumorigenic. Cancer Res. 2005;65(14):6207–19.
38. Lee HE, Kim JH, Kim YJ, Choi SY, Kim SW, Kang E, Chung IY, Kim IA, Kim EJ, Choi Y, Ryu HS, Park SY. An increase in cancer stem cell population after primary systemic therapy is a poor prognostic factor in breast cancer. Brit J Cancer. 2011;104(11):1730–8.
39. Rivera E. Implications of anthracycline-resistant and taxane-resistant metastatic breast cancer and new therapeutic options. Breast J. 2010;16(3):252–63.
40. Magni M, Shammah S, Schiro R, Mellado W, Dalla-Favera R, Gianni AM. Induction of cyclophosphamide-resistance by aldehyde-dehydrogenase gene transfer. Blood. 1996;87(3):1097–103.
41. Tang L, Bergevoet SM, Gilissen C, de Witte T, Jansen JH, van der Reijden BA, Raymakers RA. Hematopoietic stem cells exhibit a specific ABC transporter gene expression profile clearly distinct from other stem cells. BMC Pharmacol. 2010;10:12.
42. Ding XW, Wu JH, Jiang CP. ABCG2: a potential marker of stem cells and novel target in stem cell and cancer therapy. Life Sci. 2010;86(17–18):631–7.
43. An Y, Ongkeko WM. ABCG2: the key to chemoresistance in cancer stem cells? Expert Opin Drug Metab Toxicol. 2009;5(12):1529–42.
44. Zhou S, Schuetz JD, Bunting KD, Colapietro AM, et al. The ABC transporter Bcrp1/ABCG2 is expressed in a wide variety of stem cells and is a molecular determinant of the side-population phenotype. Nat Med. 2001;7(9):1028–34.
45. Hirschmann-Jax C, Foster AE, Wulf GG, Nuchtern JG, Jax TW, Gobel U, Goodell MA, Brenner MK. A distinct "side population" of cells with high drug efflux capacity in human tumor cells. Proc Natl Acad Sci U S A. 2004;101(39):14228–33.
46. Zen Y, Fujii T, Yoshikawa S, Takamura H, Tani T, Ohta T, Nakanuma Y. Histological and culture studies with respect to ABCG2 expression support the existence of a cancer cell hierarchy in human hepatocellular carcinoma. Am J Pathol. 2007;170(5):1750–62.
47. Aulmann S, Waldburger N, Penzel R, Andrulis M, Schirmacher P, Sinn HP. Reduction of CD44(+)/CD24(−) breast cancer cells by conventional cytotoxic chemotherapy. Hum Pathol. 2010;41(4):574–81.
48. Kobayashi CI, Suda T. Regulation of reactive oxygen species in stem cells and cancer stem cells. J Cell Physiol. 2012;227(2):421–30.
49. Polyak K, Weinberg RA. Transitions between epithelial and mesenchymal states: acquisition of malignant and stem cell traits. Nat Rev Cancer. 2009;4:265–73.
50. Chaffer CL, Marjanovic ND, Lee T, Bell G, Kleer CG, Reinhardt F, D'Alessio AC, Young RA, Weinberg RA. Poised chromatin at the ZEB1 promoter enables breast cancer cell plasticity and enhances tumorigenicity. Cell. 2013;154(1):61–74.
51. Smalley M, Piggott L, Clarkson R. Breast cancer stem cells: obstacles to therapy. Cancer Lett. 2013;338(1):57–62.
52. Moustakas A, Heldin CH. Signaling networks guiding epithelial-mesenchymal transitions during embryogenesis and cancer progression. Cancer Sci. 2007;98(10):1512–20.
53. Bhola NE, Balko JM, Dugger TC, Kuba MG, Sanchez V, Sanders M, Stanford J, Cook RS, Arteaga CL. TGF-beta inhibition enhances chemotherapy action against triple-negative breast cancer. J Clin Investig. 2013;123(3):1348–58.
54. Wang FY, Arisawa T, Tahara T, Takahama K, Watanabe M, Hirata I, Nakano H. Aberrant DNA methylation in ulcerative colitis without neoplasia. Hepatogastroenterology. 2008;55(81):62–5.
55. Rogers KM, Thomas M, Galligan L, Wilson TR, Allen WL, Sakai H, Johnston PG, Longley DB. Cellular FLICE-inhibitory protein regulates chemotherapy-induced apoptosis in breast cancer cells. Mol Cancer Ther. 2007;6(5):1544–51.

56. Ellis PA, Smith IE, McCarthy K, Detre S, Salter J, Dowsett M. Preoperative chemotherapy induces apoptosis in early breast cancer. Lancet. 1997;349(9055):849.
57. Buchholz TA, Davis DW, McConkey DJ, Symmans WF, Valero V, Jhingran A, Tucker SL, Pusztai L, Cristofanilli M, Esteva FJ, Hortobagyi GN, Sahin AA. Chemotherapy-induced apoptosis and Bcl-2 levels correlate with breast cancer response to chemotherapy. Cancer J. 2003;9(1):33–41.
58. Tiezzi DG, De Andrade JM, Candido dos Reis FJ, Marana HR, Ribeiro-Silva A, Tiezzi MG, Pereira AP. Apoptosis induced by neoadjuvant chemotherapy in breast cancer. Pathology. 2006;38(1):21–7.
59. Teixeira C, Reed JC, Pratt MA. Estrogen promotes chemotherapeutic drug resistance by a mechanism involving Bcl-2 proto-oncogene expression in human breast cancer cells. Cancer Res. 1995;55(17):3902–7.
60. Hahm HA, Davidson NE, Giguere JK, DiBernardo C, O'Reilly S. Breast cancer metastatic to the choroid. J Clin Oncol. 1998;16(6):2280–2 (official journal of the American Society of Clinical Oncology).
61. Miller WR, Dixon JM, Macfarlane L, Cameron D, Anderson TJ. Pathological features of breast cancer response following neoadjuvant treatment with either letrozole or tamoxifen. Eur J Cancer. 2003;39(4):462–8.
62. Wang S, Konorev EA, Kotamraju S, Joseph J, Kalivendi S, Kalyanaraman B. Doxorubicin induces apoptosis in normal and tumor cells via distinctly different mechanisms intermediacy of H(2)O(2)− and p53-dependent pathways. J Biol Chem. 2004;279(24):25535–43.
63. Merlo GR, Basolo F, Fiore L, Duboc L, Hynes NE. p53-dependent and p53-independent activation of apoptosis in mammary epithelial cells reveals a survival function of EGF and insulin. J Cell Biol. 1995;128(6):1185–96.
64. Bailey ST, Shin HJ, Westerling T, Liu XS, Brown M. Estrogen receptor prevents p53-dependent apoptosis in breast cancer. P Natl Acad Sci USA. 2012;109(44):18060–5.
65. Dowsett M, Smith IE, Ebbs SR, Dixon JM, Skene A, Griffith C, Boeddinghaus I, Salter J, Detre S, Hills M, Ashley S, Francis S, Walsh G, A'Hern R. Proliferation and apoptosis as markers of benefit in neoadjuvant endocrine therapy of breast cancer. Clin Cancer Res. 2006;12(3 Pt 2):1024s–30s (an official journal of the American Association for Cancer Research).
66. Tanei T, Shimomura A, Shimazu K, Nakayama T, Kim SJ, Iwamoto T, Tamaki Y, Noguchi S. Prognostic significance of Ki67 index after neoadjuvant chemotherapy in breast cancer. Euro J Surg Oncol J Euro Soc Surg Oncol Br Assoc Surg Oncol. 2011;37(2):155–61.
67. Sayeed A, Konduri SD, Liu W, Bansal S, Li F, Das GM. Estrogen receptor alpha inhibits p53-mediated transcriptional repression: implications for the regulation of apoptosis. Cancer Res. 2007;67(16):7746–55.
68. Aas T, Borresen AL, Geisler S, Smith-Sorensen B, Johnsen H, Varhaug JE, Akslen LA, Lonning PE. Specific P53 mutations are associated with de novo resistance to doxorubicin in breast cancer patients. Nat Med. 1996;2(7):811–4.
69. Elledge RM, Gray R, Mansour E, Yu Y, Clark GM, Ravdin P, Osborne CK, Gilchrist K, Davidson NE, Robert N, et al. Accumulation of p53 protein as a possible predictor of response to adjuvant combination chemotherapy with cyclophosphamide, methotrexate, fluorouracil, and prednisone for breast cancer. J Natl Cancer Inst. 1995;87(16) 1254–6.
70. Elledge RM, Lock-Lim S, Allred DC, Hilsenbeck SG, Cordner L. p53 mutation and tamoxifen resistance in breast cancer. Clin Cancer Res. 1995;1(10):1203–8 (an official journal of the American Association for Cancer Research).
71. King AE, Collins F, Klonisch T, Sallenave JM, Critchley HO, Saunders PT. An additive interaction between the NFkappaB and estrogen receptor signalling pathways in human endometrial epithelial cells. Hum Reprod. 2010;25(2):510–8.
72. Long MD, Thorne JL, Russell J, Battaglia S, Singh PK, Sucheston-Campbell LE, Campbell MJ. Cooperative behavior of the nuclear receptor superfamily and its deregulation in prostate cancer. Carcinogenesis. 2014;35(2):262–71.

73. Rizzo P, Miao H, D'Souza G, Osipo C, Song LL, Yun J, Zhao H, Mascarenhas J, Wyatt D, Antico G, Hao L, Yao K, Rajan P, Hicks C, Siziopikou K, Selvaggi S, Bashir A, Bhandari D, Marchese A, Lendahl U, Qin JZ, Tonetti DA, Albain K, Nickoloff BJ, Miele L. Crosstalk between notch and the estrogen receptor in breast cancer suggests novel therapeutic approaches. Cancer Res. 2008;68(13):5226–35.

74. Sisci D, Maris P, Cesario MG, Anselmo W, Coroniti R, Trombino GE, Romeo F, Ferraro A, Lanzino M, Aquila S, Maggiolini M, Mauro L, Morelli C, Ando S. The estrogen receptor alpha is the key regulator of the bifunctional role of FoxO3a transcription factor in breast cancer motility and invasiveness. Cell Cycle. 2013;12(21):3405–20.

75. Troester MA, Herschkowitz JI, Oh DS, He X, Hoadley KA, Barbier CS, Perou CM. Gene expression patterns associated with p53 status in breast cancer. BMC Cancer. 2006;6:276.

76. Cave JW. Selective repression of Notch pathway target gene transcription. Developmental biology. 2011;360(1):123–31.

77. Groth C, Fortini ME. Therapeutic approaches to modulating Notch signaling. Semin Cell Dev Biol. 2012;23(4):465–72.

78. Callahan Raafat. Notch signaling in mammary gland tumorigenesis. Journal of mammary gland biology and neoplasia. 2001;6(1):23–36.

79. Landor SKJ, Mutvei AP, Mamaeva V, Jin S, Busk M, Borra R, Gronroos TJ, Kronqvist P, Lendahl U, Sahlgren CM. Hypo- and hyperactivated Notch signaling induce a glycolytic switch through distinct mechanisms. PNAS USA 2011;108(46):18814–9.

80. Reedijk M, Odorcic S, Chang L, Zhang H, Miller N, McCready DR, Lockwood G, Egan SE. High-level coexpression of JAG1 and NOTCH1 is observed in human breast cancer and is associated with poor overall survival. Cancer Res. 2005;65(18):8530–7.

81. Reedijk M, Pinnaduwage D, Dickson BC, Mulligan AM, Zhang H, Bull SB, O'Malley FP, Egan SE, Andrulis IL. JAG1 expression is associated with a basal phenotype and recurrence in lymph node-negative breast cancer. Breast Cancer Res Treat. 2008;111(3):439–48.

82. Dontu G, Jackson KW, McNicholas E, Kawamura MJ, Abdallah WM, Wicha MS. Role of Notch signaling in cell-fate determination of human mammary stem/progenitor cells. Breast Cancer Res (BCR). 2004;6(6):R605–15.

83. Liu S, Wicha MS. Targeting breast cancer stem cells. J Clin Oncol. 2010;28(25):4006–12 (official journal of the American Society of Clinical Oncology).

84. Gonzalez-Angulo AM, Iwamoto T, Liu S, Chen H, Do KA, Hortobagyi GN, Mills GB, Meric-Bernstam F, Symmans WF, Pusztai L. Gene expression, molecular class changes, and pathway analysis after NACT for breast cancer. Clinical Cancer Res. 2012;18(4):1109–19 (an official journal of the American Association for Cancer Research).

85. Cho S, Lu M, He X, Ee PL, Bhat U, Schneider E, Miele L, Beck WT. Notch1 regulates the expression of ABCC1/MRP1 in cultured cancer cells. PNAS USA 2011;108(51):20778–83.

86. Leonessa C. ABC transporters and drug resistance in breast cancer. Endocr-Relat Cancer. 2003;10(1):43–73.

87. Mao J, Song B, Shi Y, Wang B, Fan S, Yu X, Tang J, Li L. ShRNA targeting Notch1 sensitizes breast cancer stem cell to paclitaxel. Int J Biochem Cell Biol. 2013;45(6):1064–73.

88. Qiu M, Peng Q, Jiang I, Carroll C, Han G, Rymer I, Lippincott J, Zachwieja J, Gajiwala K, Kraynov E, Thibault S, Stone D, Gao Y, Sofia S, Gallo J, Li G, Yang J, Li K, Wei P. Specific inhibition of Notch1 signaling enhances the antitumor efficacy of chemotherapy in triple negative breast cancer through reduction of cancer stem cells. Cancer Lett. 2013;328(2):261–70.

89. Campbell IG, Russell SE, Choong DYH, Montgomery KG, Ciavarella ML, Hooi CSF, Cristiano BE, Pearson RB, Phillips WA. Mutation of the PIK3CA gene in ovarian and breast cancer. Cancer Res. 2004;64(21):7678–81.

90. Jiang BH, Liu LZ. PI3 K/PTEN signaling in tumorigenesis and angiogenesis. Bba-Proteins Proteom. 2008;1784(1):150–8.

91. Winograd-Katz SE, Levitzki A. Cisplatin induces PKB/Akt activation and p38(MAPK) phosphorylation of the EGF receptor. Oncogene. 2006;25(56):7381–90.

92. Plo I, Bettaieb A, Payrastre B, Mansat-De Mas V, Bordier C, Rousse A, Kowalski-Chauvel A, Laurent G, Lautier D. The phosphoinositide 3-kinase/Akt pathway is activated by daunorubicin in human acute myeloid leukemia cell lines. FEBS Lett. 1999;452(3):150–4.
93. Clark AS, West K, Streicher S, Dennis PA. Constitutive and inducible Akt activity promotes resistance to chemotherapy, trastuzumab, or tamoxifen in breast cancer cells. Mol Cancer Ther. 2002;1(9):707–17.
94. Mabuchi S, Ohmichi M, Kimura A, Hisamoto K, Hayakawa J, Nishio Y, Adachi K, Takahashi K, Arimoto-Ishida E, Nakatsuji Y, Tasaka K, Murata Y. Inhibition of phosphorylation of BAD and Raf-1 by Akt sensitizes human ovarian cancer cells to paclitaxel. J Biol Chem. 2002;277(36):33490–500.
95. Datta SR, Dudek H, Tao X, Masters S, Fu HA, Gotoh Y, Greenberg ME. Akt phosphorylation of BAD couples survival signals to the cell-intrinsic death machinery. Cell. 1997;91(2):231–41.
96. delPeso L, GonzalezGarcia M, Page C, Herrera R, Nunez G. Interleukin-3-induced phosphorylation of BAD through the protein kinase Akt. Science 1997;278(5338):687–9.
97. Gardai SJ, Hildeman DA, Frankel SK, Whitlock BB, Frasch SC, Borregaard N, Marrack P, Bratton DL, Henson PM. Phosphorylation of Bax Ser(184) by Akt regulates its activity and apoptosis in neutrophils. J Biol Chem. 2004;279(20):21085–95.
98. Zhou BHP, Liao Y, Xia WY, Zou YY, Spohn B, Hung MC. HER-2/neu induces p53 ubiquitination via Akt-mediated MDM2 phosphorylation. Nat Cell Biol. 2001;3(11):973–82.
99. Garcia MG, Alaniz LD, Russo RIC, Alvarez E, Hajos SE. PI3K/Akt inhibition modulates multidrug resistance and activates NF-kappa B in murine lymphoma cell lines. Leukemia Res. 2009;33(2):288–96.
100. Takada T, Suzuki H, Gotoh Y, Sugiyama Y. Regulation of the cell surface expression of human BCRP/ABCG2 by the phosphorylation state of Akt in polarized cells. Drug Metab Dispos. 2005;33(7):905–9.
101. Mogi M, Yang J, Lambert JF, Colvin GA, Shiojima I, Skurk C, Summer R, Fine A, Quesenberry PJ, Walsh K. Akt signaling regulates side population cell phenotype via Bcrp1 translocation. J Biol Chem. 2003;278(40):39068–75.
102. Nakanishi T, Chumsri S, Khakpour N, Brodie AH, Leyland-Jones B, Hamburger AW, Ross DD, Burger AM. Side-population cells in luminal-type breast cancer have tumour-initiating cell properties, and are regulated by HER2 expression and signalling. Brit J Cancer. 2010;102(5):815–26.
103. Bleau AM, Hambardzumyan D, Ozawa T, Fomchenko EI, Huse JT, Brennan CW, Holland EC. PTEN/PI3K/Akt pathway regulates the side population phenotype and ABCG2 activity in glioma tumor stem-like cells. Cell Stem Cell. 2009;4(3):226–35.

Chapter 18
The Molecular Pathology of Male Breast Cancer

Rebecca A. Millican-Slater, Valerie Speirs, Thomas A. Hughes and Andrew M. Hanby

Background

Male breast cancer (MBC) is relatively rare, accounting for less than 1 % of all breast cancers in 2010 in the UK [1], however there is some evidence that the incidence rate may be on the rise [2]. Although a number of individual case reports and small case series have been published, large studies into MBC are few and far between, reflecting the scarcity of the disease. Such studies have relied on multi-centre collaboration to obtain sizeable cohorts [3–6]. At time of writing there are no clear molecular pathology readouts that are required to tailor therapy for MBC in a way they differ significantly from female breast cancer (FBC). This piece summarises the state of play with regards to the molecular pathology of MBC.

R.A. Millican-Slater
Department of Histopathology, Leeds University Hospitals NHS Trust,
Leeds, United Kingdom

V. Speirs · A.M. Hanby (✉)
St. James University Hospital, Leeds Institute of Cancer and Pathology,
University of Leeds, Leeds, West Yorkshire LS9 7TF, United Kingdom
e-mail: a.m.hanby@leeds.ac.uk

T.A. Hughes
Leeds Institutes of Molecular Medicine, Wellcome Trust Brenner Building,
St. James University Hospital, University of Leeds, Leeds, United Kingdom

© Springer Science+Business Media New York 2015
A. Khan et al. (eds.), *Precision Molecular Pathology of Breast Cancer*,
Molecular Pathology Library 10, DOI 10.1007/978-1-4939-2886-6_18

Histology and Immunohistochemistry Studies

The histology of MBCs reveals no distinct appearances that permit identification as a male originating tumour on histology alone. Morphological heterogeneity is however readily observed within MBC cohorts (Fig. 18.1).

Gene expression studies have confirmed that there is a great deal of heterogeneity amongst FBC, and there is evidence that immunohistochemistry surrogates can be used to classify FBCs into clinically-relevant different molecular subgroups [7]. Some studies have applied these immunohistochemistry surrogates directly to cohorts of MBC the findings of which are displayed in Table 18.1 [5, 6, 8, 9]. As is seen when looking at similar studies in FBC, comparison across the different studies is difficult as classifications vary for each study. In general though, a luminal A-like subtype (estrogen receptor (ER) and/or progesterone receptor (PR) positive, human epidermal growth factor receptor 2 (HER-2) negative) is the most common classification seen in MBC. With regards to immunohistochemical markers and survival, PR negativity and p53 accumulation have been reported to be associated with decreased survival in MBC (3), as has overexpression of the proliferation

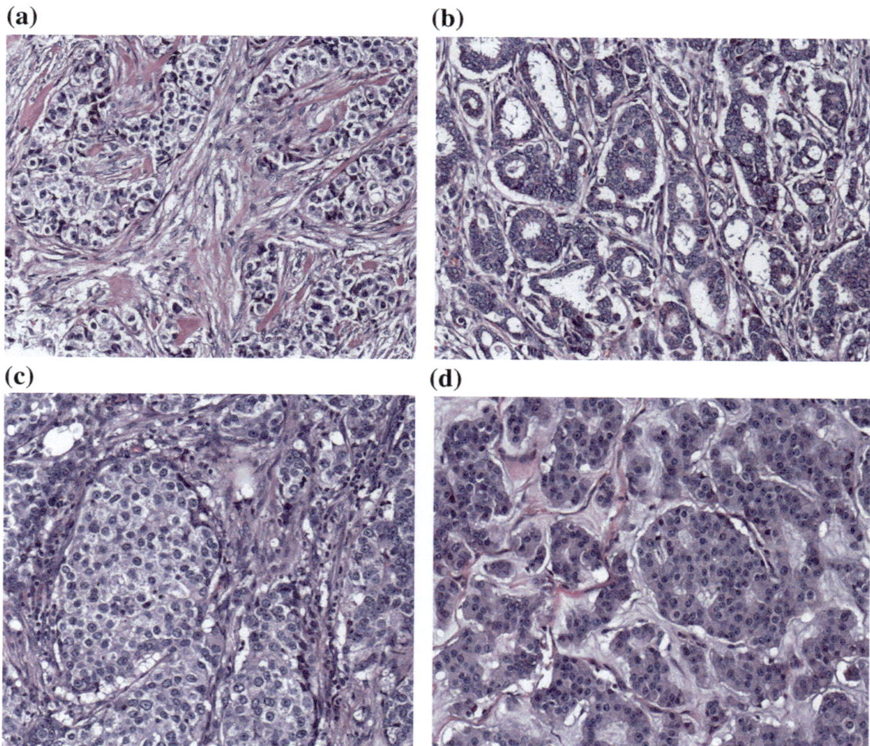

Fig. 18.1 This four-panel set of photomicrograph shows the histology displayed in sections of 4 distinct male breast cancers and demonstrates morphological heterogeneity in these tumours. All ×400

Table 18.1 Studies in which male breast cancers have been categorised into the molecular subgroups defined in FBC

Reference	Molecular subtype	IHC classification used	%
[8] $n = 130$	Luminal A	ER and/or PR positive; Her2 negative; Ki67 low	75
	Luminal B	ER and/or PR positive; Her2 positive and/or Ki67 high	21
	Her2-driven	ER and PR negative; Her2 positive	0
	Basal-like	ER, PR and Her2 negative; CK5/6, CK14 and/or EGFR positive	3
	Unclassifiable	Negative for all 6 markers	1
[9] $n = 183$	Luminal A	ER and/or PR positive; Her2 negative	81
	Luminal B	ER and/or PR positive; Her2 positive	11
	Her2-like	ER and PR negative; Her2 positive	0
	Core-basal	ER, PR and Her2 negative; CK5/6 and/or EGFR positive	1
	5-negative profile	ER, PR and Her2 negative; CK5/6 and EGFR negative	0
[5] $n = 189$	Luminal A	ER and/or PR positive; Her2 negative	68
	Luminal B	ER and/or PR positive; Her2 positive	26
	Her2-positive	ER and PR negative; Her2 positive	2
	Triple negative	ER and PR negative; Her2 negative	4
[6] $n = 203$	Luminal A	ER and/or PR positive; Her2 negative	98
	Luminal B	ER and/or PR positive; Her2 positive	0
	Her2-positive	ER and PR negative; Her2 positive	2
	Basal	ER and PR negative; Her2 negative; CK5/6 positive	0

markers cyclin A and cyclin B [7]. Androgen receptor (AR) expression in luminal A MBC has also been shown to be associated with improved overall survival compared to matched FBC [6]. Using hierarchical clustering, it was also shown that AR clustered with estrogen receptor beta (ERβ) in MBC while in FBC, estrogen receptor alpha (ERα) and PR clustered, which could indicate a difference in the biology of breast cancer between the genders (Fig. 18.2).

DNA Studies

Some studies have attempted to determine specific genomic abnormalities present in MBC and relate these to prognosis and/or compare them to FBC. One of the first of these studies used comparative genomic hybridisation (CGH) of 39 MBC and showed gains of 1q, 8q, 16p, 17q, Xq, 20q and Xp and losses of 8p, 16q, 13q, 6q, 11q and 22q [9]. This pattern was common to genomic imbalances observed in FBC. Another study looked at a cohort of 106 MBCs analysed by multiplex ligation-dependent probe amplification analyses to determine relative gene copy numbers for specific breast cancer genes [10]. A distinctive group of cancers with a poor prognosis were identified, characterized by frequent copy number gains in

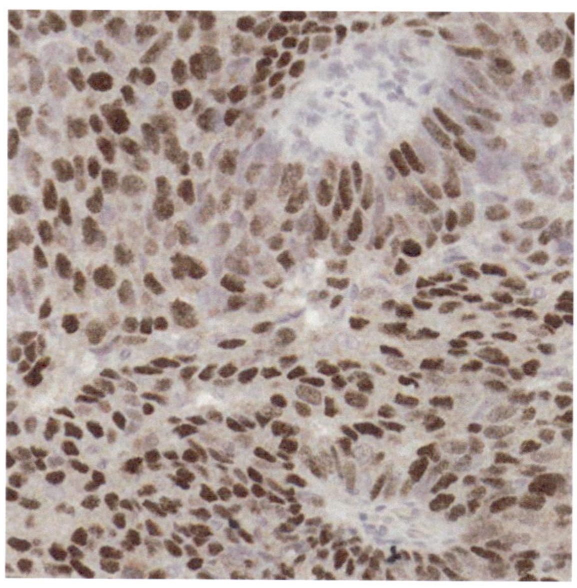

Fig. 18.2 Part of a male breast cancer showing strong nuclear staining with an antibody to the androgen receptor gene (AR). AR appears to be associated with better survival in MBC. Hierarchical clustering shows that AR clusters with estrogen receptor beta (ERβ) in MBC whereas in FBC, estrogen receptor alpha (ERα) and PR cluster

6 genes. Amplification of one of these genes, *CCND1*, was also found to be an independent prognostic factor. Interestingly, gains in some of these genes were not seen in FBC cases. Another study of 56 MBC cases found that compared to FBC, MBC was more likely to have genomic gains and less likely to have genomic losses [11]. Hierarchical clustering revealed two distinct genomic subgroups, termed male-simple and male-complex, one of which (male-simple) appeared distinct from the six subgroups identified in the FBC reference cohort. Finally, a recently published genome-wide association study (GWAS) of 823 MBC cases identified a single nucleotide polymorphism (SNP) at 14q24.1 in the *RAD51B* gene that was significantly associated with MBC risk as was *TOX3* (16q12.1) [12].

A few studies have looked at differential DNA methylation in MBC. Numerous genes have been found to undergo hypermethylation in cancer with many tumours showing hypermethylation of more than one gene. Increased methylation in the promoter region of a gene is most typically associated with reduced expression of that gene. It has been shown that promoter hypermethylation does occur in MBC with more than half of a total of 108 cases showing methylation of a number of genes that have been reported to act as tumour suppressor genes, including *MSH6*, *CD13*, *PAX5*, *PAX6* and *WT1* [13]. Methylation of these genes is uncommon or absent in normal male breast tissue. In addition, accumulation of methylated genes and an overall high methylation status correlated with a more aggressive phenotype and poorer survival. A second study analysing the methylation status of the *RASSF1A* gene, a well characterised tumour suppressor gene, in 27 cases of familial MBC and 29 cases of familial FBC showed that it was significantly more frequently methylated in MBC compared to FBC (76 % vs. 28 % respectively, $p = 0.0001$) indicating potential biological differences between the two diseases [14].

RNA Studies

Two studies have attempted to classify MBC at the transcriptional level. The first compared gene expression profiles in 37 MBC cases with 53 FBC cases matched for ER positivity and with similar clinicopathological features [15]. Differentially expressed genes were identified including some genes involved in energy metabolism, cell migration and motility, immune response, membrane transport, apoptosis and translation. They concluded that male and FBCs are quite different diseases. Interestingly, this study highlighted differences in AR pathway related genes, supporting subsequently published work at the protein level [6]. The second study looked solely at MBC cases and found that gene expression profiling of these revealed two subgroups, luminal M1 and luminal M2, which were distinct from the published FBC subgroups [16]. These differed with regards to tumour characteristics and outcome with the luminal M1 subgroup being more aggressive and associated with a worse prognosis. The same group applied computational biology to detect candidate driver genes in MBC [17] identifying 30 candidate drivers in MBC and 67 in FBC. Whilst many known drivers of breast carcinogenesis were identified in females, only 3 known cancer genes, *MAP2K4*, *LHP*, and *ZNF217*, were found in MBC. In addition, *THY1*, which is involved in invasion and related to epithelial-mesenchymal transition, was found in MBC with positivity being associated with poorer survival.

There is a small amount of literature assessing microRNAs (miRNAs) expression in MBC. miRNAs are small noncoding RNAs that alter gene expression at the post-transcriptional level. A number of miRNAs have been shown to be deregulated (some up-regulated and some down-regulated) in FBC [18]. Two studies to date have looked at miRNA expression in MBC. The first performed miRNA profiling and demonstrated that there is differential expression of several miRNAs between gynaecomastia and MBC with 17 miRNAs being overexpressed and 26 miRNAs being under expressed in the cancers [19]. The authors also reported differential expression of miRNAs between MBC cases and FBC cases. The second study analysed 319 miRNAs in MBCs and in gynaecomastia cases and found that miR-21, miR-519d, miR-183, miR-197 and miR-493-5p were most prominently up-regulated, and miR-145 and miR-497 were most prominently down-regulated in the cancer cases compared to the benign tissue [20]. With the exception of one miRNA (miR-145), there was no overlap between the results of the two studies.

Concluding Remarks

While MBC and FBC appear to be similar histologically, recent molecular pathology studies point to differing molecular landscapes between genders. Current breast cancer treatments do not differ between genders, however these emerging molecular studies suggest that men diagnosed with breast cancer could ultimately require different management and treatment strategies, especially if these molecular profiles are subsequently proven to be associated with differences in prognosis and identified gender specific targets.

Key Points

- Luminal A-like subtype (estrogen receptor (ER) and/or progesterone receptor (PR) positive, human epidermal growth factor receptor 2 (HER-2) negative) is the most common classification seen in MBC
- Hierarchical clustering shows that AR clustered with ERβ in MBC while in FBC, ERα and PR clustered, which could indicate a difference in the biology of breast cancer between the genders
- At time of writing there are no clear molecular pathology readouts that are required to tailor therapy for MBC in a way they differs significantly from FBC
- SNP at 14q24.1 in the *RAD51B* gene that was significantly associated with MBC risk
- *RASSF1A* gene is significantly more frequently methylated in MBC compared to FBC (76 % vs. 28 %)

References

1. UK, C.R. Breast cancer incidence statistics. 2013. http://info.cancerresearchuk.org/cancerst ats/types/breast/incidence/uk-breast-cancer-incidence-statistics. 1 May 2013.
2. Speirs V, Shaaban AM. The rising incidence of male breast cancer. Breast Cancer Res Treat. 2009;115(2):429–30.
3. Kornegoor R, et al. Immunophenotyping of male breast cancer. Histopathology. 2012;61(6):1145–55.
4. Nilsson C, et al. Molecular subtyping of male breast cancer using alternative definitions and its prognostic impact. Acta Oncol. 2013;52(1):102–9.
5. Ottini L, et al. Clinical and pathologic characteristics of BRCA-positive and BRCA-negative male breast cancer patients: results from a collaborative multicenter study in Italy. Breast Cancer Res Treat. 2012;134(1):411–8.
6. Shaaban AM, et al. A comparative biomarker study of 514 matched cases of male and female breast cancer reveals gender-specific biological differences. Breast Cancer Res Treat. 2012;133(3):949–58.
7. Carey LA, et al. Race, breast cancer subtypes, and survival in the Carolina Breast Cancer Study. JAMA, J Am Med Assoc. 2006;295(21):2492–502.
8. Nilsson C, et al. High proliferation is associated with inferior outcome in male breast cancer patients. Mod Pathol An Official J US Can Acad Pathol Inc. 2013;26(1):87–94.
9. Rudlowski C, et al. Comparative genomic hybridization analysis on male breast cancer. Int J Cancer. Journal international du cancer. 2006;118(10):2455–60.
10. Kornegoor R, et al. Oncogene amplification in male breast cancer: analysis by multiplex ligation-dependent probe amplification. Breast Cancer Res Treat. 2012;135(1):49–58.
11. Johansson I, et al. High-resolution genomic profiling of male breast cancer reveals differences hidden behind the similarities with female breast cancer. Breast Cancer Res Treat. 2011;129(3):747–60.

12. Orr N, et al. Genome-wide association study identifies a common variant in RAD51B associated with male breast cancer risk. Nat Genet. 2012;44(11):1182–4.
13. Kornegoor R, et al. Promoter hypermethylation in male breast cancer: analysis by multiplex ligation-dependent probe amplification. Breast Cancer Res BCR. 2012;14(4):R101.
14. Pinto R, et al. Different methylation and microRNA expression pattern in male and female familial breast cancer. J Cell Physiol. 2013;228(6):1264–9.
15. Callari M, et al. Gene expression analysis reveals a different transcriptomic landscape in female and male breast cancer. Breast Cancer Res Treat. 2011;127(3):601–10.
16. Johansson I, et al. Gene expression profiling of primary male breast cancers reveals two unique subgroups and identifies N-acetyltransferase-1 (NAT1) as a novel prognostic biomarker. Breast Cancer Res BCR. 2012;14(1):R31.
17. Johansson I, Ringner M, Hedenfalk I. The landscape of candidate driver genes differs between male and female breast cancer. PLoS ONE. 2013;8(10) e78299.
18. Zoon CK, et al. Current molecular diagnostics of breast cancer and the potential incorporation of microRNA. Expert Rev Mol Diagn. 2009;9(5):455–67.
19. Fassan M, et al. MicroRNA expression profiling of male breast cancer. Breast Cancer Res BCR. 2009;11(4):R58.
20. Lehmann U, et al. Identification of differentially expressed microRNAs in human male breast cancer. BMC Cancer. 2010;10:109.

Chapter 19
Specimens for Molecular Testing in Breast Cancer

Ali Sakhdari, Lloyd Hutchinson and Ediz F. Cosar

Background

Molecular testing can be performed on different specimen types. DNA- and RNA-based ancillary studies play an important role in identifying molecular portraits of breast carcinoma and in influencing routine therapies. Preanalytical factors including different fixatives, processing methods, and storage conditions coupled with differences in chemical and physical conditions, including time to fixation, mechanism of fixation, processing temperature and pH, storage time and conditions, all have a significant impact on the quality of the nucleic acids [1–6].

Specimen Types

Commonly used specimen types for molecular testing include fresh, frozen, formalin fixed paraffin embedded (FFPE), or alcohol-fixed samples. Nucleic acid extraction for molecular testing should be validated for each of these specimen types. Similarly, molecular assays used for clinical purposes should be limited to validated specimen types. For breast carcinoma, molecular analysis is usually performed on needle core biopsies or resection specimens, but could also include cytology samples, such as fine needle aspiration (FNA) biopsy [4, 7]. Both core biopsies and large resection specimens are usually fixed before molecular analysis is performed to allow correlation with morphology. Guidelines have been

A. Sakhdari · L. Hutchinson · E.F. Cosar (✉)
Department of Pathology, University of Massachusetts Medical School,
UMassMemorial Medical Center, Three Biotech, One Innovation Drive,
Worcester, MA 01605, USA
e-mail: Ediz.Cosar@umassmemorial.org

© Springer Science+Business Media New York 2015
A. Khan et al. (eds.), *Precision Molecular Pathology of Breast Cancer*,
Molecular Pathology Library 10, DOI 10.1007/978-1-4939-2886-6_19

introduced to standardize the processing of breast specimens [4, 5]. To achieve optimal performance, breast resection specimens should ideally be sectioned at 5-mm thickness after appropriate gross inspection and margin designation [4, 8, 9]. Preanalytical conditions may adversely impact molecular assays. The cold ischemia time should be kept to a minimum to reduce RNA and protein degradation. The optimum formalin exposure time for breast tissue specimens varies and is based on the specimen size, but in practice, the consensus is that at least 1 hour (h) of fixation per mm of tissue thickness is required [2, 6, 10, 11]. Strict adherence to these guidelines is crucial to obtain the most accurate results for predictive and prognostic tumor markers. Failure to adhere to these guidelines may significantly affect the clinical management and potentially impact the outcome.

Preanalytical Factors

There are many different parameters affecting optimal tissue preservation. Not all of them have been well studied; however, there is a wealth of evidence documenting some of the more important variables [6]. Here, we briefly touch on the more important preanalytical factors for breast specimen handling:

1. Prefixation time, which includes warm ischemia and cold ischemia time or the postmortem interval, has a great impact on the quality of the DNA and RNA in breast specimens. Optimally, cold ischemia should be less than 1 h for fluorescent in situ hybridization (FISH) and should be less than 24 h for polymerase chain reaction (PCR). In instances when a specimen falls outside of these parameters, the inclusion of an internal control gene to ascertain the specimen integrity is recommended. The latest American Society of Clinical Oncology/ College of American Pathologists (ASCO/CAP) guidelines recommend the time to fixation for breast specimens not to exceed 1 h [2, 12–14].

2. Fixation parameters:
   The following factors have been well studied:

   (a) Fixation chemistry: The mechanism of action for fixatives may be classified as cross-linkers, dehydrants, heat or acid effects, or a combination of these. In breast, as in other tissue types, 10 % neutral-buffered formalin (NBF) is the most widely used universal fixative as it preserves a wide range of tissues and tissue components [15, 16]. Unbuffered formalin fixation is not recommended as this method produces poor DNA yield and quality [17]. The amount of DNA fragmentation associated with formalin fixation is greater than that observed with alcohol fixation [16, 18].

   (b) Tissue penetration: This variable depends on the diffusibility of the fixatives. The general consensus for 10 % NBF in breast specimens is 1 mm of penetration per hour [2, 6, 19, 20]. Compared to formalin, alcohol leads to more rapid fixation, which offers better preservation of labile RNA molecules [21]. Overall the volume of fixative should be in excess of 20 times the volume of the tissue, however, this ratio can be difficult to achieve and requires proper sectioning of the large resections [22].

(c) Fixation conditions: Few studies have investigated the optimal temperature and pH necessary to preserve different nucleic acid types. However, the general consensus for the optimal fixation of breast specimens is cold temperature (optimum 4 °C, room temperature acceptable) and the use of non-acidic fixatives such as 10 % NBF. Other conditions lead to more nucleic acid degradation and reduced nucleic acid yields [6, 14, 23].

(d) Specimen size: A preferred tissue thickness enabling the appropriate formalin tissue penetration is 0.5 cm or less [5, 6, 14].

(e) Decalcification: Decalcification methods can affect DNA, RNA, and protein integrity. Methods such as PCR amplification, probe binding, in situ hybridization (ISH), and protein analysis can be adversely impacted. Decalcification using *ethylenediaminetetraacetic* acid (EDTA) solution, especially in combination with ultrasound when available, is superior to other methods of decalcification [12, 24–27].

(f) Duration of fixation: Although there is some variability in the recommendations for the fixation time of different tissue types [28–30], the revised ASCO/CAP guidelines recommend 6–72 h of fixation for breast tissues [4, 9].

3. Postfixation parameters: Relatively, few studies address the issue of quality control and assurance metrics for the appropriate storage of paraffin blocks [31, 32]. In particular, the storage time of FFPE blocks has been shown to adversely affect the nucleic acid quality. Formalin fixation and residual water exposure can have detrimental effects on nucleic acids, especially RNA [19, 21]. This specifically applies to tissue blocks that are older than 5 years for DNA studies and older than 1 year for RNA studies [4, 6, 9, 20]. Therefore, it is necessary to consider these adverse effects when selecting the blocks for molecular studies. As for the stored sections from FFPE tissue blocks, guidelines recommend molecular testing within 6 weeks for clinical purposes [4, 9].

Fixative Types

NBF (10 %) is the preferred and most widely used fixative, and molecular assays have been optimized for this fixative. It has been shown that formalin fixation forms chemical cross-links between proteins, DNA, RNA, and other macromolecules and leads to fragmentation of DNA that adversely affects molecular testing in a length-dependent manner. Molecular analyses that require amplicons approaching 1000 base pairs (bp) are usually successful when nucleic acids are extracted from fresh or frozen tissue samples, but are far less reliable in formalin-fixed specimens. Consequently, most assays are designed to utilize DNA sequences shorter than 300 bp to obtain satisfactory results [6]. In addition, random nucleotide base changes introduced by formalin fixation may be detected by more sensitive assays, especially in samples with low DNA concentration, and this may lead to false-positive results [6, 33, 34]. Any breast tissue specimen collected for molecular testing (cytology samples, needle biopsies, resection specimens) should be immersed in a sufficient volume of 10 % NBF as soon as possible (time to fixation ideally within 1 h). Several studies have shown that a delay greater than 1 h may lead to erroneous results in *HER2* FISH testing [2, 10]. Resection specimens should be sectioned through the tumor upon receipt. Cold ischemia time, type of fixative, and the time the sample was placed in fixative must be documented. Evidence suggests that the optimal duration of fixation for 10 % NBF is between 6 and 72 h [4, 8]. Alternative fixatives containing heavy metals such as mercury chloride (B-plus, B5, and Zenker) or acid zinc formalin and acidic solutions (Bouin and bone decalcifier) have detrimental effects on nucleic acids. This is also true for unbuffered formalin, because spontaneous oxidation of formalin, in time, produces formic acid. Heavy metals can have inhibitory effects on enzymes, which are routinely used in molecular assays. For instance, heavy metals inhibit DNA polymerases through competition with magnesium, an essential cofactor for polymerase activity [35]. On the other hand acidic solutions can "nick" the DNA backbone producing tiny fragments and cause depurination, making them unsuitable for testing [6]. If a sample gives a negative result in the absence of internal control elements, testing should be repeated on an alternate sample, such as different tissue block or specimen [4, 9].

Detection of *ERBB2* (*HER2*) Gene Amplification by In Situ Hybridization (ISH) Assay

ERBB2 (*HER2*) gene status may be assessed by various ISH methods including fluorescence or bright field in situ hybridization. These are molecular cytogenetic techniques that identify *HER2* gene amplification [1, 4]. Reverse transcriptase real-time PCR assays employed by Oncotype Dx also provide information about *HER2* gene mRNA levels, but are not routinely used to make treatment decisions for HER2 targeted therapy. A variety of factors influence the performance of these assays. Time to fixation will have a different effect depending on the specific nucleic acid analysis platform [2, 12, 36]. A cold ischemia time of more than one hour leads to reduced FISH signals [2]. RNA-based assays are even more sensitive to this variable [37–39]. *HER2* testing can be compromised by overfixation as well. The current ASCO/CAP guidelines recommend using 10 % NBF with tissue fixed for 6–72 h [4]. Needle core biopsies fixed for less than 1 h or resections fixed for less than 6 h should not be tested [4, 14]. Fixation with alcohol results in DNA condensation and this may influence FISH interpretation and should be considered when alcohol fixative is used [28]. On the other hand, DNA cross-linking, which commonly occurs with formalin fixation, may prevent probe penetration and binding to target DNA resulting in faint signals [6, 12]. Enzymatic digestion times for ISH can be modified to optimize the probe signal intensity. Overdigestion with proteases may result in split or fragmented signals that can lead to misclassification as gene copy number gain [4, 14].

Other Routine Molecular Assays

Aside from the *HER2* gene FISH testing, there are several other prognostic and predictive gene sets in breast cancer. Reverse transcription polymerase chain reaction (RT-PCR) is a relatively recent approach to detect *HER2* gene amplification in breast cancer. This approach has also been utilized in well-known and widely used FDA approved assays, such as Oncotype Dx (Genomic Health Inc, Redwood City, California), MammaPrint (Agendia, Amsterdam, the Netherlands), and PAM50 (Nanostring Technologies Inc., Seattle, Washington) . All 3 tests can provide an overall risk assessment of breast cancer recurrence [40–43]. These assays have benefited greatly from standardization of fixation practices, designed to ensure consistent results for *HER2* and estrogen receptor (ER) and progesterone receptor (PgR) and other ancillary studies [43, 44].

Oncotype DX is a multiplex, 21-gene, RT-PCR assay optimized for quantification of RNA extracted from FFPE tumor tissue that predicts the likelihood of disease recurrence (recurrence score- RS) in women with stages I or II, hormone receptor-positive, lymph node-negative, invasive breast cancer [41, 45].

MammaPrint is a 70-gene expression profile that was initially developed using oligonucleotide expression array (25,000 genes). Analysis consisted of consecutively collected tumor specimens from a cohort of women with stage I or II breast cancer who had undergone definitive surgery only without systemic therapy and with at least 5-year clinical follow-up [46, 47]. Originally, Mammaprint assay was limited to fresh tissue for assessment, but recently specimens fixed in 10 % NBF have been validated [48]. These assays heavily rely on careful primer design to minimize the effects of RNA degradation [48].

Prediction Analysis of Microarray (PAM) 50 is a 50-gene breast carcinoma subtype predictor, which was initially developed using microarray and quantitative RT-PCR. PAM50 measures the expression levels of 50 genes in surgically resected breast carcinoma samples. The risk of recurrence (ROR) can be determined in both patients without previous systemic therapy, and with systemic therapy. The PAM50 gene set is therefore used for gene expression-based subtyping of breast carcinomas and for probability of disease recurrence [49–51].

Other Molecular Assays

Other than commonly used molecular assays, there are some other methods that have gained popularity in recent years. As mentioned in the previous section, RT-PCR can be used to test for the *HER2* gene status in breast carcinoma specimens. When proper fixation protocols are followed, studies have shown a concordance rate of 92–94 % between FISH and RT-PCR. Some studies even proposed that RT-PCR may represent a better methodology than FISH, especially for equivocal samples by IHC [52–54]. *HER2* gene amplification is highly associated with HER2 mRNA overexpression, and quantification of HER2 mRNA by RT-PCR shows strong agreement with *HER2* gene amplification by FISH [55]. Compared with FISH, which offers semiquantitative values, RT-PCR offers quantitative values [44]. Despite these advantages, the labile nature of RNA introduces the risk of false negative results and therefore is not widely accepted as a clinical test to assess *HER2* gene status. This method is also limited by the need for a nearly pure invasive tumor cell population, which may require expensive and specialized methods, such as laser capture microdissection (LCM). Microarray-based expression profiling has similar limitations. In addition, this method provides only a semiquantitative assessment of gene expression, and sensitivity and specificity are limited by the nature of the probes included in the platform [56, 57].

Various DNA-based methods can be used to test for gene copy status in breast carcinoma specimens. Comparative genomic hybridization (array CGH) and single nucleotide polymorphism (SNP) array analysis have provided a wealth of data on gene copy number aberrations in breast cancer and have helped to identify potential therapeutic targets for subgroups of breast cancer patients. However, these array technologies do not provide any information about structural genomic aberrations. SNP array can provide information about nucleotide base pair variations [58, 59]. These array technologies require high quality DNA and consequently FFPE tissues may be unsuitable for these methods. Therefore, gene copy number information has been primarily derived from fresh or frozen tissue [60]. For these reasons and the high cost, these methods have not been adopted into routine clinical practice.

MicroRNAs

MicroRNAs are endogenous, small noncoding RNAs, which regulate gene expression by directly binding to the untranslated regions of the target messenger RNAs and may act either as tumor suppressor or oncogene [57, 61–64]. Levels of specific miRNAs differ between normal and malignant breast tissue and among tumors of varying histological grade, molecular subtype, lymph node status, and hormone receptor (HR) status [65, 66]. In addition, miRNAs have been linked to breast cancer invasion, proliferation, and metastasis [67–69]. Different miRNAs have been shown to be associated with aggressiveness of breast cancer or work as a tumor suppressor [1, 61]. The available miRNA technologies are not without limitations, such as the susceptibility to degradation associated with all types of RNA. Because of their smaller size, miRNAs are relatively less affected by the damaging effects of formalin fixation and can readily be extracted from FFPE tissue [70]. miRNAs have been discussed in greater detail in chapter 13.

Future Directions

Next-generation sequencing (NGS), also known as massively parallel sequencing, has been rapidly gaining popularity in clinical testing. The Cancer Genome Atlas (TCGA) project has revealed a spectrum of diverse genomic anomalies through exome and whole genome sequencing [58, 71]. NGS is changing our understanding of the molecular traits of tumors at the genomic, transcriptomic, and epigenetic levels [72, 73]. The data from whole genome sequencing can provide a global view of individual tumor biology by integrating a variety of molecular information [73, 74]. The ability to distinguish between driver and passenger mutations is helpful in determining which genes are important in tumor development and therapeutic resistance [75]. Genetic heterogeneity in breast cancers has been confirmed and further reinforced by NGS methods [75, 76]. NGS can be used to analyze the entire genome or to target the gene regions containing high-frequency mutations. The latter targeted approach can provide high-level sequencing coverage and allows detection of low level mutations. The value of NGS in clinical testing is further emphasized by the capacity to sequence small specimens with scant tumor cells, such as samples obtained by FNA. In contrast to traditional Sanger sequencing, NGS also has the advantage of multigene panel testing using as little as 10 nanograms/microliter of DNA [77, 78]. With proper design, these systems are less prone to the adverse effects of formalin fixation and associated DNA fragmentation. The availability of customizable multigene panels has enabled the identification of mutations that may serve as early indicators of disease and may be used to monitor disease progression and therapeutic response [75]. Clinical predictors based on the molecular signature and detection of the vulnerabilities of an individual's tumor to facilitate precision medicine represent promising opportunities, such as personalized therapy, to improve cancer care [79–81].

Key Points

- Commonly used specimen types for molecular testing include fresh, frozen, FFPE, or alcohol-fixed samples.
- Preanalytical factors including different fixatives, processing methods, and storage conditions coupled with differences in chemical and physical conditions, including time to fixation, mechanism of fixation, processing temperature and pH, storage time and conditions, all have a significant impact on the quality of the nucleic acids.
- Different molecular assays can be utilized in breast pathology including in situ hybridiziation (ISH), reverse-trascription polymerase chain reaction (RT-PCR), Comparative genomic hybridization, single nucleotide polymorphism array, microRNA assessment and next generation sequencing.

References

1. Cornejo KM, et al. Theranostic and molecular classification of breast cancer. Arch Pathol Lab Med. 2014;138(1):44–56.
2. Khoury T, et al. Delay to formalin fixation effect on breast biomarkers. Mod Pathol. 2009;22(11):1457–67.

3. Tong LC, et al. The effect of prolonged fixation on the immunohistochemical evaluation of estrogen receptor, progesterone receptor, and HER2 expression in invasive breast cancer: a prospective study. Am J Surg Pathol. 2011;35(4):545–52.

4. Wolff AC, et al. Recommendations for human epidermal growth factor receptor 2 testing in breast cancer: American society of clinical oncology/college of American pathologists clinical practice guideline update. J Clin Oncol. 2013;31(31):3997–4013.

5. Wolff AC, et al. American society of clinical oncology/college of American pathologists guideline recommendations for human epidermal growth factor receptor 2 testing in breast cancer. Arch Pathol Lab Med. 2007;131(1):18–43.

6. Srinivasan M, Sedmak D, Jewell S. Effect of fixatives and tissue processing on the content and integrity of nucleic acids. Am J Pathol. 2002;161(6):1961–71.

7. Zoon CK, et al. Current molecular diagnostics of breast cancer and the potential incorporation of microRNA. Expert Rev Mol Diagn. 2009;9(5):455–67.

8. Hammond ME, et al. American society of clinical oncology/college of American pathologists guideline recommendations for immunohistochemical testing of estrogen and progesterone receptors in breast cancer. Arch Pathol Lab Med. 2010;134(6):907–22.

9. Wolff AC, et al. American society of clinical oncology/college of American pathologists guideline recommendations for human epidermal growth factor receptor 2 testing in breast cancer. J Clin Oncol. 2007;25(1):118–45.

10. Apple S, et al. The effect of delay in fixation, different fixatives, and duration of fixation in estrogen and progesterone receptor results in breast carcinoma. Am J Clin Pathol. 2011;135(4):592–8.

11. Yaziji H, et al. Consensus recommendations on estrogen receptor testing in breast cancer by immunohistochemistry. Appl Immunohistochem Mol Morphol. 2008;16(6):513–20.

12. Bass BP, et al. A review of preanalytical factors affecting molecular, protein, and morphological analysis of formalin-fixed, paraffin-embedded (FFPE) tissue: how well do you know your FFPE specimen? Arch Pathol Lab Med. 2014;138(11):1520–30.

13. Khoury T, Liu Q, Liu S. Delay to formalin fixation effect on HER2 test in breast cancer by dual-color silver-enhanced in situ hybridization (dual-ISH). Appl Immunohistochem Mol Morphol. 2014;22(9):688–95.

14. Rakha EA, et al. The updated ASCO/CAP guideline recommendations for HER2 testing in the management of invasive breast cancer: a critical review of their implications for routine practice. Histopathology. 2014;64(5):609–15.

15. Bramwell NH, Burns BF. The effects of fixative type and fixation time on the quantity and quality of extractable DNA for hybridization studies on lymphoid tissue. Exp Hematol. 1988;16(8):730–2.

16. Douglas MP, Rogers SO. DNA damage caused by common cytological fixatives. Mutat Res. 1998;401(1–2):77–88.

17. Ross JS. Clinical implementation of KRAS testing in metastatic colorectal carcinoma: the pathologist's perspective. Arch Pathol Lab Med. 2012;136(10):1298–307.

18. Yagi N, et al. The role of DNase and EDTA on DNA degradation in formaldehyde fixed tissues. Biotech Histochem. 1996;71(3):123–9.

19. Sanchez-Navarro I, et al. Comparison of gene expression profiling by reverse transcription quantitative PCR between fresh frozen and formalin-fixed, paraffin-embedded breast cancer tissues. Biotechniques. 2010;48(5):389–97.

20. Ben-Ezra J, et al. Effect of fixation on the amplification of nucleic acids from paraffin-embedded material by the polymerase chain reaction. J Histochem Cytochem. 1991;39(3):351–4.

21. Evers DL, et al. The effect of formaldehyde fixation on RNA: optimization of formaldehyde adduct removal. J Mol Diagn. 2011;13(3):282–8.

22. Start RD, Cross SS, Smith JH. Assessment of specimen fixation in a surgical pathology service. J Clin Pathol. 1992;45(6):546–7.

23. Noguchi M, et al. Modified formalin and methanol fixation methods for molecular biological and morphological analyses. Pathol Int. 1997;47(10):685–91.

24. Alers JC, et al. Effect of bone decalcification procedures on DNA in situ hybridization and comparative genomic hybridization. EDTA is highly preferable to a routinely used acid decalcifier. J Histochem Cytochem. 1999;47(5):703–10.
25. Reineke T, et al. Ultrasonic decalcification offers new perspectives for rapid FISH, DNA, and RT-PCR analysis in bone marrow trephines. Am J Surg Pathol. 2006;30(7):892–6.
26. Brown RS, et al. Routine acid decalcification of bone marrow samples can preserve DNA for FISH and CGH studies in metastatic prostate cancer. J Histochem Cytochem. 2002;50(1):113–5.
27. Arber JM, et al. The effect of decalcification on in situ hybridization. Mod Pathol. 1997;10(10):1009–14.
28. Lindeman NI, et al. Molecular testing guideline for selection of lung cancer patients for EGFR and ALK tyrosine kinase inhibitors: guideline from the college of American pathologists, International association for the study of lung cancer, and association for molecular pathology. Arch Pathol Lab Med. 2013;137(6):828–60.
29. Greer CE, Lund JK, Manos MM. PCR amplification from paraffin-embedded tissues: recommendations on fixatives for long-term storage and prospective studies. PCR Methods Appl. 1991;1(1):46–50.
30. Ferrer I, et al. Effects of formalin fixation, paraffin embedding, and time of storage on DNA preservation in brain tissue: a BrainNet Europe study. Brain Pathol. 2007;17(3):297–303.
31. Masuda N, et al. Analysis of chemical modification of RNA from formalin-fixed samples and optimization of molecular biology applications for such samples. Nucleic Acids Res. 1999;27(22):4436–43.
32. von Weizsacker F, et al. A simple and rapid method for the detection of RNA in formalin-fixed, paraffin-embedded tissues by PCR amplification. Biochem Biophys Res Commun. 1991;174(1):176–80.
33. Wong C, et al. Mutations in BRCA1 from fixed, paraffin-embedded tissue can be artifacts of preservation. Cancer Genet Cytogenet. 1998;107(1):21–7.
34. Gillespie JW, et al. Evaluation of non-formalin tissue fixation for molecular profiling studies. Am J Pathol. 2002;160(2):449–57.
35. Gaydosh L, DeLeon V, Golden T, Warren J, Roby R. Metal ions as forensically-relevant inhibitors of PCR-based DNA testing. In: American academy of forensic sciences: 65th anniversary meeting program; 2013.
36. Greer CE, et al. PCR amplification from paraffin-embedded tissues. Effects of fixative and fixation time. Am J Clin Pathol. 1991;95(2):117–24.
37. Yildiz-Aktas IZ, Dabbs DJ, Bhargava R. The effect of cold ischemic time on the immunohistochemical evaluation of estrogen receptor, progesterone receptor, and HER2 expression in invasive breast carcinoma. Mod Pathol. 2012;25(8):1098–105.
38. Portier BP, et al. Delay to formalin fixation 'cold ischemia time': effect on ERBB2 detection by in-situ hybridization and immunohistochemistry. Mod Pathol. 2013;26(1):1–9.
39. Li X, et al. The effect of prolonged cold ischemia time on estrogen receptor immunohistochemistry in breast cancer. Mod Pathol. 2013;26(1):71–8.
40. Paik S. Development and clinical utility of a 21-gene recurrence score prognostic assay in patients with early breast cancer treated with tamoxifen. Oncologist. 2007;12(6):631–5.
41. Paik S, et al. A multigene assay to predict recurrence of tamoxifen-treated, node-negative breast cancer. N Engl J Med. 2004;351(27):2817–26.
42. Bueno-de-Mesquita JM, et al. Validation of 70-gene prognosis signature in node-negative breast cancer. Breast Cancer Res Treat. 2009;117(3):483–95.
43. Kittaneh M, Montero AJ, Gluck S. Molecular profiling for breast cancer: a comprehensive review. Biomark Cancer. 2013;5:61–70.
44. Kaklamani V. A genetic signature can predict prognosis and response to therapy in breast cancer: oncotype DX. Expert Rev Mol Diagn. 2006;6(6):803–9.
45. Paik S, et al. Gene expression and benefit of chemotherapy in women with node-negative, estrogen receptor-positive breast cancer. J Clin Oncol. 2006;24(23):3726–34.

46. van't Veer LJ, et al. Gene expression profiling predicts clinical outcome of breast cancer. Nature. 2002;415(6871):530–6.
47. van de Vijver MJ, et al. A gene-expression signature as a predictor of survival in breast cancer. N Engl J Med. 2002;347(25):1999–2009.
48. Sapino A, et al. MammaPrint molecular diagnostics on formalin-fixed, paraffin-embedded tissue. J Mol Diagn. 2014;16(2):190–7.
49. Parker JS, et al. Supervised risk predictor of breast cancer based on intrinsic subtypes. J Clin Oncol. 2009;27(8):1160–7.
50. Nielsen TO, et al. A comparison of PAM50 intrinsic subtyping with immunohistochemistry and clinical prognostic factors in tamoxifen-treated estrogen receptor-positive breast cancer. Clin Cancer Res. 2010;16(21):5222–32.
51. Dowsett M, et al. Comparison of PAM50 risk of recurrence score with oncotype DX and IHC4 for predicting risk of distant recurrence after endocrine therapy. J Clin Oncol. 2013;31(22):2783–90.
52. Kulka J, et al. Detection of HER-2/neu gene amplification in breast carcinomas using quantitative real-time PCR—a comparison with immunohistochemical and FISH results. Pathol Oncol Res. 2006;12(4):197–204.
53. Susini T, et al. Preoperative assessment of HER-2/neu status in breast carcinoma: the role of quantitative real-time PCR on core-biopsy specimens. Gynecol Oncol. 2010;116(2):234–9.
54. Vinatzer U, et al. Expression of HER2 and the coamplified genes GRB7 and MLN64 in human breast cancer: quantitative real-time reverse transcription-PCR as a diagnostic alternative to immunohistochemistry and fluorescence in situ hybridization. Clin Cancer Res. 2005;11(23):8348–57.
55. Pusztai L, et al. Gene expression profiles obtained from fine-needle aspirations of breast cancer reliably identify routine prognostic markers and reveal large-scale molecular differences between estrogen-negative and estrogen-positive tumors. Clin Cancer Res. 2003;9(7):2406–15.
56. Geyer FC, Reis-Filho JS. Microarray-based gene expression profiling as a clinical tool for breast cancer management: are we there yet? Int J Surg Pathol. 2009;17(4):285–302.
57. Calin GA, Croce CM. MicroRNA signatures in human cancers. Nat Rev Cancer. 2006;6(11):857–66.
58. Reis-Filho JS. Next-generation sequencing. Breast Cancer Res. 2009;11(Suppl 3):S12.
59. Tan DS, et al. Getting it right: designing microarray (and not 'microawry') comparative genomic hybridization studies for cancer research. Lab Invest. 2007;87(8):737–54.
60. Nakao K, et al. A predictive factor of the quality of microarray comparative genomic hybridization analysis for formalin-fixed paraffin-embedded archival tissue. Diagn Mol Pathol. 2013;22(3):174–80.
61. Foekens JA, et al. Four miRNAs associated with aggressiveness of lymph node-negative, estrogen receptor-positive human breast cancer. Proc Natl Acad Sci USA. 2008;105(35):13021–6.
62. Bartel DP. MicroRNAs: genomics, biogenesis, mechanism, and function. Cell. 2004;116(2):281–97.
63. Caldas C, Brenton JD. Sizing up miRNAs as cancer genes. Nat Med. 2005;11(7):712–4.
64. Wang L, Wang J. MicroRNA-mediated breast cancer metastasis: from primary site to distant organs. Oncogene. 2012;31(20):2499–511.
65. Blenkiron C, et al. MicroRNA expression profiling of human breast cancer identifies new markers of tumor subtype. Genome Biol. 2007;8(10):R214.
66. Iorio MV, et al. MicroRNA gene expression deregulation in human breast cancer. Cancer Res. 2005;65(16):7065–70.
67. Huang Q, et al. The microRNAs miR-373 and miR-520c promote tumour invasion and metastasis. Nat Cell Biol. 2008;10(2):202–10.
68. Ma L, Teruya-Feldstein J, Weinberg RA. Tumour invasion and metastasis initiated by microRNA-10b in breast cancer. Nature. 2007;449(7163):682–8.

69. Tavazoie SF, et al. Endogenous human microRNAs that suppress breast cancer metastasis. Nature. 2008;451(7175):147–52.
70. Ibberson D, et al. RNA degradation compromises the reliabiliy of microRNA expression profiling. BMC Biotechnol. 2009;9:102.
71. Russnes HG, et al. Insight into the heterogeneity of breast cancer through next-generation sequencing. J Clin Invest. 2011;121(10):3810–8.
72. ten Bosch JR, Grody WW. Keeping up with the next generation: massively parallel sequencing in clinical diagnostics. J Mol Diagn. 2008;10(6):484–92.
73. Curtis C, et al. The genomic and transcriptomic architecture of 2,000 breast tumours reveals novel subgroups. Nature. 2012;486(7403):346–52.
74. Voelkerding KV, Dames SA, Durtschi JD. Next-generation sequencing: from basic research to diagnostics. Clin Chem. 2009;55(4):641–58.
75. Desmedt C, et al. Next-generation sequencing in breast cancer: first take home messages. Curr Opin Oncol. 2012;24(6):597–604.
76. Radovich M. Next-generation sequencing in breast cancer: translational science and clinical integration. Pharmacogenomics. 2012;13(6):637–9.
77. Sanger F, Nicklen S, Coulson AR. DNA sequencing with chain-terminating inhibitors. Proc Natl Acad Sci USA. 1977;74(12):5463–7.
78. Parkinson NJ, et al. Preparation of high-quality next-generation sequencing libraries from picogram quantities of target DNA. Genome Res. 2012;22(1):125–33.
79. Bieche I, Lidereau R. Genome-based and transcriptome-based molecular classification of breast cancer. Curr Opin Oncol. 2011;23(1):93–9.
80. Miller WR. Controversies in breast cancer 2009. Breast Cancer Res. 2009;11(Suppl 3):S1.
81. Cameron D. Proceedings of controversies in breast cancer held in Edinburgh UK, 7–8 September 2009. Breast Cancer Res, 2009. 11 Suppl 3: pp. S1–25.doi:10.1186/bcr2442

Index

Note: Page numbers followed by *f* and *t* indicate figures and tables respectively

© Springer Science+Business Media New York 2015

A. Khan et al. (eds.), *Precision Molecular Pathology of Breast Cancer*,
Molecular Pathology Library 10, DOI 10.1007/978-1-4939-2886-6

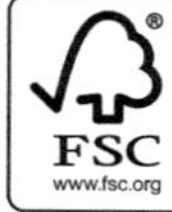